"At a time when kids are being prescribed more and more medications to treat symptoms, Dr. Shetreat-Klein turns the prevailing paradigm on its head by outlining how fresh food, rich soil, and contact with nature can reverse the growing epidemic of chronic childhood illness. Filled with fascinating science and hands-on advice, her book gives you all the tools you need to get your kids healthy and keep them that way."

—Andrew Weil, MD, author of *True Food* and
*8 Weeks to Optimum Health*

"Delves into research that suggests that spending time around farms, parks, and other green spaces can benefit children in surprising ways, protecting against allergies, enhancing immune function, and potentially even improving attention span and academic performance."

—*The New York Times*

"The text is full of scientific information presented in a fun and in-formative way, giving concrete evidence that good food can transform one's life."

—*Publishers Weekly*

"Carefully researched and compellingly written . . . A must-read!"

—Mark Hyman, MD, director, Cleveland Clinic's Center for
Functional Medicine, author of the #1 *New York Times* bestseller
*The Blood Sugar Solution*

"*The Dirt Cure* is an exhilarating book that had me cheering from page one. Don't go to the pediatrician without it!"

—Christiane Northrup, MD, author of *Goddesses Never Age*
and *Women's Bodies, Women's Wisdom*

"If you are a parent, or planning to be one, *The Dirt Cure* is your nutritional bible. You can save your kids from a vast array of physical/emotional chronic illnesses, now, when they're still young, and for the rest of their (longer and healthier) lives."

—David Edelberg, MD, author of *The Triple Whammy Cure*

"A tour de force prescription for creating a more nourishing environment to fight and prevent chronic disease in kids and adults, *The Dirt Cure* combines cutting-edge science and medicine with common sense to illustrate the intimate, visceral connection between the health of the natural world that surrounds us—our terrain—and our own health. As the environment sickens, so do we. As the environment thrives, so do our children, and so do we."

—Robert K. Naviaux, MD, PhD, codirector, Mitochondrial and Metabolic Disease Center (MMDC), UCSD School of Medicine

"This is a reader-friendly book, and Shetreat-Klein powerfully lays out the case for why bleach, hand sanitizers, fluoride, ibuprofen, and acetaminophen aren't all they're cracked up to be. She convincingly argues the case for a dirt-filled but chemical-free life."

—*Booklist*

# THE
# DIRT
## CURE

*Healthy Food, Healthy Gut,*
*Happy Child*

## MAYA SHETREAT-KLEIN, MD

with Rachel Holtzman

**ATRIA** PAPERBACK

New York   London   Toronto   Sydney   New Delhi

This publication contains the opinions and ideas of its author. It is intended to provide helpful and informative material on the subjects addressed in the publication. It is sold with the understanding that the author and publisher are not engaged in rendering medical, health, or any other kind of personal professional services in the book. The reader should consult his or her medical, health, or other competent professional before adopting any of the suggestions in this book or drawing inferences from it.

The author and publisher specifically disclaim all responsibility for any liability, loss or risk, personal or otherwise, which is incurred as a consequence, directly or indirectly, of the use and application of any of the contents of this book.

**ATRIA**
PAPERBACK

An Imprint of Simon & Schuster, Inc.
1230 Avenue of the Americas
New York, NY 10020

First Atria Paperback edition May 2017

**ATRIA** PAPERBACK and colophon are trademarks of Simon & Schuster, Inc.

For information about special discounts for bulk purchases, please contact Simon & Schuster Special Sales at 1-866-506-1949 or business@simonandschuster.com.

The Simon & Schuster Speakers Bureau can bring authors to your live event. For more information or to book an event contact the Simon & Schuster Speakers Bureau at 1-866-248-3049 or visit our website at www.simonspeakers.com.

Manufactured in the United States of America

10  9  8  7  6  5  4  3  2  1

Library of Congress Control Number: 2016287081

ISBN 978-1-4767-9697-0
ISBN 978-1-4767-9698-7 (pbk)
ISBN 978-1-4767-9699-4 (ebook)

*I dedicate this book to the sacred:*
*to rocks; to seeds, soil, and sunshine; to wind, water, and wilderness;*
*to plants, trees, and all living beings seen and unseen.*

# CONTENTS

## PART IV. STEP THREE: PUT IT ALL TOGETHER

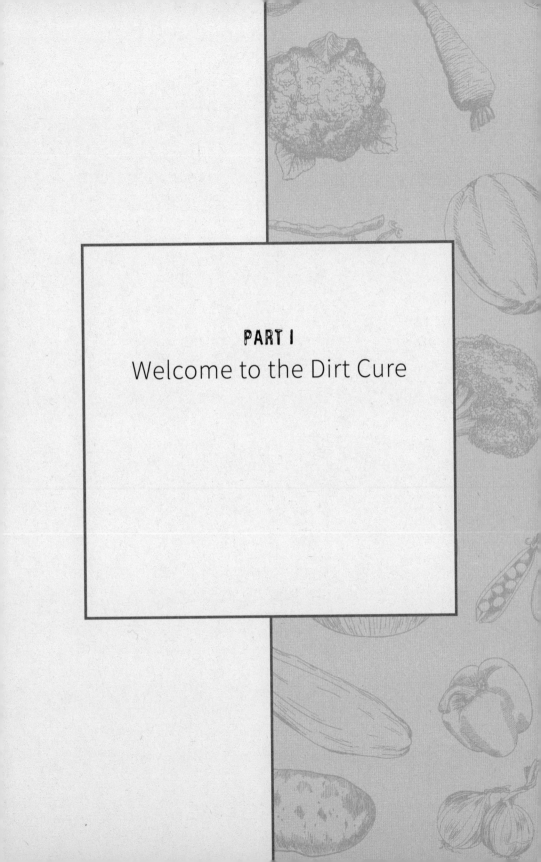

## PART I
# Welcome to the Dirt Cure

*Look deep into nature, and then
you will understand everything better.*
—ALBERT EINSTEIN

It's a particularly nerve-racking time to be a parent. With every new study, we're reminded that the incidence of children with diseases and behavioral disorders like ADHD, autism, learning disabilities, anxiety, depression, epilepsy, bipolar disorder, and Tourette's syndrome is through the roof. During the last decade in the United States, children ages 3 to 17 with developmental disabilities increased by double digits. The incidence of conditions like autism increased by as much as *78 percent.*[1] Starting as young as two, 11 percent of school-aged kids and 20 percent of teens carry diagnoses of ADHD—a 41 percent rise over the past decade. During that same period, the number of children medicated with stimulants or antipsychotics more than tripled.[2] A recent study showed that in the United States, one out of every five children has been diagnosed with mental illness, costing us $247 billion a year.[3]

As if that's not enough to swear off procreating altogether, we're also seeing an unprecedented rise in cases of food allergies, eczema, asthma, inflammatory bowel disease, and other autoimmune conditions,[4,5,6] particularly in the United States. For several years, type 1 diabetes diagnoses have increased 6.3 percent annually in children five years and younger.[7] And so-called normal maladies like colic, chronic ear infections, poor sleep, and constipation have become all too common. (When did pooping once a week become normal?!) But most of all, why is it that no matter how educated and wealthy our society, how medically advanced, how successful at eradicating infectious diseases, our kids are only getting sicker?

As a pediatric neurologist, I think about these alarming statistics on a daily basis because I care for these children in my private practice. For many of my patients, I'm what you could call a "last stop." Most of the families who come to my office—often having traveled a great distance—arrive after struggling down a long road of unsuccessful treatments by traditional methods. Like many patients, they've been given conventional medications for their symptoms, suffered side effects, and taken more medication to manage the first medication's side effects. Worst of all, they've been told that their children are simply untreatable. That they are going to be chronically sick for life.

I don't see their situations as helpless or hopeless. Then again, I'm not your typical doctor. And that's partly because I was once one of those panicked parents without answers.

On my youngest son's first birthday, seemingly out of nowhere, he had his first episode of wheezing. It lasted a week, and it continued on and off for the next ten months. Despite numerous prescriptions from his pediatrician—antibiotics, steroids, and nebulizers—his symptoms would improve for only a few days. Then his nose would start running again and his breathing difficulties resumed. He perpetually erupted in mysterious itchy rashes. Simultaneously, his cognitive development plateaued. Though he had said his first words early at eight months, he stopped acquiring language the moment he began to have trouble breathing. He tripped frequently and no longer held out his hands to catch himself; his face and head hit the ground more times than we could count. Most frightening, no doctor could offer any approach that might reverse his course. If I—a doctor myself—wasn't getting answers from physicians, then who was?

Over the course of these ten terrifying months, I began to do my own research, asking those questions that no one else seemed to be asking: How had my son's body become so sick? We learned early on that dairy made him gassy, so he had been drinking soy milk instead. Could changing his diet again be the key to helping him?

Though our team of doctors discouraged us from pursuing this path, by then I recognized I was on my own in this journey. After tracking down an allergist willing to test him and not dismiss the possibility that his symptoms could be connected to food, we determined through both skin and blood testing that my son was severely allergic to soy. Within one week of entirely eliminating soy—including the ubiquitous soy oil found in pretzels and other snack foods, and in almost everything cooked in restaurants—my son's constant running noses, coughing, and wheezing disappeared. More amazing still, his language promptly began to improve after being stalled for months.

**I know it's hard to believe. I could hardly believe it myself. My son's sick body had led to a sick brain; and as his body became healthier, so did his brain.**

Meanwhile, I felt terribly guilty. I had been feeding my son what I thought was a pretty healthy diet, and it turned out that his food had been making him sick. The hardest part was not that no one believed that his food was affecting his health. It was that no one seemed to think he was *sick* at all. It was "just some asthma," and "developmental delay." But what about those is normal?

**Somehow, when no one was paying attention, chronic illness became the new "normal" for children.** Instead of catching the occasional bug with clear onset and recovery, many children get sick, get a little better, and get sick again. And the illnesses evolve. These kids—maybe even your own kids—go from colic at six weeks to eczema at six months to chronic ear infections at one year to tubes or a tonsillectomy at three years to an ADD diagnosis at six. Many kids have medication lists that would rival those of senior citizens: steroid cream for eczema; H2 blockers for gastric reflux; antihistamines for allergies; anti-inflammatories for migraines; Miralax for constipation; stimulants for ADHD and learning disabilities; SSRIs for depression; mood stabilizers for anxiety . . . sometimes all prescribed at the same time! And more and more kids take insulin for type 1 diabetes or metformin for type 2 diabetes; thyroid medication for hypothyroidism; antiepileptics for seizures; antipsychotics for explosive behavior or anxiety; and steroids or other immune modulators like chemotherapeutics for a wide range of autoimmune diseases that have become shockingly common in children.

Meanwhile, we live in a world of hand sanitizers, antibiotics, and steroids, as well as pesticides, chemical fertilizers, and GMOs. These advances were supposed to solve society's ills, yet even as lives have been saved, somehow children have become sicker than ever before.

We've been told dirt is bad, germs are bad, bugs are bad, and weeds are bad. And we've taken all the necessary precautions against these interlopers. We bleach away germs, we inoculate our kids against microbes, we treat infections with antibiotics and Tylenol, we poison household and garden pests, and spray weed killer to achieve perfect lawns and crops. We've done everything "right."

Still, our children are struggling. **Could we be missing something?** Consider: The latest research shows that children exposed to bleach actually have *more, not fewer* infections—including a 20 percent higher risk of coming down with the flu.[8] Hand sanitizers contain triclosan, which disrupts endocrine function and increases risk of eczema, allergies, and asthma,[9] even cancer.[10] Research also shows that good old soap does as good a job as sanitizers anyway.[11] And study after study shows that repeated courses of antibiotics— especially in children—have a detrimental impact on future health, from obesity to allergies to autoimmune disease.[12] **We're starting to understand that short-term gains from technology may not be the best solutions to complex problems posed by nature.**

As conservationist John Muir said, "When one tugs at a single thing in nature, he finds it attached to the rest of the world." Each technological and industrial advance has set off unintended consequences that have negatively affected our children's health and development in unforeseen ways.

Simply put, we have overlooked that the most fundamental ingredients kids need to be healthy and happy come from nature. Our bodies evolved with the natural world; we recognize all of the elements on a cellular level. And nutrient-dense food—infused with sunshine, fresh air, and clean water, rich with vitamins, minerals, phytochemicals, and beneficial bacteria all derived from the soil— provides integral building blocks from nature critical for children's bodies and brains.

Remember the adage "You are what you eat"? Well, it should really be "You are what your food eats." We eat plants and animals. Animals eat plants. And what do plants "eat"? Sunshine, air, water . . . and dirt. Yes, dirt, that stuff we got yelled at for rolling around in as kids. If we are what our food eats, we are only as healthy as the soil our food is grown in. Food is a direct manifestation of soil fertility: the many minerals that come from the rocks, animal scat, bacteria, bugs, worms, and fungi that work together to feed our soil. So it stands to reason that just as we are in a direct, dynamic relationship with our food, *we are simultaneously in relationship also with soil and the natural world.* And unless we take care of soil and the natural world, soil and the natural world can't take care of us by providing dense nutrients.

**It turns out that all the things that are messy and dirty in the world, the very things we thought we needed to control or even eliminate to stay alive, are actually the very elements necessary for robust health.** Research says that bacteria, fungi, parasites, insects, weeds—and living, nutrient-dense soil full of all of those elements—play direct and critical roles in the health of our food, and by extension, the health of our children. Instead of developing new antibiotics, doctors are beginning to treat chronic disease using the opposite approach: bacteria, parasites, soil, even—wait for it!—stool.

You don't have to be a scientist to know that spending a few hours outside exploring does wonders for any child. We all know that kids thrive when they are connected in all ways to good, old-fashioned dirt. Research supports this: Kids who take walks in parks or play in green playgrounds have improved attention spans and better test performance—and are happier and calmer—than their peers who spend their time in less natural environments. Spending time in the forest boosts children's immune system function measurably.[13] **Dirt and nature reach into children's bodies and minds through their food and play.**

So what did this mean I needed to do for my son? To remedy the damage caused by the steroids and antibiotics he had been prescribed—which had thrown the healthy critters in his gut out of balance and dysregulated his immune system—he ate fresh produce directly from our garden, rinsed but with traces of soil still clinging to it. I gave him fermented probiotic foods like pickles, yogurt, kefir, and ruby red sauerkraut to repopulate his microbiota. I made him healing bone marrow broths infused with shiitake and maitake mushrooms, astragalus, and ginger to rebuild his gut, restore his immune system, and help him absorb nutrients. I added immune-regulating spices to his diet, such as turmeric and black cumin seeds. I included brain-enhancing foods like broccoli and Brussels sprouts grown in our vegetable garden, egg yolks from our pastured backyard chickens, omega-3-rich sardines and anchovies, and occasionally, rich, balancing dark chocolate. He spent tons of time outdoors, playing in parks, walking in the woods, and getting messy exploring nature.

As his body healed with these foods, my son quickly reached milestones that had been delayed for the better part of a year. He gained new words, became steadier on his feet, and was much happier. **His transformation awakened me to just how powerful the connection is between nutrient-dense foods and children's physical and emotional health.**

Now I want to show you how you can help your own children.

In the biblical story of creation, Adam is built from dirt. People may say it's figurative, but science is telling us that same story in a different way: We are only as good as the dirt our food is grown in and our kids play in. In *The Dirt Cure* we'll explore the science about nutrient-dense foods that can heal kids' ills—from eczema to ear infections to anxiety to ADHD—and keep your healthy kids (really, truly) well. We'll talk about what destroys soil fertility, how to avoid foods grown that way, and how to find the most abundantly nutritious food from the best sources. And then I'll help you develop a plan for the most wholesome diet possible for your child, including tips for how to prepare foods deliciously so that he or she will eat and reap the benefits. By the end, you'll see that your children's health really does come straight from the soil.

# CHAPTER I
## Where True Health Begins

I love to work with soil. During my pediatrics residency, I gained local notoriety for the melons, tomatoes, peppers, cucumbers, arugula, and beans that burst from the small raised bed I'd built next to our hospital housing. Even though our new apartment in the Bronx overlooked a park, I had yet to find a space of my own where I could *grow*.

Miraculously, I found an office for my practice that had a lot behind the building. The grumpy landlord confirmed that the building did indeed have a "backyard" and agreed to include it in my lease. Key to padlocked gate in hand, I emerged into a desolate space nothing like the verdant Eden I'd imagined. Between the dying tree, the mass of thigh-high weeds and vines as thick as small tree trunks (not to mention sizable piles of what appeared to be petrified dog excrement), I had my work cut out. Despite all the overgrowth aboveground, the hard-packed, dusty earth revealed little below—no "potato" bugs, spiders, or garden snakes, and, worse, not one worm. I could barely fathom how to help this sick land get well.

I enlisted an extra set of hands—Jesse, a young artist who wanted to plant a permaculture food forest in each borough of New York City. We spent the next few months working side by side, covered in dirt, using straw, broken cardboard boxes, and a hilariously named manure called Chickity-Doo-Doo to build soil that would retain moisture and nutrients and invite worms and bugs. Over time, the terrain began to heal. As the soil became rich and substantial, worms returned, which meant that their invisible communities—beneficial bacteria and fungi and organic matter in the soil that fed the plants—were returning, too. We installed laying hens and honeybees as residents. My plants—beans, melons, kale, tomatoes, kiwi, berries—grew abundantly. I learned that even urban gardens invited delicious edible wild plants like dandelion greens and lamb's-quarters. When pests came, I resisted the (powerful) urge to poison them with pesticides. Instead, we picked off what we could, but more important, fed the soil with kelp, bone meal, and rich, black compost from kitchen and garden scraps . . . and the pests decreased considerably. While pests never disappeared altogether, the plants were able to mount an effective defense without my help and live in equilibrium with various critters. I discovered that a nourished terrain rich in microbes and minerals yielded healthy, resilient plants.

This brought to mind a famous old rivalry between two scientists: Louis Pasteur, father of "germ theory" and pasteurization, and his colleague Claude Bernard disagreed about which played a bigger role in disease: the germ or the person who had the germ. Pasteur pinned human disease on the presence and action of certain germs. According to his theory, the fewer microbes the body is exposed to, the better. Bernard said that a person's internal environment plays the more important role in health. He maintained that most common microbial diseases are caused by organisms *present in the body of a normal individual*. Normally, these microbes help with cellular and metabolic processes—unless the body is out of balance, which allows these same microbes free rein to cause illness. For Bernard, the health of the host—and not the power of the microorganism—instigates most disease. And the story goes that Pasteur conceded on his deathbed: "The microbe is nothing. The terrain is everything."

In the tradition of Pasteur, my own medical training taught the paradigm that disease could strike anyone at any time, which I call the "sitting duck" theory. In that sense, disease is bad luck and the ideal preventive steps would be to eliminate exposure to as many microbes as possible with the strongest treatments available. This philosophy has been a guiding principle of modern medicine, and has extended into animal husbandry, agriculture, and food production. While incorporating practices like hand washing with soap and quarantining the ill has indeed helped to reduce the risk of spreading infection, the story is actually more complex.

My garden experience broadened this picture by illustrating the truth in Bernard's theory. There, healing the terrain—indeed, adding *more* microbes, bugs, and worms—powerfully strengthened plants in the face of stressors like infection and pests. Any number of pests could be attacking the plants in my neighbor's garden just ten feet away without making much of a dent in my plants. The most effective strategy was not declaring war on bugs. **I learned that a balanced terrain acts as powerful protection from whatever challenges nature doles out.** This unexpectedly resonated for me as a physician. These observations from the plant world translated to my work with children.

In my practice, as in my garden, the health of a child's inner terrain reflects the health of the child's outer terrain. In other words, the elements of nature make all the difference to a child's resilient health. For this reason, growing healthy children cannot occur in a sterile terrain, but only a richly diverse one.

**Germ theory pits microbe against terrain, but we are learning that in large part, diverse and abundant microbes *are* our terrain**. To maintain health, both plants and children need to be in contact with—not protected from—the full array of living elements: sunshine, truly fresh food, soil, all sorts of microbes, even critters. Both need to be actively nourished with living food, minimal toxins, rich in dirt. Their health depends on it.

## THE BODY IS ALWAYS LEARNING

Our bodies are not intended to be islands. We are built to be challenged. Indeed, these challenges come from every one of our diverse interactions with nature—food, dirt, microbes, animals, people—as well as synthetic chemicals, pharmaceuticals, heavy metals, and the like. Our bodies are complex information processing centers, and each interaction serves as another bit of information that educates the body. Every small challenge teaches our bodies what to do when bigger challenges come along. This is why it's normal—even important—for kids to be exposed to the outside world and to get occasional runny noses, fevers, coughs, and so on. As they recover from these mild infections, kids' bodies and immune systems begin the lifelong process of learning to navigate the world in all its complexity.

Somehow, we've lost trust in the body's ability to heal itself. Instead, we use frequent rounds of Tylenol, ibuprofen, and antibiotics at the first hint of symptoms because we are afraid the body won't know what to do. Paradoxically, each time we unnecessarily interfere with our bodies' natural survival mechanisms—even out of a desire to protect—the body becomes less able to recover on its own. A body that is constantly shielded from fighting and recovering from small illnesses may not respond effectively when bigger challenges inevitably arise. How could it? If you want your child to learn to play the violin, you can't bring someone else in to practice the violin for him (or slap his hand away every time he tries to practice on his own!). **Allowing children to overcome small illnesses without interfering strengthens their immune systems. It also provides opportunities for the body to evaluate whether challenges are benign or dangerous, when to live and let live, and when to pick a fight. These are skills critical for your child's lifelong health.**

Take fever. We're so fearful of the body malfunctioning that we've come to mistake the body's healthy immune response for something inherently dangerous. Some of the sickest kids I see—like those with severe chronic disorders—rarely get fevers. But this isn't necessarily a good thing. Fevers allow the immune system to expel organisms and compounds from the body. These kids don't even mount a response. Even my own son—with all of his "runny noses" and coughing— never developed a fever as a young child. He ran his first fever when he was *seven*. And when he finally did, we were thrilled. I understand it sounds weird, but his immune system finally could do what it was supposed to do: fight and overcome infection.

I'm not suggesting that kids should live in misery when they're sick. But avoiding all exposures or interfering with the body's normal response is not the answer. This book will discuss ways you can strengthen your child's body and immune system to enhance his or her ability to recover.

## Fever: The Body Knows What to Do to Heal

Fever itself is not a disease; it's a remedy to disease. Fever is a component of a complex inflammatory cascade that the body launches in response to infection. Fever acts as a natural "antibiotic," raising internal temperature to make it inhospitable for unhealthy elements. Yet during the past 30 years, many parents have come to believe that they must immediately administer antipyretics—fever-lowering medications such as acetaminophen or ibuprofen—for any fever or no fever at all.[1] Yet according to the American Academy of Pediatrics, fevers below 104°F are not damaging. In fact, fevers may well allow children to get over infections more quickly.[2] Antipyretics reduce the body's purposeful rise in temperature and also interrupt the inflammatory response that helps to vanquish the infection.

Sometimes fevers reflect dangerous infections, in which case your child may appear very ill and should be evaluated and treated by a medical professional. Otherwise, the best approach is to support the immune system and keep your child comfortable with cool cloths, lukewarm baths, hydration, and plenty of rest.[3] I recommend giving your child elderberry syrup, thyme-infused honey, a cup of licorice tea, and loads of chicken soup infused with sliced gingerroot, maitake and turkey tail mushrooms, and astragalus root to promote immunity and fight infection. Yarrow tea or tincture can help initiate sweating, which can mitigate a high fever without interfering with the immune system's job. A mug of peppermint tea or a compress dunked in ice water infused with a few drops of peppermint essential oil is also soothing.

## LET'S GET (REALLY, TRULY) HEALTHY

What does it mean to be healthy? Many people define being healthy simply as "not being sick." Yet health is more than the absence of illness; it's the dynamic relationship between us—our bodies and minds—and the world around us. *Homeostasis* is a term that describes the tendency of the body to maintain internal equilibrium by normalizing function at every moment and at every level. It's the driving force that keeps everything from heart rate to blood sugar to white blood cell levels in balance with the world around us. When our internal terrain is in alignment with our external terrain, we are healthy. When it's out of alignment, we become sick. And by the time severe illness rears its head, there likely have been ongoing signs that things were out of balance for some time.

Yet more and more, these ongoing problems that indicate children are not in balance are not recognized as problems. For example, I might ask, "How many ear infections has your child had in the past year?" The answer is usually something along the lines of, "Oh, no more than normal." Or "How often does your kid poop?" "The normal amount." **Beware: The prevailing definitions of normal may not be all that normal.**

For example, one really smart, lovely mom came in with her five-year-old daughter for learning disabilities. I asked about her child's stool, and she said, "Oh, it's normal." But her child volunteered enthusiastically, "I clog the toilet every time I poop!" Her mom recoiled: "Honey, the doctor doesn't need to know that!" I told her that's exactly what I need to know. Not only did this little girl clog their toilet, her mom carried a plastic knife in her purse so she could break up her poop to avoid clogging toilets at other people's houses. "I call her my super pooper!" she declared. She represents her child's stool as "normal," yet she carries a sharp utensil in her bag to slice up her kid's poop. That's how thoroughly we can justify our kids' conditions as normal—even to ourselves!

Similarly, parents often say no when I ask whether their child has any medical history. I review all the systems: eyes, ears, nose, throat, lungs, heart, belly, skin, and so on? *Nope. He almost never gets sick; he's really healthy!* So I've learned to collect medical history backward, by asking if their child has ever been on common medications like antibiotics. *Oh, no more than normal.* "How many times is normal?" *Maybe six or seven times a year.* "How about steroid cream?" *Oh, yes, he needs that for his eczema all winter long.* "Allergy medication?" *Of course, he takes those every spring and fall or he can't breathe!* Three plus medications and counting in a "healthy" child—that's how blurred the line between healthy and unhealthy has become. Each of these is a warning sign that a child's body is out of balance.

Our normalizing of chronic illness in kids has extended to all kinds of problems: recurrent headaches, eczema, allergies, asthma, gastric reflux, anxiety, depression, explosive behavior or irritability, chronic diaper rash, "ants in the pants," trouble sleeping, or trouble gaining or losing weight. Even families in constant struggle due to their children's health conditions may deny that their children have a "chronic illness" until symptoms become so severe that they're forced to visit numerous doctors or the hospital. **The new normal for children's health has become chronic illness, with chronic symptoms and chronic medications to treat them.**

What if I told you that these conditions aren't healthy or "normal"? That some kids never get ear infections, ever? That skin inflammations like eczema and even diaper rash are ways that the body—especially the gut—asks for help? Despite what we've been led to believe, babies with eczema aren't born with a topical steroid deficiency! ADHD isn't a stimulant deficiency. And constipation isn't a Miralax deficiency. Each of these conditions is a symptom of a depleted and overloaded body—a body in distress.

**Every symptom happens for a reason.** Sometimes the reason remains a mystery, but often we can act as detectives to uncover triggers by asking: Why is this happening? What recently changed for my child? What might be my child's triggers? How can I alter these triggers to change the course of his or her health? Often it has to do with the interaction between what's inside our bodies—including our genes—and the world outside our bodies.

## Signs of a Dysregulated Body

Here are two ways we know that the body isn't working as it should:

1. A child begins to struggle when exposed to foods, trees, or flowers with which we evolved, side by side, for thousands of years. When the familiar becomes so unfamiliar that the body treats it as a potentially deadly enemy, the body is out of balance with its environment.

2. The most fundamental and necessary functions of a child's body—eating, breathing, pooping, sleeping, running, laughing, speaking, thinking, learning, playing, and, most important, healing—are disrupted.

### Healthy Children Are Resilient

The best evidence that a child is healthy becomes clear *after* a child gets sick. After a bout with an illness like the flu, healthy kids go right back to normal—usually with rest, time, and a little TLC. They are back to their active, curious selves before you know it and they can stay that way *the majority of the time*.

The most important manifestation of health is "resilience," a term used in biology and economics to mean that something or someone has the ability to meet a challenge, adapt, and thrive. Also called grit, it's the vital capacity to cope with the constant unpredictability in our world—to recover from challenges small and large and come out better and stronger on the other end. Remember homeostasis, our system's tendency to always move toward balance? The ability to maintain homeostasis reflects the body's overall resilience. All of this happens literally on a cellular level in organelles called the mitochondria. (More on that later.)

Luckily, raising happy, healthy, resilient children doesn't require elaborate measures. In fact, the body—in all of its sophistication and complexity—is capable of doing the heavy lifting. The body is built to withstand the trials that life throws our way—intense exercise, occasional lack of sleep, microbes, even some toxins. A well-nourished child who's allowed to interact with diverse exposures becomes naturally resilient.

## YOUR GENES ARE NOT YOUR DESTINY

Why do so many parents accept as normal that their kids suffer from chronic maladies? It may be because we ourselves suffer from similar conditions, so we assume it's our family heritage. I've heard from many parents that there's nothing to be done about a condition or even that it's "normal" because it "runs in the family" and "everyone has it." What if I told you that many chronic conditions that you thought were "genetic" are not necessarily written in stone? What if you could alter your child's genetic destiny?

Your DNA dictates your genetic vulnerabilities. The actual DNA sequence—the genome passed down from grandparents to parents to children—is relatively stable, changing only in rare cases of a mutation. But DNA is more dynamic than anyone previously imagined. As children grow and develop, parts of the genome activate and deactivate at strategic times and in specific locations. This process happens even on a seasonal basis: Many inflammatory conditions worsen in the winter because genes promoting inflammation upregulate and genes suppressing inflammation downregulate.[4] Children's cells—down to their DNA—respond constantly to changes in the world around them. And it turns out that exposures to both natural and man-made compounds can induce epigenetic changes that are also passed down from generation to generation.

Your child's DNA interacts with one particularly complex and powerful exposure every day, many times a day. **For better or worse, every bite of food your child ingests—along with soil nutrients, microbes, or synthetic chemicals from the farm where it was grown or raised, traces from its packaging or the pan in which it was prepared—can influence his or her gene expression.** Often these powerful influences on their genes are temporary, altering their metabolic function only for as long as the nutrients, microbes, or other exposures persist in their bodies. But when this back-and-forth between their genes and their experiences in the outside world produces sustained changes in the way DNA works, it's called epigenetics.

Epigenetics (literally "above genetics") means that food, infections, toxins, and even experiences alter the way DNA is expressed in our appearance, function, and overall health. Through epigenetic modification, life exposures can silence or activate genes in enduring ways, even through generations. One simple example of the epigenetic impact of food in the insect world: Worker bees have no ovaries, but queen bees—who are genetically identical—do. This is because worker bees eat honey, which turns on the no-ovary gene, while queen bees eat royal jelly, which turns it off. Toxins can influence our genes as well. Pregnant mice who ate food laced with bisphenol A (BPA), a toxic plastic that lines the cans of food we buy, gave birth to babies with altered gene expression. The babies developed what's called an *agouti* phenotype: odd yellow fur instead of their normal brown, along with a higher risk for obesity, diabetes, and cancer. What's more, this effect unexpectedly impacted the next generation of mice as well. Their grandbaby mice also had the same odd yellow fur and health risks, even though their moms hadn't ever directly been exposed to BPA. On the other hand, pregnant mice whose food contained BPA plus folate did *not* express the abnormal *agouti* phenotype because folate "silenced" the toxic effects of BPA on the gene. These mice had regular brown babies and grandbabies that carried no increased risk of disease. Think of it: exposures from their food—both good and bad—influenced their gene expression, over generations.

Think of your DNA as an ongoing instruction manual for how to build and maintain your body, which remains in use every moment of every day. The cells and enzymes responsible for helping the body to grow, replenish, and repair continuously refer to those instructions. The manual itself rarely changes, but *how it's read* does. Nutrients, microbes, and synthetics that enter our bodies—largely but not exclusively through food—can signal which sets of instructions our cells should follow. It's like putting sticky notes on some pages of the manual, while leaving others unread. So you might carry the genetic predisposition for things like cancer, mental illness, ADHD, or obesity, but it's by no means a sure thing that those portions of your DNA will be expressed. Nutrients flag important areas at certain times; thus many "on" and "off" labels come from food. Epigenetics even helps to determine seemingly random events in our children's physiology, such as timing of maturity: when a young woman begins to menstruate, for instance, or when pubertal growth spurts happen in a boy. **Genetic predisposition may make your child more vulnerable to disorders, but that's not the final word.**[5]

What does this mean for us? Genetics may predispose a child to certain disorders, even the timing of life cycle events, but our exposures—good and bad—have the final say. It's been said about certain diseases that "Genes load the gun; environment pulls the trigger." To a degree, these variations are explained by epigenetics.

Consider identical twins—often they start off looking so much alike that no one can tell them apart. But as time goes on, their interaction in the world can change their appearance. Maybe it's through the nutrients in their food, microbes, or toxins they're exposed to, or life experiences. Some of these operate on a metabolic level and disappear after the exposure. But other factors change how their respective blueprints are read. Even though they have the same exact underlying genetic code, many twins no longer look exactly the same—on the inside or the outside—as they age. So now they'll differ not only in their physical characteristics, but also in their health. One may develop cancer, while the other doesn't. One may suffer from an autoimmune disease, and the other won't.

In one study, researchers examined the conventional wisdom that identical twins with identical DNA would develop the same medical and neurological conditions, especially one with known genetic links, such as autism. Yet they discovered that both identical twins developed autism in just under 70 percent of the cases.[6,7] Another identical-twin study noted that less than 40 percent of autism risk in twins could be attributed to genetics alone, while shared environmental influences may account for as much as 55 percent of risk.[8]

These and subsequent studies have acknowledged the role of epi-genetics.[9]

Scientists have spent years trying to identify the "autism gene," "diabetes gene," or "ADHD gene," but they've so far been stumped in the pursuit of this magical "one-disease, one-gene" model. Genes can occasionally be singled out as indicating a high risk for develop-ing autism or other disorders, such as specific forms of epilepsy, or other neurological or chronic diseases. Causes of these disorders, however, are considerably more complex than the DNA we bring to the table.

While our knowledge of epigenetics is still young, what's exciting is that epigenetic changes can be *reversible*. And not just for future generations—but right here, right now, for your kids—especially dur-ing early periods of rapid development. There's still much to learn about which epigenetic exposures achieve desired outcomes. But I've seen children who are sick with some of the most severe or seemingly intractable conditions improve significantly—in enduring ways my training said wasn't possible—when we change their food and en-vironment. Epigenetic modification offers the possibility of durable healing.

Now you know that your child's health is fluid, not static. The potential for transformation—not to mention prevention—always exists. Together, our job is to create the opportunity for shifts toward better balance within ourselves and with the world around us. So now let's embark on a journey to explore ways for your child to be better, stronger, and more resilient.

## GETTING STARTED: A CLEAN SLATE

*The real voyage of discovery consists,*
*not in seeking new landscapes, but in having new eyes.*
—MARCEL PROUST

Forget everything you've been told about your child's health up until now—good or bad. I want you to get in touch with your intuition, your inner-knowing about your child. No expert—no matter how smart or highly trained—will ever know your child as you do. **You are the expert on your child.** Whenever I hear parents preface an observation about their child with "This may not mean anything, but . . ." or "I don't know, but . . ." I immediately tell them, "You *do* know!" And so do you. The key is to trust your instincts.

I want you to regard your child with new eyes. We're thinking beyond *what* your child has been labeled with: "constipation," "ADHD," "asthma," "hypothyroidism," "epilepsy," or "eczema." They're really just descriptions of these symptoms themselves. We're now asking *why* your child isn't well, not just *what* you need to fix. Calling chronic symptoms "diseases" permits doctors to medicate away symptoms without ever searching for or addressing the cause.

To illustrate: Let's say someone you know died and you wanted to know why. If you look at death certificates, you'd find many that list "cardiac arrest" as the primary cause of death. That's kind of like saying they died of "death syndrome." It's a description of what that person experienced, but it doesn't provide insight as to *why*. Similarly, for many chronic conditions, the diagnosis describes what but not why. And if pharmaceutical meds quell symptoms satisfactorily, many docs see no need to look deeper.

## Looking Deeper

ADHD is a real-life example of how a group of simultaneously occurring symptoms may be misconstrued as a disease. ADHD is really a description of a constellation of symptoms. While the symptoms can be very real, the diagnosis doesn't tell us anything about the root cause. One child can have ADHD symptoms for different reasons than another does. ADHD is not caused by a specific gene, nor is it an inherent brain disorder—or if it is, it's many different brain disorders! It's a set of symptoms caused by a variety of factors. Some children exhibit symptoms due to reactivity to food and food chemicals,[10] others due to toxic exposures,[11] still others become symptomatic when their blood sugar drops about an hour after breakfast or right before lunch. Other kids are in a learning environment that's wrong for them and when moved to a more appropriate setting or get a new teacher, *poof!* Huge improvement. The reason for symptoms may not always be obvious, but there is always a reason.

Reflux is another example. Most babies who frequently spit up are diagnosed with "reflux." Instead of asking what the trigger may be, doctors are often quick to prescribe H2 blockers to reduce acid in the stomach—what my colleague Dr. Sidney Baker calls the "Name It–Blame It–Tame It" approach. When doctors turn the symptom into the disease ("reflux") without asking why, they can prescribe a pill to treat and control the disease. But reflux is not a disease; it's a *symptom*, often caused by food reactivity (most commonly, difficult-to-digest cow's milk proteins in formula or breast milk).[12,13,14] One study found that of the 33 percent of refluxing infants and children who didn't respond to reflux medication, *all of these children's symptoms improved when they stopped all cow's milk proteins.*[15] (The other 66 percent of infants and children were not given the opportunity to trial off dairy.) Another study showed that removing cow's milk–protein based formula improved reflux even when the baby tested negative for cow's milk allergy.[16] You might say, "Who cares if the baby takes medicine so long as he or she is feeling better?" First, adequate stomach acid is necessary for breaking down proteins that may trigger an allergy, which otherwise only further activate the gut's immune system. Second, stomach acid acts as a line of defense against potential pathogens. Third, stomach acid is necessary for absorbing calcium, magnesium, and zinc; therefore, use of these medications can cause nutritional deficiencies at a time when demand is very high.[17]

Even when a child must start medication—which in some cases may be a lifesaver because things have gotten that bad—we must continue to investigate and address underlying causes. The goal is to preclude the need for long-term medication. Ideally, we avoid starting medication at all.

Healing or "curing" is rarely part of the prevailing medical lexicon based in pharmaceutical medication. This is because any cure must come from the body itself. I repeat: *Any cure comes from the body itself.* The role of pharmaceuticals, among other treatment approaches, is to help the body get back on its figurative feet. **But when a child's body is depleted and improperly nourished, it cannot heal.** Under these circumstances, ongoing pharmaceuticals become necessary to force a physiological response that the body can't create on its own. If a child's body has the resolve to make this leap to healing, medication can be stopped and the child thrives. Otherwise, the child is called "chronically ill."

A body nourished by nutrient-dense food and nature will have the building blocks to heal itself. To a great degree, you can influence these variables with how you interact with your living environment and what you eat. That's right: Your food, drink, and contact with nature offer exceptional tools both for healing and maintaining health and happiness.

This is what I call the "Dorothy" moment. At the end of *The Wizard of Oz*, Dorothy realizes that the almighty wizard didn't actually have all of the answers, and that she herself had the power to get home on her own all along. In this case, you and your child may well already have the answers to how to be resilient and well. My job is to help you find them. It's time to shed preconceived notions, start looking with fresh eyes, and begin asking, "Why?"

## Keeping a Journal

I've included the checklist below to help you take an inventory of your child's health and to get an idea of where there might be room for improvement. Whether your child is struggling to flourish or has chronic issues, this step will allow you to begin to see what true health looks like—and help not just your child, but your entire family—reach it.

## A Healthy Child

- **Sleep:** Goes to sleep at night in less than 30 minutes, with infrequent nighttime waking, and wakes up rested.
- **Stool:** Has formed bowel movements one or more times daily (which aren't painful, don't clog the toilet, and don't make the entire house smell).
- **Diet:** Eats a variety of foods, including vegetables and fruit.
- **Digestion:** Has little to no gas, few stomachaches, and no "colic." Grows normally.
- **Infections:** Gets occasional coughs and colds, but infrequent ear infections (or croup, or strep) over his or her entire childhood.
- **Skin:** Has clear skin, not rough, "sensitive," or itchy. No frequent rashes. And no red ears or blotchy cheeks that persist for more than five to ten minutes after being hot or cold.
- **Eyes:** They look clear and bright, with no dark circles, redness, or swelling.
- **Energy:** Has the stamina to keep up with other children.
- **Resilience:** Gets occasional fevers with illness that resolve with minimal or no intervention. Doesn't suffer from allergies, asthma, or other chronic conditions.
- **Behavior:** Has infrequent tantrums. No violent behavior or destruction of property and is able to recover fairly quickly.
- **Focus:** Is reasonably able to concentrate, learn, and remember for a child his or her age.
- **Mood:** Can engage in and enjoy life.

Without getting caught up in labels or a diagnosis, make your own list applicable to your child by adding any symptoms of concern. As you follow the recommendations I'll make throughout this book—adding healing foods and practices, eliminating those that are potentially damaging—refer back to this list and note how your child evolves with the changes. My goal is for you to see your child in almost every item on the "healthy" list—and in fewer and fewer on the "needs improvement" one.

## CHAPTER 2

# Learning to Listen to the Body: What Symptoms Tell You

O ur society has followed Pasteur's theories to the extreme, focusing attention almost exclusively on attacking the "microbe"—whether germ or disease—rather than on strengthening "terrain," the health of the individual who has developed the disease. Yet our internal terrain is largely responsible for our susceptibility to illness. **Why** does this child get ear infections every month? **Why** all of these strep infections? **Why** does this child get a bad case of the flu and these others don't? **Why** does this child recover easily from an episode of Lyme disease, while another child becomes so chronically ill that her parents say, "She hasn't been the same since . . ."

These differences reflect the child's terrain: how resilient they are, and how well they maintain homeostasis in the face of challenges. This depends to some degree on genetic vulnerabilities, but even more so, it depends upon their internal resources and their exposures. When the body's reserve is tapped out, we start to see symptoms, which indicate that the body is in distress.

### Symptoms Are the Body's Way of Asking for Help

The body constantly communicates what it needs and how we might support it. And it does this primarily with symptoms. Sometimes the body can manage these challenges on its own without needing intervention. Other times, though, the body needs help. And when we ignore the body's messages, they may become progressively louder—more intense, frequent, or unmanageable—until we no longer can ignore them.

Children's symptoms provide clues that enable you to determine what is making their body sick. Even conditions like eczema, asthma, migraines, ADHD, and seizures aren't diseases themselves, but really just symptoms.

Instead of considering symptoms as annoyances to suppress, take rashes, insomnia, and tummy aches as clues that alert you to the need for help. Become a detective. I can share with you my experience of talking to the body in its own language, so that you know how to tune in when symptoms arise.

## BUILDING A CASE: IDENTIFYING SYMPTOMS

When I began in private practice, I saw how children's myriad symptoms would either be medicated, ignored, or written off as just "who they are." A child might be referred to me for headaches, but no one had considered that his chronic eczema or seven annual ear infections might be related. When I questioned whether one girl's once-a-week bowel movements might be addressed more effectively, her mother replied, "Her doctor has tried everything already; she says that's just Jamie." When I called one child's pediatrician and wondered aloud whether his ADD might be connected to his astronomical number of ear infections, she said, "Listen, sometimes an ear infection is just an ear infection." Yes, maybe. But are 15 ear infections just 15 ear infections? Are 25 ear infections just 25 ear infections? Where does it end?

I saw this interconnection of symptoms as a parent, too. When my son was reacting to soy, he had symptoms of asthma as well as a chronic runny nose, rashes, and developmental plateau. But our (otherwise very caring) pediatrician didn't put those symptoms together. In fact, he didn't think much of them. To him, my son was just a "reactive" kid. He said: "That's just him. Some kids are like that." Ultimately, it felt like a total cop-out. It wasn't until I started asking **why?** that we began our road to healing.

Conventional medicine doesn't explore the complex connections between closely networked systems of the body (digestive, immune, nervous, endocrine). Most docs aren't looking at problems in a big-picture way and are trained to see things only within their area of specialty: asthma is a lung problem; eczema is a skin problem; constipation is a gut problem; ADHD is a brain problem. But the body is one complete system. Nothing happens in isolation. Gut and immune system. Lungs and skin. The brain is connected to the rest of the body. Sounds obvious, I know, but then why are we treating children as though they are bundles of disembodied symptoms? A child with epilepsy may come to my office with severe constipation, eczema, asthma, and poor growth, in addition to seizures. This child might be visiting a gastroenterologist, a dermatologist, a pulmonologist, and a neurologist. But no one considers the whole child.

By peeling back the layers like an onion, symptom by symptom, we can eventually heal the child from gut to brain. So when a child presents with migraine headaches and the parent says, "He has a lot of gas [or stomachaches or constipation]"—that's where we start. A colleague of mine once said, "I went into neurology to deal with the brain, not the other end!" But I can't imagine how I could successfully treat children *without* asking about digestion and stool. Together, a child's physical symptoms tell a story. When addressed comprehensively, even difficult neurological symptoms—such as seizures, tics, OCD, explosive behavior, or anxiety—can improve. We must pay attention to *all* the body's ongoing symptoms.

## Suppressing Symptoms Can Damage the Body

Think about the last time you got a prescription for your child. Maybe it was steroid cream for eczema or antibiotics for a sore throat. Or over-the-counter medicines—Tylenol for fevers, Pepto-Bismol for diarrhea, or Robitussin for coughing. The message we get is clear: We're being good, caring parents by relieving symptoms that cause our children discomfort. And most doctors—myself included—were trained to treat (read: suppress) the symptoms of illness with medication instead of addressing the underlying problem that puts the body out of balance.

By suppressing symptoms though, medications put our body's communication on mute. While medications sometimes allow us to be more comfortable, they also permit us to ignore our body's distress communication. Yet muting our body's emergency broadcast systems doesn't eliminate the impending crisis. Persistent imbalances in the body eventually translate to recurrent clinical symptoms if they're not addressed.

Medication also affects our body's ability to manage future challenges. If a child doesn't practice violin before her recital, she can't play well in her performance. Similarly, the immune system is a quick study but can only learn when given the chance. In this way, even infections can serve as an important opportunity. Consider every fever, cold, or sore throat an opportunity for the immune system to learn to respond better next time. Tylenol, ibuprofen, or antibiotics can interrupt that opportunity to learn by shutting down our bodywide innate immune response. When we constantly interfere with or take over each difficult situation, the body can't develop and hone the skills that allow it to fight infections on its own.

Medication is not the solution to getting well. Healing the root cause of one's symptoms is. In my practice, I can count on one hand the number of times I write a prescription for medication in a given month. And even when I start a patient on meds, I'm always thinking of how we will wean the child off of them.

## PHARMACEUTICAL MEDICINE: IS IT REALLY HEALING?

During the past hundred-plus years, our society has made impressive medical and technological advances. Antipyretics, antimicrobials, and antibiotics have enhanced our ability to reduce children's deaths from infection and spare them discomfort and pain. As use of these treatments has crescendoed, however, kids have been growing steadily sicker.[1,2,3]

Even though the United States holds only 5 percent of the world's population, it's responsible for *75 percent* of global prescription drug use. And these prescribed medications have consequences. Selective serotonin reuptake inhibitors (SSRIs) used for depression carry a black box warning because they can increase the risk of suicidal thoughts and behaviors in children and young adults who are started on high doses.[4] Aside from insomnia and suppressed appetite, ADHD medications such as Ritalin or Adderall can lead to addiction, anxiety, and occasionally psychosis.[5]

A 14-year-old girl named Phoebe came to my practice because she felt foggy. She was taking Focalin for poor attention, Trazodone for the insomnia she experienced from Focalin, and Zoloft for the depression she experienced after starting the Trazodone. When I asked Phoebe's pediatrician to consider gradually reducing her medication over time to help with the fogginess, the doctor replied, "Let's just leave things as they are. She's finally doing so well."

In my early days of practice, I treated children as young as six years old who had been put on three or more psychoactive medications daily. By a strange logic it made sense—each medication answered a need that another medication created. They might take an antiepileptic for seizure disorder, a stimulant for attention issues due to an antiepileptic side effect, and an antipsychotic for aggressive behavior triggered by the stimulant. *Take note: Sometimes the drugs themselves actively contribute to children's illnesses.*

Indeed, sometimes the very tools we use to combat infection later can contribute to autoimmune and inflammatory disorders.[6] Following their discovery in 1928, antibiotics are thought to have saved 100 million lives since World War II. Yet antibiotics, commonly prescribed in repeated rounds to infants and children, carry a greater threat to children's long-term health than to adults' because they disrupt the balance of bacteria in children's developing digestive tracts just at their most vulnerable. In exchange for the very real accomplishment of improved control over infectious disease, antibiotics have contributed to the observed rise in a variety of complex diseases—from "immune-mediated" diseases to metabolic disorders to possible cancer.[7]

And it's not just prescribed medications we're talking about—widely used medications, even those sold over the counter for colds, coughs, fevers, and other common symptoms—can be detrimental to our children's bodies and immune systems. We consider medications like acetominophen and ibuprofen—things we can pick up at the grocery store and even many gas stations—as totally safe. Yet they're not. The use of acetaminophen-containing meds like Tylenol can increase the risk of developing asthma, allergies, and eczema,[8,9] especially when given in the early years of life—and may increase the risk of a child developing ADHD when exposed in utero.[10] Why? The acetaminophen in Tylenol binds to a powerful antioxidant called glutathione, which acts as a garbage truck for our cells, carting away free radicals and toxins as part of the body's detoxification process. But acetaminophen irreversibly binds glutathione and reduces its cell-scrubbing abilities, especially in areas demanding high glutathione, like the brain and liver.[11,12] Acetaminophen toxicity has replaced viral hepatitis as the most common cause of acute liver failure and is the second most common cause of liver failure requiring transplantation.[13] Yikes. And beware: The FDA has strengthened warnings on good old ibuprofen and other nonsteroidal anti-inflammatory (NSAID) medications because they can increase risk of heart attack and stroke by as much as 50 percent.[14]

In addition to these concerns, these medications interfere with the body's mounting a robust immune response to vanquish whatever is causing trouble. Consider: A fever is your body's innate "antibiotic"— a natural antimicrobial response that reflects the immune system mobilizing in ways more complex and often more powerful than pills. By acting as the superhero that swoops in to "save the day" every time, medication can weaken the ever-learning immune system by preventing it from building relationships with the organisms that come its way. What results is that immune T cells don't evolve to develop tolerance and an immune imbalance ensues.[15] The memory-based T cells that remember and search for previous threats become paranoid, and begin to see enemies where there are none. This sets the stage for allergies, asthma, and autoimmune disease.

Medication can be critical at times to address crises. But our society's overreliance on pharmaceutical treatments has created a dangerous cycle. We are liberally administering medications for isolated symptoms as a replacement for determining root cause. And doctors, skilled as they are at targeting a treatment to a symptom, are less adept at considering the ramifications of drugs on all systems of the body *over time*. For instance, parents too often complain that their doctors have disregarded troubling side effects in their children so long as their prescribed medication successfully treated the symptom of interest. Or they denied that the side effects really were side effects—even when the very symptoms were listed right on the insert of the commonly used medications to treat asthma, ADHD, allergies, and other disorders.

TIP ————————————————————————

Take a moment to read the side effect profile of any medication you are thinking of administering to your child. Always ask your physician what the risks of this treatment are so you can make an educated choice. If your doctor claims that there are none, get a second opinion. All treatments carry some risks.

Doctors also don't do a good job of utilizing the precautionary principle when assessing the long-term effects that medications may have: Even without definitive proof, could a medication or medical treatment—even if it's helpful now—potentially cause health problems down the road? This is particularly important in infants and children. For example, one study of more than 65,000 adults showed that those who took frequent stimulants (for ADHD or other reasons) were 60 percent more likely to develop Parkinson's later in life than those who didn't take them frequently.[16] This study was in adults. What long-term impact might daily stimulants have on the developing brains of children? We don't yet know, but information like this implies we should be very cautious.

## HEALING FROM THE INSIDE OUT

Is your relationship with your body a two-way street? Chances are that you take much more than you give, whether you insist that your body keep up with your usual tasks when it's not feeling well or ask it to perform without the optimal fuel or rest. Your expectation of your body is likely high while your community with it is low. And this is what our society teaches children to do as well. Most parents expect that their children's illness and convalescence should take no longer than a brief 24-hour window so that the kids can get right back to school, parents can get to work, and so on.

Now it's time to give back. Before you can ask your body to perform—or even heal—you must nourish and care for it. And the primary way to do that is with the food you eat. Food is inherently different from medication because it offers the body the tools necessary to heal *itself*.

All of the materials our bodies require to function—from repairing DNA to building muscle and replenishing red blood cells—come from the vitamins, minerals, amino acids, and other raw materials in food. This is true even for healthy children—those blessed with "good genes" and vibrant health right now. The foundation for a long, healthy life starts in childhood. Ideally your child won't ever run into any of the issues we've discussed. And if your child isn't as resilient as you believe he or she can be, you're about to learn how to create a new normal for them.

## CHAPTER 3
# Healthy Body, Healthy Brain

When my daughter was in kindergarten, she had stomachaches all the time. We were constantly getting calls from school because her tummy hurt. We thought maybe it was emotional, or that she was hungry. We tried different things—more snacks, resting in the nurse's office—and sometimes she felt better, sometimes she didn't. The occasional stomachaches persisted and became more frequent. She started to complain of occasional headaches. Then, her third-grade teachers noticed her poor focus. We wondered whether she might have a learning disability. It took the principal asking, "Do you think she has a food allergy?" to awaken me to that possibility. (Talk about the shoemaker's kids going barefoot!)

We removed dairy and gluten—common allergenic foods—for a couple of weeks, and the tummy complaints stopped. To confirm our hypothesis that she was reacting to food, we reintroduced gluten. After a "hard-core" gluten day—bagel for breakfast, pasta for lunch, pizza for dinner—she felt like she had the flu for about 24 hours. But my husband still wasn't convinced. So we tried again—removing and then reintroducing those foods. Sure enough, she got sick again. Dairy seemed to be less of a problem for her, but we removed gluten for good. Her performance in school skyrocketed to straight As; focus and learning became non-issues. But every once in a while, she'd come home from school and I'd see her nose twitching like a little rabbit. "What'd you eat today?" I'd ask. "Oh, someone gave me a cookie," she'd say. Or "I ate pretzels at snack." The days she had this tic were always the days she'd eaten gluten, and we never saw it as long as she adhered to her gluten-free diet.

But the questions remained:

- *How did something that simply gave her a stomachache morph into something that affected her focus and cognition, and eventually triggered tics, a neurological dysfunction?*
- *Is it possible that food affects the body from the digestive system to the immune system to the nervous system?*
- *If food affects the nervous system, does that mean that problems we once thought were just "brain problems" really stem from something else going on elsewhere in the body?*

Buckle your seat belt; we're about to turn things upside down.

## YOUR BODY'S OWN TERRAIN: THE GUT

The gut doesn't get a lot of glory. It's mostly associated with a certain amount of embarrassment compared to more glamorous organs like the brain. But your gut produces three quarters of your body's neurotransmitters and holds two thirds of your immune system to boot. Yep, your stomach acid, your tonsils, your appendix, your spleen, and all the lymph nodes that line the wall of your intestines make up the huge immune system of the gut.

The gut is one of the most complex and important parts of the body. In a sense, it acts as the soil from which everything else in the body is nourished. And like rich soil, our guts house abundant nutrients and diverse microbes for our bodies to be healthy. Open at both ends (mouth and anus), our intestinal tract is uniquely part of both the external and internal terrain of the body. As a result, almost anything can get in—the gut is awash in food, microbes, toxins, dirt . . . you name it! But it's also largely concealed inside the body, communicating intimately with organs and even the brain. The gut is the interface between our inner and outer world.

Let's explore some of what's inside. Here's stomach acid, which isn't as malevolent as those antacid commercials would have you believe; quite the opposite. Along with saliva and bile, stomach acid disables harmful pathogens, neutralizes some toxins, and helps to break down large molecules of food into smaller, more easily absorbable forms. In fact, protein can only be broken down by stomach acid.

Next, there's a microscopic universe of a hundred trillion microbes—including mostly viruses, as well as bacteria, fungi, and yeast. These two to four pounds of organisms living in the gut compose our microbiome, which supports digestion, especially of carbohydrates, regulates immunity, aids in flushing toxins, and manufactures nutrients like vitamin K and the range of B vitamins.[1] The gut microbiome is all about balance and tolerance. Like a rich soil, our gut is healthiest when bathed in abundant nutrients and diverse microbes—the more biodiverse, the better. Fewer types of microbes in the gut makes it more likely that one type of organism will dominate improperly, which can lead to gas, bloating, inability to absorb nutrients, and even severe gastrointestinal infections.

Then there's the specialized "skin" that is the gut wall, which acts as a bouncer that guards the very exclusive club that is our insides. These epithelial cells decide what can enter the bloodstream and what can't, ideally allowing in what nourishes us and protecting us from entities ranging from unwanted microbes to toxic agents.

For reasons we'll explore later, sometimes the gut can become more permeable or "leaky," allowing foreign molecules, microbes, and toxins to enter circulation. These immunological triggers float through the bloodstream, activate the immune system,[2] and make kids vulnerable to allergies, sensitivities, and—in some cases—autoimmune diseases like celiac disease and type 1 diabetes.[3]

*My child eats healthy food and still has health problems. Why?*

Good question. No matter how nourishing the food, if your child's gut can't absorb nutrients, he or she won't benefit from that food. Soothe the gut with the inner gel of aloe vera (not whole leaf), deglycyrrhizinated licorice powder, and bone broths. Add prebiotics to feed the microbiome by way of burdock, chicory, and garlic, and natural probiotics through yogurt, kefir, and fermented vegetables like sauerkraut, pickles, and dilly beans. Avoid nutritionally empty processed foods and additives like polysorbate 80[4] and carrageenan[5] that actively damage the gut.

## THE IMMUNE SYSTEM BEGINS IN THE GUT

Beyond digestion, our intestinal tract also has a built-in information-processing team housed in organs throughout the gut. Yep, your tonsils, stomach acid, appendix, spleen, and all the lymph nodes that line your intestinal wall make up the huge immune system of the gut. Even the appendix, long thought to be a useless remnant, performs diverse immune functions, including safe-housing critical gut microorganisms to replenish our supply when needed.[6,7] Together, this gut-associated lymphoid tissue (GALT) comprises more than 70 percent of the body's immune system.[8]

Our digestive police force constantly samples gut contents and patrols for "suspicious characters"—everything from potentially damaging microbes to toxins. Millions of immune cells act as sentinels to detect whether anything untoward is going on at any moment. The immune system acts as one unit with the gut and its microbiome: any disruption—by foods, additives, pesticides, toxins, problematic microbes, even antibiotics, steroids, or other meds—impacts the whole body.

Take colic. Numerous studies suggest that colicky babies—those that cry incessantly for periods of time (or all the time) for no known reason—improve considerably with the administration of the probiotic *Lactobacillus reuteri*.[9] For anyone who has had to contend with a colicky baby, consider how powerful the organisms in our gut are to improve such tremendous distress!

## MICROBIAL BIODIVERSITY

The "hygiene hypothesis," which proposes that kids today live in overly sanitized environments thanks to things like bleach and Purell, has been long used to explain the rise in children's allergies. The thought was that urban immune systems do not get exposed to enough bacteria and other microbes that prime the immune system to be healthy. This hypothesis is partly based on studies showing that children raised on farms have fewer allergies and asthma attacks.[10] Playing outside, digging for worms, planting vegetables, and essentially coming into contact with plenty of dirt and livestock are actually good things. Not just good—essential!

Bacteria, viruses, parasites, and fungi play a critical role in developing and maintaining a healthy gut and immune system. Another explanation for the rise in allergies has been called the "old friends hypothesis,"[11] because allergic children lack a diversity of these friendly microbes in their guts. To evaluate these theories, scientists compared microbial samples from an urban apartment to those from a rural farm. Shockingly, they found that the two environments actually had similar numbers of microbes. What differed, however, was the *diversity* of bacteria.[12] The microbial sample from the urban apartment was limited, while the microbial sample from the farm was rich with varied microbes. A study of an Amazonian indigenous tribe free of chronic illness—isolated entirely from modern life—revealed the most diverse number of microbes ever documented in humans.[13] A healthy gut is filled with diverse microbes: the more kinds, the better. **Biodiversity makes the difference between balance and dysregulation**.

### A Bit on Bugs

We all know that infections following exposures to microbes can be deadly. But can they also be beneficial? How could bacteria, viruses, and parasites—the stuff of dirt, things that we meticulously avoid—actually make our kids healthy? Consider this: Strains of *Clostridia*, a gut bacterium that can make you sick under certain circumstances, may reverse peanut allergy in mice.[14] That's right: Bacteria in the gut had the power to stop a severe—even fatal—immunogenic reaction. In an August 2014 study, scientists decimated the gut bacteria in the mice and then exposed them to peanut allergens, which triggered a strong immune response. These mice produced peanut-targeting antibodies at significantly higher levels than mice with normal levels of gut bacteria. But when *Clostridia* were introduced, these mice's immune cells generated high levels of a protective signaling molecule called interleukin 22 (IL-22), which suppressed the allergic response. In other words, the immune system partnered with certain strains of bacteria to quiet a severe allergic response.

Similarly, *H. pylori*—the villainized bacterium associated with increased risk of ulcers and stomach cancer—once was found in the stomachs of almost everyone. By the turn of the twenty-first century, however, only 6 percent of the population carried *H. pylori*. Yet paradoxically, its eradication has seen increases in reflux, Barrett's esophagus, and esophageal cancer.[15] Without *H. pylori*, the balance of appetite-regulating hormones leptin and ghrelin changes, and the risk of childhood hay fever, allergies, and asthma increases.[16] **Chances are that something about us has changed rather than these bacteria being good or bad. Microbial balance and biodiversity are key.**

Certain parasites may also be beneficial. A recent study actually showed that parasites communicate with bacteria in the gut to regulate immunity. A colleague of mine who works with immigrants has seen many children from Ethiopia who tested positive for parasites. Though they were asymptomatic, he treated their "infections." To his surprise, many promptly developed asthma, eczema, and other allergic conditions. He decided to stop treating for parasites in asymptomatic patients, and he stopped seeing these problems. Science backs up his observations.[17] People who live in areas highly endemic for parasite infections have a lower risk of developing types 1 and 2 diabetes.[18,19] Scientists are even investigating parasite eggs as a treatment for multiple sclerosis, inflammatory bowel disease, celiac disease, type 1 diabetes, rheumatoid arthritis, and asthma.[20] **Our bodies evolved with these "old friends."**

Even viruses play a beneficial role as part of the "microvirome."[21] A 2014 landmark study in the journal *Nature* has revealed that some viruses can step up to take over immune-regulating roles of the microbiome when our gut bacteria is dysregulated—precluding any of the normal gut and immune disruption typically seen after antibiotics.[22] Another *Nature* paper showed that latent infection following certain common viruses similar to cytomegalovirus or Epstein-Barr virus (which causes mononucleosis) protected mice from dying from deadly infections like bubonic plague.[23] And it gets weirder. People who have had mumps as children may halve the risk of developing ovarian cancer later in life, possibly because the immune system patrols for those cells better.[24] Measles virus, too, is being explored as an unexpected darling of the oncology world as an oncolytic[25]—cancer killer—for difficult-to-treat cancers like osteosarcoma, leukemia, glioblastoma, and others.[26,27,28,29] Infection with measles and mumps in childhood has also been associated with lower risk of cardiovascular disease in adulthood.[30] **Ultimately, our bodies are part of a superorganism in which the immune system is not a killer, but a balancing force that shapes homeostasis.**[31]

Believe it or not, even stool is proving an effective treatment for some conditions. Academic hospitals across the country are using Fecal Microbial Transplant (FMT)—yes, enemas infused with donor stool—as a treatment for recurrent *Clostridium difficile*, an opportunistic infection arising from antibiotic overuse, with great success.[32] **The benefits of microbial biodiversity in stool—as with soil—cannot be easily imitated by synthetic pharmaceuticals.**

Ultimately, we share our bodies, including genomic information, with our organisms. They really become "part of us." We want neither too much of any one organism, nor too few; the key is balance. **We are in constant relationship with the diverse microbial world around us and within us. That rich microbial diversity is a defining ingredient of our children's health.**

## THE BRAIN IN THE GUT, THE GUT IN THE BRAIN

The gut actually functions like a brain in your body along with the brain in your head. That's right, the gut and brain work together as one nervous system. So it makes sense that food and digestive imbalance can cause problems in the brain. The gut and its microbes release more neurotransmitters than the *entire central nervous system.* Just like neurons in the brain, the gut even has its own "entero-neurons" that communicate with the rest of the nervous system—and ultimately the brain.

It makes sense. Think about a "gut-wrenching" experience—an emotional response that you feel deep in your belly. What about gut reactions or "butterflies in your stomach"? Consider this: People with significant concussions or brain injuries experience a breakdown of gut health, leading to the development of conditions like ulcers—even without direct trauma to their digestive systems.[33] Other studies show that the brain plays a role in changing the bacteria in the gut. For example, mice that were subjected to a social stressor for six days had altered gut flora composition compared to unstressed mice.[34] Even food choices change your gut microbiome: For example, people who ate a high-fat/low-fiber diet transformed their disordered gut microbiome within ten days of switching to a low-fat/high-fiber diet.[35]

What about the other way around? Indeed, the gut also influences the brain.

## FROM FOOD TO THOUGHT: THE GUT-IMMUNE-BRAIN CONNECTION

Gut and brain are in constant communication with each other, thanks to our internal messaging systems. The vagus nerve originates deep within the gut and pelvis, innervating diaphragm, lungs, and heart all the way up to the brain stem. This complex electrical web connects the gut to the internal organs to the brain, and the brain to the gut and organs. In a sense, this is like a (very rapid) gut-brain dial-up connection. The vagus nerve modulates crucial functions like digestion, steady heart and respiratory rate, even inflammation, and transmits information up and down the body. So, for example, cells in the gut send all manner of messages to the brain via the vagus nerve regarding what microbes and other entities of interest are detected in the gut, and whether there is distress that must be addressed.

Immune cells in the gut (and elsewhere) release cytokines to communicate with other immune cells. In a sense, immune cells act as the body's "police," stationed throughout the gut, looking for signs of danger. These cells patrol the digestive system, casing suspicious food proteins, microbes, and toxins. An immune cell that encounters something amiss sounds the wireless alarm by releasing cytokines that warn other immune cells all over the body, activating them and releasing cytokines in turn. These messages cross the blood-brain barrier to activate the brain's immune system. Why do cytokines have this privilege? *Survival.* Imagine you accidentally eat something rancid. Your brain must be made aware immediately so that it can quickly react—stop eating the food, drink water, vomit, or otherwise detoxify. Cytokines can even act as neurotransmitters at times. The system is so sensitive that even one abnormal bacterium entering the gut has the potential to change the way the brain fires within a couple of hours.[36]

So neurotransmitters (from the gut's entero-neurons) or cytokines (from immune cells) that originate in the gut influence other systems in our body, including the central nervous system (CNS). And when you influence the CNS, you're affecting learning and memory, clear thinking and focus, sleep patterns and mood. A major message being transmitted in this conversation between gut, immune, brain, and microbes is TOLERANCE. If they lose tolerance to each other, we lose tolerance to ourselves, which can lead to allergies and autoimmune disease.

Normally, all this communication is a really good, healthy thing. It means all our parts and systems are working together to ward off potentially harmful invaders of all kinds. But when the gut is repeatedly calling the brain with emergencies, the brain doesn't just listen, it *changes.* In a 2011 study, researchers sterilized the guts of living mice to be free of organisms.[37] Over time, these animals showed significantly diminished brain function; their learning, cognition, and memory plummeted.[38] So did the production of brain growth factors necessary for plasticity. The mice's behavior changed, too: They started exhibiting anxiety behaviors. But when the researchers added back the bacterium lactobacillus, all those factors normalized except the anxious behavior. They added back another bacteria, bifidobacterium, and anxiety behaviors also improved. Throughout, researchers had done nothing to the brain directly—only the gut.

This study has since been repeated several times in several different ways. All point to the same conclusion: Housing diverse bacteria—in balance—is the difference between a healthy body and a dysregulated one.[39] Moreover, a thriving microbiome promotes learning, memory, and good mood. Conversely, bad news in the gut can mean bad news for the brain. We see parallel reactions in kids. Anxiety, aggression, depression, insomnia, trouble focusing or learning, even tics and seizures can be traced back to an unhealthy gut.

What happens when the gut *doesn't* do what it's supposed to do? When it's out of balance—due to reduced stomach acid (sometimes from H2 blockers) or improper microbiome (often disrupted by antibiotics or steroids)—pathogenic microbes or improperly digested proteins may activate the immune system. This "riffraff" triggers an inflammatory response from immune cells, creating a war zone in the gut. The inflammation damages the gut wall "protectors"—epithelial cells linked by tight junctions—so the lining becomes leaky, or vulnerable to permeability.[40] All this disrupts your child's ability to effectively digest and absorb nutrients. As a result, your child may suffer from belly pain, gas, bloating, constipation, diarrhea, or even failure to thrive.

That means that some toxins, bacteria, and harmful microbes can now enter into circulation with impunity. So what begins as a gut issue can involve the body and brain, too. The increased permeability, or leakiness, of the gut barrier allows unrecognized entities to enter systemic circulation.[41] The immune system then releases cytokines that instigate inflammation throughout the body and CNS. Inflammation isn't always a bad thing; it's necessary to fight invaders so that they don't overwhelm the body and even helps to prune away connections in the brain that are no longer needed. But when the immune system is constantly signaling SOS and the *whole body*—gut, lungs, tonsils, skin, and even ear canals—is in a constant state of alert with inflammation everywhere? *That's* when it becomes a problem. And with excessive systemic inflammation come all sorts of symptoms, including but not limited to irritable bowel syndrome or inflammatory bowel disease, asthma, enlarged tonsils and adenoids, eczema, and ear infections.

Can inflammation that starts in the gut really affect your ears? Yes. Children's tympanic canals have a diameter narrower than a strand of hair, and the smallest amount of inflammation causes it to swell, blocking the normal flow of fluids and leading to infection due to stasis.[42] Chronic ear infections reflect inflammation elsewhere.

But that's not all. Cytokines that travel to the brain trigger the brain's own protectors—the microglia—to go on alert. These specialized immune cells, which outnumber neurons in the brain three to one, normally function in a restorative way—from pruning unused connections producing proteins that nourish neurons to releasing growth factors that stimulate new connections to form. But cytokines activate the microglia from "restorative mode" to "warrior mode."[43] They attack the perceived enemy, but in the process damage the very neurons they normally protect.

Such episodes may be tolerated for a limited period. Sometimes, though, the body chronically releases cytokines as an ongoing response to gut microbial imbalances, inflammatory food additives and chemicals, toxins, immunogenic foods, or even inoculations that trigger temporary inflammatory reactions. And sometimes, these microglia can become "stuck" as warriors—a state called microglial activation—and can't return to restorative mode. This process can even begin in utero if a mother has an infection or chronic inflammation herself.[44,45] Chronically activated microglia have been implicated in neurological disorders[46] ranging from sensory integration disorder, autism,[47] seizures,[48,49] ADHD, and Tourette's[50] early in life to schizophrenia, glaucoma, chronic pain syndromes,[51] Alzheimer's, and Parkinson's disease later in life.[52] Understanding what can trigger microglial activation, why cells get stuck in warrior mode, and what can turn it off, appears to hold badly needed answers to chronic intractable brain disorders.

All health begins in the gut. Most people think of the brain as the top of the totem pole, but in many ways, it's downstream from other organs. The gut—the body's soil—calls many of the shots. An unhealthy gut—or depleted soil—leads to an unhealthy immune system, endocrine system, and nervous system. These lead to disordered focus, cognition, behavior, sleep, and mood, among other symptoms. It's why, if not addressed, a child's disrupted gut can trigger an allergy or reactivity and eventually present as stomachaches, asthma, ear infections or croup, and later morph into troubling neurological dysfunction.

Many of the children who come to see me aren't there to discuss their digestive symptoms. In fact, most parents don't understand why I'm asking questions about poop when they want to tell me about their kid's intractable seizures or asthma or ADHD or autism. But once I explain how it's all connected, they have "Aha!" moments. "You mean to tell me that her asthma is related to her gas and bloating?" or "His constant night-waking could be related to his constipation?"

When Anika came to my practice, she had attention issues and asthma so severe it had landed her in the hospital on several occasions. She was teeny for her age, but her parents had been told that was "her pattern." One of my first questions was whether she had ever been tested for celiac disease, an autoimmune reaction to gluten that damages the small intestine lining that prevents the absorption of food nutrients. Children who have ADHD, seizures, or even autism symptoms test positive for celiac significantly more often than children without neurological issues.[53,54] And these children may present with only neurological issues and no gastrointestinal issues.[55] In this case, Anika's numbers were off the charts. The lab couldn't even measure them. Her parents were stunned to learn that the key to all of her neurological, lung, and growth issues had all begun in her gut, probably much earlier in her life.

## THE SCOOP ON POOP

You know how you can tell a lot about a person by what they throw away? Poop is no different. It's a window into your body.

I ask every child about their stool: how often they go, if it hurts, if it's easy to clean afterward, if they have a lot of gas or stomachaches or bloating. One kid I treated said he went to the bathroom as seldom as possible. I asked him why. His response: "It takes too long to wipe. I hate it." It took him nearly an entire roll of toilet paper just to clean himself because his stools were so pasty. He'd never had a solid, formed stool! But he was coming in to see me for severe OCD, tics, and anxiety. In his case—as with many kids whom I see—his gut flora was out of balance from a highly processed diet and many rounds of antibiotics.

A critical element in this very anxious boy was a need to balance his autonomic nervous system. Digestion is modulated by the sympathetic and parasympathetic nervous systems and is influenced by the "fight or flight" response. When a perceived threat activates the sympathetic nervous system, digestion shuts down because you don't have time to sit and poop if you're running away from a lion. When the threat passes and the "calming" parasympathetic nervous system kicks in, normal digestion should resume. But chronic stress or anxiety—an issue for many kids—plays havoc with gut motility. Constipation, diarrhea (or both) ensues.

Some parents say, "What's the big deal if my kid goes every third day? That's just his pattern." First, even in the absence of explicit complaints, children are uncomfortable walking around full of stool all the time. Second, children rarely withhold stool for no reason. Holding stool means something is awry in the gut. Third, poop is the body's waste. We have to take out the garbage! Countless families relate stories of their children having increased seizures, more tantrums, worse behavior, or heightened anxiety when they're constipated. Regulated bowels—which includes passing formed stool easily one or two times daily—is a key component of regulated brain and behavior.

Our waste exits through our colon. The colon is thrifty; it inspects outgoing material to make sure nothing leaves that shouldn't. The small intestine has already absorbed minerals, fats, sugars, and so on. But the colon asks, "What about these water molecules? Or this magnesium? Let's keep it." Great. But this inspection can quickly turn into an episode of *Hoarders*. If poop sits at this final outpost for longer than usual, the colon reabsorbs things that aren't good for the body, like lead, mercury, arsenic, pesticides, or other rejected odds and ends. When you don't take out the garbage regularly, it creates an unpleasant environment in your home by emitting unpleasant smells and attracting vermin. In the gut, retaining stool leads to flatulence, bad breath, disrupted microbes, and increased toxicity. So rule number one: Take out the garbage every day.

## LET'S STOP BUGGING OUR BUGS

Building a healthy internal terrain starts early. In order to understand why so many children have less diverse bacteria than they should, let's look at the biggest offenders to gut health:

- **Antibiotics:** These powerhouse pills can wipe out some infections in the short term, but they can also wipe out microbial communities in the gut (and elsewhere) with impunity. Particularly when overused, antibiotics damage the gut microbiome and disrupt the immune system. Some antibiotics can cause significant toxicity to the energy makers of the cell called the mitochondria.[56]
- **Toxicants:** By definition, toxic substances hurt our bodies in ways large and small, impairing digestive, immune, endocrine, reproductive, and neurological health. A recent study from Harvard School of Public Health and New York's Mount Sinai Medical Center reports that the increase in neurobehavioral disorders such as ADHD, autism, oppositional defiant disorder (ODD), sensory processing disorder, and dyslexia can be attributed to a host of toxicants.[57] These can appear in processed

food as allergens, dyes, artificial ingredients, nanoparticles, BPA, and countless other additives; chemicals like pesticides and herbicides; heavy metals in the water and soil; pollution and mold in the air; and even stress. We'll be talking about these things in more detail in chapters to come.

- **C-section deliveries and formula:** Both of these can be life-saving under certain circumstances. That said, children born via C-section and/or not breast-fed have different microbiomes and immune health than their vaginally born, breast-fed peers. Studies comparing gut flora of babies born vaginally to those delivered by C-section show that the former appropriately have vaginal flora healthfully colonizing their guts—that's the way babies normally seed their intestinal tracts, folks!—whereas C-section babies' guts are colonized primarily by skin flora.[58] During a C-section, mothers are given a dose of peri-surgical antibiotics, which further impacts the diversity of bacteria that might be transmitted.

  On average, children who are breast-fed have lower rates of colds, ear infections (particularly recurrent), gastroenteritis, respiratory syncytial virus (RSV) (a 75 percent reduced risk), allergies, celiac disease, obesity, types 1 and 2 diabetes, and cancer, and they have better cognition and development.[59] Breast milk infuses the gut with a "glycobiome"—prebiotics that promote *Bifidobacter longum,* desirable gut bacteria that coat the gut and powerfully protect against harmful bacteria.[60] Babies are born with an inherently "leaky gut," but *B. longum* acts to make the gut wall impermeable.[61] *But it exists only in the guts of breast-feeding infants,*[62] *and only for as long as they are drinking breast milk.*[63] Breast milk also enhances immune function by transmitting fragments of maternal microRNA (miRNA), which talk directly to the baby's genes that promote immunity.[64] Formula-fed babies don't receive these and other benefits.

- **Parents' gut health:** That's right. If either you or your partner suffer from ongoing digestive issues such as heartburn or reflux, burping, gas, constipation, diarrhea, irritable bowel syndrome

(IBS), food sensitivities, or allergies, or if you have been treated with repeated antibiotics, even as children, your gut microbiome may be disrupted. You may have transmitted this to your child at birth, but remember that it doesn't end there. You continuously share flora with your child because you live together. That goes for adoptive parents, too! Consider this an incentive to improve your own gut health.

None of these factors alone is *the* cause of allergy, inflammation, or other illness. It's not "or," it's "and, and, and." Many factors build the gut, immune system, and brain. Obviously, many children born by C-section and fed formula have immune systems that develop normally and grow up to be healthy. Their bodies may have to work harder to get there, though, and along the way, they may be more vulnerable to whatever stressors they encounter. Conversely, children born vaginally and fed breast milk may encounter stressors great enough to overcome these benefits. Either way, knowing this information is necessary as you seek solutions for improving—or simply maintaining—your child's health. And you'll see that our bodies have the amazing ability to adapt, regenerate, and heal.

Just as the body can change for the worse, it can also change for the better. A body given the tools to reverse damage will mend and become *more* resilient than before. These tools can include fermented foods or bacteria-friendly probiotics that bring the gut back into balance as well as nutrients that boost your own detoxifying powers. And as a result, we can transform our children's bodies and brains.

**Health is a function of a healthy terrain. A healthy terrain is dirty, messy, complex, and doesn't come in a pill or package. It's a process that begins with eating and living in alignment with the natural world. It's the very messiness of the natural world that makes us resilient, which is the key to robust health.**

## CHAPTER 4

# Time to Clean Up

**W**e parents spend a lot of time telling our kids to "clean up": their rooms, their toys, their backpacks. And while kids' bodies do need dirt and microbes, they also need to clear what they don't need. To identify what needs to be cleaned from the body's terrain, you first need to understand the body's natural detoxification system.

Imagine the body as a basin that fills with the good (like food and its nutrients), the "bad" (infectious illnesses like strep and flu), and the ugly (toxins and allergens from our food and environment). **Every moment, our bodies take in vast amounts of exposures from food we eat, air we breathe, toiletries and materials on our skin, and water we drink and bathe in.** A healthy body accepts and benefits from nourishing input, and flushes poisons and waste: from every cell, through lymphatics, to liver, spleen, kidneys, and gut, and eventually through urination, defecation, perspiration, coughing and sneezing, tears, and even vomiting if necessary.

But sometimes the basin doesn't drain as well or as quickly as it should. By that, I'm not referring to how frequently your kid pees or poops (though that is an important component). I'm talking about how effectively your child flushes toxins that interfere with normal function. Here, cleaning things up and moving out makes all the difference between staying healthy and getting sick.

## THE DRAIN: HOW WE CLEAN UP

Our basins should process everything that comes into contact with our bodies, expelling what we don't want. But if the drain stops working well, the basin fills. Eventually, what happens in the basin doesn't stay in the basin. Instead of excreting damaging compounds through normal physiological mechanisms like urination and defecation, a full basin overflows with toxins. And that is when we start to see symptoms.

Initially, overflow can present with mild symptoms like hives, headaches, or constipation. **If we disregard the symptoms that reflect minimal overflow, however, the problems can amplify into something more severe.** These symptoms might look different in different children, depending on their genetic vulnerabilities: a "skin" kid might get eczema; a "brain" kid might express symptoms of ADHD, migraines, or seizures; a "gut" kid might have constipation, inflammatory bowel disease (IBD), or reflux; and a "lung" kid might have asthma, croup, or chronic pneumonia. And so on. **Many times, a child's seemingly unrelated symptoms may share the same underlying problem: an overfull basin and inefficient drain.**

## What Is a Toxin?

A toxin is a compound that damages our bodies either alone or cumulatively. Just as our health is a dynamic relationship with the world around us, toxicity, too, is a relationship between all of the potentially damaging compounds we see each day and how well our bodies can process them. Dose matters, number of exposures matter, and the genetics and previous exposures of the person matters. Minuscule levels of many potentially damaging compounds can accumulate in the body and act synergistically to be exponentially more toxic than any one exposure by itself. Ultimately, exposure is not one-size-fits-all. **One thing is for certain: Children are more vulnerable.**[1] Science is still catching up to the complex ways that different compounds accumulate in the body to disrupt children's bodies during periods of rapid development.

## The Body's Detoxification System

In reality, our bodies are far more complex than a simple basin and drain. Our basin is our physical, emotional, and spiritual landscape, and the drain is our ability to cleanse ourselves of substances on all of these levels. Our physical stressors come from outside the body—medications, pesticides, herbicides, plastics—and from inside the body—hormones, metabolic by-products, and stress.

Many environmental toxins are fat-soluble, rendering them easily absorbed and stored in the body's fatty tissues (including the brain), but simultaneously difficult to excrete. The body works constantly to clear toxins. Detoxification occurs in two phases, with the overall aim of making toxins water-soluble so they can be excreted through urine or perspiration (why *not* to use antiperspirants!). Others remain fat-soluble and are bound by bile (by way of the gallbladder and liver) and ultimately are excreted in stool (which is why bowel movements must happen regularly!).

Phase 1 of detoxification mainly uses oxygen and liver enzymes to prepare toxins for excretion. Phase 2 involves binding—or "conjugating"—the toxins that have completed phase 1 to an array of nutrient compounds, allowing the body to expel them. The good news is that our bodies are designed to process and excrete compounds that can be damaging to us. Every cell in the body works constantly to clear toxins, which creates demand for an ongoing supply of both nutritional and energetic resources. This high demand is why nutritional depletion is dangerous. All of the elements necessary for detoxification come from our food and water. **What we eat can either promote rapid and efficient detoxification, or slow it down.**

## Not All Basins Are Created Equal

Often I hear people say, "If food X or toxin Y is so bad, then why doesn't everyone get sick from it?" The simplest answer is that our basins, drains, and cumulative exposures vary. Everyone has a unique set of strengths and vulnerabilities. You may have read interviews with centenarians who credit their longevity to cigars and whiskey, and you think, *I never smoked a day in my life. I buy organic food and clean with baking soda and vinegar instead of the toxic stuff. And my kid is still sick!* Why is one person's cigar another person's throat cancer? Or one kid's peanut another kid's anaphylaxis?

To some extent, this comes down to our individual genetics. Some people are fantastic detoxifiers all around; they have no problem producing all the liver and metabolic enzymes necessary to clear toxicants effectively. They benefit from what I call "cigar and whiskey genes" (or "Coke and Twinkie genes"). They have big basins, nice open drains, and their genes can take insult after toxic insult in stride. The body's ability to detoxify partly depends on our DNA. Small differences in our genes, called "polymorphisms," can affect our detoxification system's liver enzymes (CYP), methylation enzymes (including MTHFR and COMT), and many others. These mini-mutations are not severe enough to cause disease directly, but can create particular vulnerabilities that are unmasked by our diet and environmental exposures.

In a state of abundant nutrition from nutrient-dense food grown in rich soil and diverse microbial exposure, these polymorphisms may be nonissues. But your vulnerabilities become problems when you are poorly nourished and exposed to toxins. In one study, for example, pesticide exposure doubled risk for Parkinson's disease . . . but only in those with a particular liver enzyme polymorphism. Having the polymorphism or the pesticide exposure alone didn't increase the risk.

(Depending on a child's polymorphisms, phase 1 may be slow, so toxins build up. Or phase 1 may be very fast, but phase 2 can't keep up, creating a pileup of partially metabolized—but still damaging—toxic metabolites. You may already know whether you are a fast or slow phase 1 metabolizer by way of the "caffeine test": If you're one of those people who drinks caffeine at lunch and experiences heart palpitations or stays up until 2 a.m., then phase 1 is probably slow. If you drink coffee right before bed and fall asleep with no problem, then phase 1 is on the faster side. Either extreme means your system needs extra support.)

What you eat plays a critical role in your detox capacity. Consumption of partially hydrogenated vegetable oils, charbroiled meats, Tylenol, pesticide residues, and certain food preservatives like BHT (commonly found in chips, cookies, cereals, and vegetable oil) are just some exposures that muck up detoxification. On the other hand, adequate ingestion and digestion of protein from quality meats, eggs, seeds, nuts, and legumes enhance detoxification capacity, as do phytochemicals found in cruciferous vegetables like broccoli, cauliflower, and Brussels sprouts; teas; spices like turmeric, rosemary, thyme, peppermint, or black cumin; as well as berries, citrus, onions, garlic, and even olive oil. A healthy microbiome facilitates detoxification.[2] We'll talk more specifically about all the building blocks of a healthy terrain—and in turn, efficient detoxification—throughout this book.

**While individual polymorphisms can dictate risk for developing diseases, metabolic and epigenetic interactions with nature confer potential for healing. Even children who can't be "cured" of their condition have potential to improve their health or even quality of life in measurable ways.**

## Recognizing Symptoms of Toxicity

A child with rashes or chronic hives or eczema or ear infections or constipation or gassiness or even cavities is *a child at risk*. No, these "benign" conditions won't kill your child, but they sound an alarm that you should heed: "Total load is building. Demand outweighs resources. Alert!" You do not necessarily need to panic when a new symptom appears, but you do need to pay attention. Even mild symptoms tell us that the body is out of balance, which means the body is vulnerable. Vulnerability means decreased resilience. **Decreased resilience means that the next inevitable insult or stressor that comes your child's way—an illness, toxic exposure, stressful event—may trigger a chronic condition.** That's what you want to avoid.

Symptoms of initial toxicity can include:

Headache

Coughing, wheezing, and shortness of breath

Eye, ear, nose, or throat irritation

Chills or fever

Dizziness, vertigo, unsteady gait

Nausea

Hair loss

Rashes

Weakness or fatigue

Chronic pain

Depression

Infertility in women and men (or frequent miscarriage)

Neurological dysfunction, including poor memory, concentration, low tone, learning disorders, sensory dysfunction, ADD, and others (when toxicity is advanced)

Cancer (when toxicity is advanced)

## MEET THE MITOCHONDRIA

What is happening in the body when the basin is filling with toxins? Much of the damage happens at the level of the cell. Cells make up the organs like the heart, brain, lungs, gut, and so on. Mitochondria are the energy makers of each cell, producing fuel for all cellular functions, among many other critical tasks.[3] When all is well, mitochondria produce energy, the cell runs optimally, and we feel great. When mitochondrial function is disrupted, however, one of three things happens:[4] cells die that shouldn't (which can lead to degenerative conditions like Parkinson's or Alzheimer's), cells don't die that should (which can lead to proliferative conditions like cancer), or cells simply function suboptimally (which has been implicated in autism, epilepsy, ADHD, allergies, asthma, diabetes, metabolic syndrome, and other chronic conditions). Mitochondria also act as sentinels that sample various compounds—good, bad, and ugly—that make their way into the cell. And depending on the level of stress these compounds impose upon the cell, mitochondria decide whether the cell will live or die. In this way, these amazing organelles are arbiters of cell life, cell death, and resilience.

When the cell is under stress—let's say during infection with the flu—it issues emergency defense orders called the cell danger response (CDR) that enable cell survival.[5] CDR is why you'd likely feel extremely fatigued and ill as your body fights the flu effectively. Luckily, CDR usually serves its purpose within days to weeks—as with a successful recovery from the flu—and everything goes back to normal.

Under certain circumstances, mitochondria can get stuck in a permanent danger mode, especially when bombarded by exposures like allergenic foods, food additives, drugs, pesticides, heavy metals like lead, mercury, arsenic, or aluminum; volatile organic compounds (VOCs); or air pollutants. Even inoculations require temporary activation of the cell danger response to produce durable, persistent immunity.[6] But if an exposure triggers a siege state from which cells can't easily recover, clinical symptoms morph from acute to chronic. A chronic siege state increases our nutritional demands and renders our cells even more vulnerable to toxic exposures.

Chronic symptoms related to damaging exposure can manifest in any organ(s)—lungs, gut, immune, endocrine (for instance, thyroid or reproductive systems). Children, however, are particularly vulnerable to neurologic effects—mood, cognition, behavior, focus—due to rapid brain development and the very high density of mitochondria in the brain. For instance, children who are exposed to pesticides have a higher risk of ADHD, learning disabilities, and cancer.[7,8] Children exposed to lead are more likely to have aggressive behavior as well as myriad learning issues. Children who live close to coal plants, highways, and other sources of pollution in early life are more likely to be diagnosed with autism.[9,10] Pollution of all kinds, especially combined with particular genetic vulnerabilities, can literally poison children.

The good news is that most people with mitochondrial dysfunction do not have inherently broken mitochondria. As sentinels, mitochondria continually respond to exposures—both good and bad. This means that under improved circumstances, chronic symptoms of all kinds—asthma, eczema, ADHD, and on—can quiet for good. Even seemingly permanent conditions like autism can improve when the cell danger response quiets.[11] Mitochondria, cells, and organ systems can recover, with the help of plants, nature, and dense nutrition from food. This is how children improve, move beyond this siege state, and regain their resilience.

## HOW FULL IS YOUR BASIN?

My 15-year-old patient Sarah came to me with intractable menstrual migraines so severe that no medication helped. She missed school frequently. "I know why I get them," she said, reciting what other doctors had told her. "They're *hormonal*."

"Okay," I said. "But most women have the same monthly hormonal surges and don't get migraines. Why are you different?" One reason was that Sarah's basin was overfull from daily exposures—largely from her diet—allowing her monthly hormonal surge to overwhelm her detoxification mechanisms, leading to migraines.

To treat, we reduced problematic exposures while increasing her intake of nutrient-dense foods and herbs—which emptied her basin and expanded her drain. Our first stop was her diet, composed largely of Diet Coke and processed foods. When I explained the damning science behind the chemicals she was consuming—which we'll explore here shortly—she reluctantly agreed to change her diet. One month later, she was no longer reluctant. Her migraines had decreased by 75 percent. After another month, Sarah was headache-free and medication-free for the first time since she turned 12.

For already vulnerable children, all it can take is one more stressor for a basin to overflow, which depletes, burdens, or damages innate healing mechanisms, and ultimately triggers illness. Some risks include:

- Processed foods containing preservatives, dyes, and other additives, as well as sugar and synthetic fats

- Conventionally grown foods treated or packaged with chemicals that stress the body: GMO, glyphosate, antibiotics, pesticides, plastics, and more
- Food grown in depleted, sick soil instead of nutrient-dense soil
- Repeated treatment with antibiotics, steroids, acetaminophen (Tylenol), or reflux medications
- Receiving vaccines while ill or on antibiotics

Foods and medications that cause the basin to overflow give rise to symptoms. By heeding these alerts when they're mild, you may be able to prevent an illness from ever developing at all.

# TAKE HOME

1. Healthy, nourished cells flush most nasty exposures. This also depends partly on our individual genetics, or polymorphisms, as well as on previous exposures.
2. Symptoms arise when cells become overwhelmed in this process.
3. You can help your child's systems by minimizing exposures to toxins: pesticides and herbicides, heavy metals, air and water pollutants, fluoride, food additives, plastics, synthetic fragrances, and highly processed sugars and foods.
4. Don't spend all of your time feeling fearful of encountering inevitable toxic residues. Avoid what you reasonably can, but the key to healthy minds and bodies is to enhance resilience by nourishing the body with good things—food, plants, germs, dirt—so that our bodies are well prepared when faced with challenges.

## ACTION STEP: Cleaning Out the Basin (and Keeping It Clean)

To move toward optimal wellness . . .

1. **Remove from the body what hinders mitochondrial and cellular health, and**
2. **Add what supports it, beginning with the food you eat.**

Unfortunately, eating nourishing food isn't as straightforward as you may think. That's because not everything you eat is actually *food*, which loves and nourishes your body. It's time to forget everything you think you know about food—all the health claims and dos and don'ts. It's time to regard your food with new eyes.

# PART II

—

## STEP ONE: Heal

—

*Avoiding Foods That
Are Not Really Food*

*Let your food be your medicine and your medicine be your food.*
*Anyone who does not understand that concept,*
*how can he understand the diseases of man?*

—HIPPOCRATES

Two hundred years ago, we knew exactly what we were eating because we grew a good portion of the food ourselves. Then the Industrial Revolution came along and our agrarian society of self-sufficient food producers began its insidious transformation into a nation of urban consumers. Just a century later, our knowledge of how to grow food, discern its quality, and prepare it has disappeared.

As we've become less self-sufficient, we've also become sicker. Our outsourced food is produced, processed, and depleted by industry. Even "whole foods" like meat or milk in a sense have become "processed foods" based on how the animals were raised or the food was processed before arriving at our table. Additives—from flavoring agents to dyes to preservatives—further stress vulnerable children in ways that aggravate or trigger chronic illness. **We're allowing industry to safeguard our children's food, and, by extension, their health.**

Food's impact on children's health and development is tremendous. The food we eat communicates with our bodies intimately, from our digestive tract to our immune cells to our mitochondria, down to our very DNA. And the kind of food we eat determines whether this epigenetic communication will be loving or damaging. Our DNA then responds in kind by either: (1) upregulating a complex array of enzymes and other proteins that enable cells to function optimally, or (2) initiating production of inflammatory components that trigger a cell danger response. There is one main guiding principle. **Nutrient-dense foods nourish us on a cellular level, which can transform ailing cells into thriving ones.**

It can feel daunting to reduce processed food. It's difficult to take enjoyable foods from children, particularly when they already struggle with other issues. But most parents in my practice say that changing to better foods ultimately made life much easier for their families. The improvements they witnessed after changing their diets convinced them never return to old habits like using junk food as a bribe to mollify picky eaters or tantrumming children. Just a few simple changes can make an enormous difference in your child's life.

**We must once again become participants in the story of our food.**

## CHAPTER 5

# Food Allergens and Sensitivities:
# How "Healthy" Foods Can Hurt

If you're a parent, grandparent, teacher, babysitter, coach, neighbor, or anyone who provides food to children, then you've probably had to navigate the growing epidemic of food-allergic children. And if you're a health-care practitioner, therapist, or school nurse, you've seen first-hand just how many kids have special dietary needs.

Epipens (for severe allergic responses) are now prescribed at phenomenal rates. More and more classrooms have large signs posted in the front: ALL SNACKS MUST BE PEANUT- AND TREE NUT–FREE. Many children have more than one food allergy. When my food-allergic son was three years old, he was known at the playground for lisping, "Does it have dairy or egg or soy?" when food was offered to him. A friend of mine wanted to bring freshly baked cookies to welcome her new neighbors, but was so overwhelmed by the children's copious food allergies that she gave up and instead brought flowers.

## WHAT'S THE DEAL WITH ALL THESE ALLERGIES?

It's the million-dollar question, the one I'm asked publicly during Q&As and privately by colleagues and friends when we chat about their kids. "We ended up in the ER when my daughter ate a snack containing peanuts. Her throat swelled up and she couldn't swallow," said a friend from college. A neighborhood friend stopped me in the store: "My son had a rash around his mouth and was acting completely out of control; it turned out he was severely allergic to milk." "My twelve-month-old was vomiting and crying incessantly, and we were thinking the worst," my friend from residency confessed. "The allergist discovered she'd developed a severe egg allergy."

Parents discuss it quietly with one another: "I don't remember any kids having allergies when we were little." Back then, it was notable if even one kid had a food allergy. What's changed?

There are dramatically more food allergies now than there used to be. Between 1997 and 2011, food allergies in children rose by *50 percent*. One in 13 children has food allergies, and deadly allergies are on the rise. Children in cities are at the greatest risk. One study showed that 10 percent of children raised in an urban environment developed a food allergy to eggs, milk, or peanuts by age five and that 55 percent would develop food sensitivity.[1] The authors of the study stated that the cumulative risk of food allergy likely would have been much higher if additional commonly allergic foods had been included. How have children's bodies changed over the past three decades for so many foods to cause inflammatory responses? And what does having an allergy indicate about your child's health?

There's no simple cause. Many factors contribute to the problem.

But growing data say our children are allergic because we have sanitized them. We've attacked microbes with hand sanitizer, antibiotics, steroids, pasteurization, irradiation, and even with more and more inoculations. We've taken our germ-free obsession so far that we've even sanitized dirt. Pesticides, herbicides, antifungals, and antibiotics kill critical microbes in the soil and coat our food.

**It comes down to this: Our attempts to control the messy complexity of nature have had unintended consequences for children's health.** According to germ theory, microorganisms are unequivocally dangerous. The subsequent war we launched against germs, carried out with the best of intentions, has fundamentally changed our children's internal and external terrains. In the meantime, it's becoming clear that exposure to microbes—in tremendous variety—is pivotal to our children's immediate and lifelong health.

It starts at birth, or even before. Newborns' guts colonize with bacteria by swallowing vaginal secretions, rife with diverse microbes, as they are pushed through the birth canal. Now, more children than ever before—greater than 30 percent in the United States[2]—are born by C-section, causing them to miss out on that important bacterial colonization. These babies are at increased risk of allergies, asthma, autoimmune disease, and even cancer.[3] Breastfeeding, too, supports the microbiome and immune system in unique, long-lasting ways.[4] Babies who drink formula are more likely to have increased infections and allergies among other issues.[5,6] Antibiotic use in infancy and childhood, and even pregnancy and birth, can contribute to food allergy by creating imbalances of gut microbiome that sensitize the immune system to improperly overreact.[7,8]

Even attempts to eliminate childhood viral illnesses appear to have unintended consequences. Just as bacteria are critical to children's immune regulation, viruses appear to compose a protective "microvirome"—similar to our microbiome—that is essential to gut health.[9] Previously common childhood viruses like measles and mumps reduce allergy and even teach the immune system to target cancer, for example.[10,11] Viruses are still deemed unequivocally "bad."

Yet our immune cells are social, and seem to have a quota for the number of organisms they want to meet and greet each day. Without a stream of diverse microbes to identify, they become crotchety and paranoid, and target what does come through every day, like food. Meanwhile, children's early immune systems are primed to be more reactive by the adjuvants in their inoculations.[12] Adjuvants—which include aluminum and thimerosal, among others—are intentionally designed to amplify the immune response as a way to induce lifelong, protective antibodies to certain viral illnesses. According to some studies, however, the adjuvants may sensitize some percentage of children's immune systems to other exposures as well, such as foods, or even plant pollens.[13] In other words, children's immune systems are intentionally amped up while simultaneously they are introduced to new food after new food, which may play a role in developing food reactivity. Based on this scientific literature, you may consider **avoiding introducing new foods to infants and children within two to**

**four weeks of inoculations to reduce the risk of developing food reactivity.**

## LATENT FOOD REACTIVITY

Most of us consider food reactivity to be relevant only to children afflicted with spontaneous hives or anaphylaxis. But *every* child's health, mood, and behavior can be affected by food. As a pediatric neurologist, I think of food reactivity differently than many allergists. Allergists define allergies strictly based on a very specific reaction that includes physiological markers (IgE antibodies, release of histamine) and a particular reaction (typically immediate, including vomiting, anaphylaxis, hives, swelling of the lips and face, and rash). A positive skin test and the IgE blood test, even when very low, each offers clues about which foods trigger systemic and neurological symptoms. Both, along with clinical observations, have value. **The trouble is that a negative test doesn't prove that a specific food is not causing a troublesome issue.** Foods interact with our immune system in many ways, and the symptoms don't always look like the welt-covered kid exposed to peanuts. Very real, very serious reactions to food manifest in children's guts, skin, lungs, and nervous systems, though many parents and physicians don't recognize these symptoms as food reactions. In fact, "innocent" conditions that our children experience every day—constipation, constantly runny noses, recurrent croup, chronic ear infections, mysterious rashes and daily headaches, to name a few—often are directly related to food reactivity.

Sometimes parents connect the dots in spite of their doctors. Parents say: "Johnny curls into a ball in pain for a day or two after eating gluten, but his labs are fine so his doctor says he doesn't have wheat allergy or celiac." Or, "When Sadie eats cheese, she's gassy for days and then ends up with either ear infections or croup, but my doctor says that's not a sign of allergy." Call it what you will, these kids are reacting to their food.

Also called "non-IgE-mediated" food reactivity or "sensitivities," these reactions have real impacts on health and quality of life. And data suggest what parents observe. Some examples: Reactivity to food affects gut motility—which can cause constipation or diarrhea or "irritable bowel syndrome."[14] Food allergies cause inflammation and swelling of the middle and inner ear, including the eustachian tube, blocks fluid flow and promotes bacterial growth in the middle ear,[15,16] and can also lead to vertigo and Ménière's disease when the inner ear is involved.[17] Removing the food culprit can reduce or eliminate symptoms—from the annoying to the serious.[18]

You are the best expert on your child. Many doctors only accept parents' observations if a skin or blood test "proves" it, but these tests have limited efficacy and don't always tell the whole story.

## TIP

### Is Your Child Reactive to Food?

**Eliminate a food** you think creates a negative response or symptom for at least a month.

**Trust your intuition.** If you observe that your child is more aggressive, congested, rashy, or just plain sick after eating certain foods—and if symptoms improve without them—avoid that food. You don't need permission.

**Be scientific.** Document symptoms before, during, and after eliminating a food by using a daily journal, photos, videos, teacher reports, or other relevant measures. If the symptom is behavior or a tic, develop a rating scale of 1 to 10 to measure daily how often you see it.

**Reintroduce.** If you're not sure, add the food (best on the weekend) to see if symptoms return.

NOTE: Sometimes symptoms improve, but not the one you expect. Improvement can also be subtle. *But don't eliminate whole, healthy foods "just in case" without clear improvement.*

## Food Reactivity: Examples of Ways That Children Can React

1. Allergy: True allergy implies that the reaction is IgE based, an antibody responsible for the classic histaminergic allergic reaction that includes hives, itchiness, agitation, swelling, breathing difficulties, vomiting, and anaphylaxis. Many doctors recognize this as the only category of food reaction.

2. Sensitivity or Intolerance: Food sensitivity spans the remainder of most food reactions. A skin prick test or blood test won't provide the whole picture. From gluten to dairy to egg to any other food or drink, sensitivities can trigger an array of symptoms from digestive upset, fatigue or hyperactivity, inattention, explosive behavior, and anxiety, to rash/eczema/sensitive skin, headaches, and more.

3. Celiac: An autoimmune condition in which IgA and IgG antibodies are triggered by gliadin (a protein in gluten-containing grains), celiac can present with diverse and varied symptoms including abdominal discomfort, bloating, bad breath, failure to thrive, migraines, ADHD, or even seizures. Contrary to popular belief, children can present with only neurological or mood symptoms, and no digestive or growth issues.

4. Lactose Intolerance: Lactose is a sugar found in milk. When children's symptoms after eating dairy are gastrointestinal alone—limited to gas, bloating, and diarrhea after eating or drinking dairy products—lactose intolerance may be the reason. However, any other symptoms (vomiting, increased mucus, rashes or itchiness, constipation) indicate that a milk allergy or sensitivity may be a cause.

5. Sensitivity to A1 Casomorphins: Some people have a variant digestive enzyme that breaks down certain milk proteins into a biologically active fragment called a "casomorphin." Instead of breaking the protein down into amino acids and

absorbing them, casomorphins can cause a "drugged," morphinelike state after drinking milk, as well as constipation, allergy, increased risk for SIDS, and exacerbations of behaviors associated with autism and schizophrenia.[19] Milk from goats and some cow breeds, like Jerseys and Guernseys, contain safer A2 caseins that don't break down into casomorphins in people with that variant enzyme.

6. Fructose Malabsorption (FODMAPS): Children who have abdominal discomfort, bloating, and gas after eating foods like honey, fruit, and some grains and dairy products may have difficulty absorbing fructose.

7. Polyphenol Sensitivity: Fruits and vegetables that are red or purple—like apples, grapes, berries, and tomatoes[20]—contain certain antioxidants that can be difficult for some children to process. These children may exhibit bright red ears and cheeks, dark circles under their eyes, difficulty sleeping, and hyperactive or highly emotional behavior.

## BRAIN ALLERGIES?

Why is it so important to identify "instigators" in your child's diet, regardless of an allergy diagnosis?

A body exposed to a reactive food is burdened, and struggling to be healthy. Remember that the immune system patrols the intestinal tract, the blood, the skin, even the brain. When food is identified as an enemy, immune cells ratchet up the inflammatory response throughout the body and the brain every time that food comes through.

When I started my work as a pediatric neurologist, I was stunned to discover that changing a child's diet could transform that child's health. This was true not just for kids with eczema, asthma, constipation, diarrhea, or gas, but even for difficult-to-treat kids with ADHD, migraines, autism, Tourette's, OCD, and seizures.

Ten-year-old Ella had missed a quarter of the school year due to abdominal migraines—she'd failed countless medications and been hospitalized repeatedly. I tested her blood for allergies, and while she showed only the most minimal allergy possible to milk, I felt it was worth having her avoid dairy completely for a one-month trial. After much convincing—"What could milk possibly have to do with my problems?"—Ella stopped dairy. Her abdominal migraines reduced by 75 percent and we were able to address the remainder of her events with botanical and nutritional remedies. She did not miss one day of school the following year for this issue.

Milo's degenerative seizure disorder meant he had hundreds of daily seizures that could be suppressed only with powerful sedation in the pediatric intensive care unit. When sedation was lifted, he returned to having 30 seizures a day. Even though he was on a ketogenic diet—very high in fat (butter) and protein (eggs) with no carbohydrates—we trialed him off dairy and eggs based on blood tests that showed he was significantly reactive. For the first time, he went two weeks completely seizure-free and thereafter experienced a considerable decrease to weekly seizures, rather than many times daily.

Clearly, children are reacting to foods in unexpected ways—often unbeknownst to themselves or the people around them. Because health-care providers and parents only expect traditional symptoms of hives, swollen lips, and itchy mouth, they can miss other kids who react differently. **The good news, however, is that you have more control over your child's health than you realize.** You can change your child's diet to improve conditions both common and rare, which may help you to mitigate the need for long-term medications with all of their associated expense and side effects.

I learned about the powerful effects of food on the brain by accident when I first entered practice. A two-year-old twin, Tony, was nonverbal and on the autism spectrum, although his sister was developing normally. On their first visit to see me, Tony screamed continuously as his mother described her concerns. His ears and cheeks were bright red and his belly bloated. His stools were loose, and he had chronic, severe diaper rashes. When I asked about his diet, his mother hesitated. "He doesn't really eat," she said. Tony was not underweight, however, so I encouraged her to share what he did consume. "Well . . . he mostly drinks milk." His mother revealed that Tony was drinking eight 8- to 10-ounce bottles of milk per day, flavored with strawberry syrup "to convince him to drink them." Otherwise, all he'd eat was Doritos and ramen noodles. These three "foods" are reservoirs of MSG, food additives, trans fats, and genetically modified corn.

I recommended that he stop dairy—not because I expected him to have a positive behavioral change by eliminating dairy, but because he was drinking so much cow's milk that he couldn't possibly get the sort of diverse nutrition a growing two-year-old required. Pediatric training teaches that toddlers shouldn't drink too much milk; it can lead to anemia by causing microscopic hemorrhages in the gut that lead to chronic loss of tiny amounts of blood. We talked about alternative foods such as almond and coconut milk, so that she could reduce and then eliminate dairy over a week's time. When his mother left that day, I wasn't at all sure that she was onboard, or that in the chaos of chasing her twins during our appointment, she had even grasped what I had recommended.

When Tony's mother called three weeks later, however, she asked me so many questions about his diet that I had to stop her to ask for an update on Tony's condition. She said, "I removed dairy three weeks ago. Since then he has gained fifty words, stopped throwing tantrums, and eats three square meals a day." Before our next visit, she decided independently to remove gluten and discovered that his belly lost its bloat. He potty trained within the week. Though this intervention is by no means this effective a treatment for every child with autism, Tony eventually shed his diagnosis and successfully moved to a mainstream classroom.

After this startling success, I began to look more carefully at the diets of my other neurology patients. An angelic-appearing five-year-old girl named Sarah came to my office for an assessment for ADHD. Her patient mom said with humor but no small amount of despair, "My daughter is like the Energizer Bunny on crack." Indeed, this little girl was so restless and internally agitated that she would have climbed the walls of my office clear to the ceilings if she could have. Notably, the child herself did not look happy to be in perpetual motion; it seemed as if she couldn't stop herself from moving. I found that she had a strong history of dairy-reactive red flags—croup, chronic ear infections, eczema, constipation. She also ate a tremendous amount of dairy and craved it like an addict. I advised a trial 100 percent off dairy and to take some steps to clean her diet, though overall it was healthy.

A month later, the family returned. Sarah sat in my office, startlingly calm and relaxed. No more eczema or constipation. Best of all, her mother said, "She can still be the Energizer Bunny sometimes. But she is no longer the 'Energizer Bunny on crack.'" Dairy was confirmed as the culprit when her siblings, home from college, had taken their baby sister out for ice cream: The hyperactive symptoms returned with a vengeance, then dissipated a few days later.

Other patients of mine have gone from endless difficulty reading basic words to suddenly reading chapter books during their month off dairy. Intractable tics have remitted. A growing number of studies have shown that dairy-allergic children with epilepsy can experience a dramatic remission of seizures—including normalization of their EEGs after stopping dairy in some cases.[21,22] Others became seizure-free after removing gluten from their diets and were able to reduce or be weaned off medication. A little boy with egg allergy no longer screamed about every itchy tag and tight waistband after his diet was changed. And my own son, who had reacted to soy with a developmental regression, flourished when we removed soy from his foods.

In order to help your child truly get well, step one is to remove reactive foods (and associated chemicals) so that your child's body is not constantly irritated by them. After healing and nourishing your child, you may find it possible to reintroduce once-problematic foods (not the processed ones!) as the body becomes balanced and resilient.

TIP ————————————————————————————

Removing troublesome foods can be the first step toward complete resolution of symptoms for a significant number of kids. Even if a child's condition isn't "cured" by removing a problematic food, the change can mitigate symptoms (for example, getting a full night's sleep!), allow for lower doses of medication, and improve quality of life.

————————————————————————————

## ARE THESE FOODS HEALTHY OR NOT?

Often, allergic children react to foods typically considered "healthy," like dairy, soy, wheat, eggs, peanuts, tree nuts, shellfish, even citrus. This is one of the hardest facts about allergy for parents (never mind grandparents!) to fathom—"Not milk! Really?" Inevitably, when we review abnormal lab results, parents will respond, "But I thought X was healthy!" So how does a seemingly wholesome food become a trigger of unhealthy symptoms?

Let me clarify here that food itself is not the enemy. In theory, milk is just milk, eggs are just eggs, wheat is just wheat, soy is just soy. Our bodies have evolved with these foods for millennia. The problem is twofold: first, food is grown, raised, produced, and manufactured in ways that deplete nutrients and our health. Second, children's guts and immune systems have become dysregulated and are prone to react. These foods essentially taunt children's immune systems . . . and their bodies react in surprising and detrimental ways.

Take peanuts. They were traditionally eaten boiled, fried, or raw in eastern Asia and Africa, where allergies to peanuts are far less common than in the United States or Europe. But as a result of aspects of mass production, they're almost entirely eaten dry roasted now. Dry roasting takes advantage of the Maillard reaction—that yummy caramelizing effect that happens when cooking at high temperatures—but also creates advanced glycation end products (AGEs), which in turn stimulate the allergic response more significantly than raw peanuts.[23]

Children are also exposed to substances found in and on food that should never appear there. In 2014, the *Annals of Allergy, Asthma & Immunology* published a report of a little girl who was allergic to antibiotics and milk, but had an anaphylactic response to—of all things— blueberry pie. Testing revealed that she had no allergy to any specific ingredient of the pie.[24] The culprit? *Antibiotics applied to the blueberries.* Banned in Europe, the antibiotic streptomycin is used in the United States and Canada on certain crops to prevent bacteria, fungi, and algae. (Disturbingly, we are exposed to antibiotics not only through produce and animals, but also in the resulting runoff into our water supply.)

Soy is another example. I had always been under the impression that soy was healthy, but while researching to help my son, I learned that more than 90 percent of soy and as much as 85 percent of corn in the United States is genetically modified,[25] which can make it more allergenic by exposing us to unanticipated proteins,[26,27] by disturbed gut flora or digestive enzymes, or other means.[28,29,30] High pesticide use on the crop damages our cells, bacteria, even our DNA,[31,32] and heightens the risk of health conditions like asthma, celiac, neurological illness, and cancer.[33,34,35,36] Furthermore, those pesticides can actually bind nutrient uptake from the soil into the plant,[37] which reduces the availability of nutrients we can derive from food. Even the way we prepare and eat soy may render it an irritant to an already reactive immune system. My son, for example, reacted not just to soy but also to soybean oil (used in most restaurants and many prepared foods). Allergists (and the FDA) say that only proteins can cause allergies; because they're removed by the oil-refining process, restaurants don't disclose it as an ingredient. Yet when my son consumed soybean oil, his asthma attacks were as severe as if he had eaten tofu. And when it comes to problems in our food chain, soy is by no means the only culprit.

As you'll see in the upcoming chapters, everything about our food has changed drastically. It's now more common than not to see food that's been hybridized and standardized, pasteurized, irradiated, sprayed with pesticides, administered antibiotics, genetically modified, and from microbe- and nutrient-depleted soil. Many of these interventions are thought to be "necessary" because producing food on a large scale increases the risk of contamination considerably. The "new" food may be good for efficiency, prolonged shelf life, reliability, and quantity, but it isn't very good for plants, for animals, or for us.

Ultimately, food has changed faster than our physiology can evolve to keep up. When food became an industrial commodity rather than a source of nourishment and balance, we gained the luxury of eating the same very handsome foods all year round with little interruption. But the way our food is now raised, produced, and processed—from animals and their milk and eggs to fruits, vegetables, grains, and other plants—is making us sick.

**Simply put, food was never meant to be a commodity on this grand a scale.**

### Dairy

Most milk comes from cows that eat grain-based feed in a tiny stall and not grass in a pasture. Milk cows are dosed with antibiotics to help them grow faster and with hormones to produce more milk. Milk has been pasteurized and homogenized, which alters its structure and components. Since today's typical store-bought milk differs significantly from milk that previous generations got straight from the udder, it shouldn't surprise us that children's bodies regard dairy products differently, too.

Science confirms what I've seen in my practice for years—that dairy-containing foods can trigger ailments from ear infections to migraines to seizures to ADHD, and exacerbate allergies, asthma, IBS, ulcers, and Crohn's disease.[38] One study correlated ADHD with cow's milk intolerance as well as other allergic conditions, skin infections and prescriptions for antiasthmatics, respiratory or topical steroids, antibacterials or antifungals.[39] Indeed, these are the children who might come to my office simultaneously on Miralax for constipation, frequent antibiotics for chronic ear infections or impetigo, antihistamines for allergies, inhaled steroids for asthma, topical steroids for eczema, and stimulants for attention deficit. Yet the authors of the study did not conclude by suggesting that future research might include a trial off of cow's milk to potentially mitigate the constellation of neurological, allergic, and infectious symptoms. Rather, they focused on the fact that asthma and allergy sufferers should not be deterred from taking their medication.[40] **Chronic medication may mask symptoms, but altering diet can virtually eliminate some or all symptoms.**

Dairy consumption and cow's milk allergy can even play a role in seizure activity for some children sensitive or allergic to dairy. As with ADHD, cow's milk allergy, eczema, and asthma are more common in children with epilepsy[41,42] and should be considered red flags for food allergies even in a child who's exhibiting primarily a neurological syndrome. More than one study suggests that removal of dairy from the diets of children with epilepsy can lead to lessening of seizure activity, EEG abnormalities, and other behavioral and cognitive symptoms. A child with skin positivity to dairy showed sustained improvement in seizures and EEG following removal of dairy from his diet.[43] In a follow-up study, three unmedicated children with partial cryptogenic epilepsy tested positive to dairy. These children had problems with sleep, handwriting, or behavior. When dairy was removed from their diets, their seizures, EEG abnormalities, and other issues lessened. All of these problems returned shortly after dairy was reintroduced, and then improved again upon removal of dairy.[44] Another study showed that children who have rolandic epilepsy (a syndrome in which children typically have seizures during sleep, often associated with temporary inability to speak) had fewer events upon removal of dairy.[45] It's no panacea, but it's certainly worth exploring.

Many parents of children with autism describe a range of symptoms that exacerbate after milk ingestion, and dramatically improve—from behavior to cognition—after they remove it from their diet. One study found a high incidence of immune markers to dairy proteins in autism spectrum disorder.[46] Another study reproduced this finding, but also determined that those antidairy antibodies tricked the body into having autoimmune reactions following infections like strep.[47] A few studies have explored removal of dairy alone from the diet; some studies have noted significant improvement in autistic symptoms upon the removal of both dairy and gluten from the diet.[48,49] While there is no definitive "diet for autism," many families notice improvement during a trial off problem foods.

So which children should stop dairy? You want to watch for a constellation of symptoms because each child presents differently. I've treated dairy-sensitive kids in my practice who are drinking three 8-ounce glasses of milk a day to "get calcium"—with their doctor's encouragement—but suffer from eczema, constipation, asthma, or croup, and the inability to focus. A child who is allergic or intolerant to dairy might have dark circles under his eyes or red cheeks and ears. He might be "spacey" or, conversely, explosive or hyperactive, especially after drinking a big glass of milk.

Many doctors pooh-pooh parents' observations that dairy seems to make their children worse. "Never mind that," they're told, "just make sure he's getting enough milk for calcium." Yet these kids are treated with topical steroids to reduce their eczema, antihistamines for chronic congestion, laxatives for intractable constipation, inhaled steroids for asthma, and Ritalin to enhance focus. Meanwhile, some of these medications further compromise the balance of intestinal flora that's critical for these children's health, making them more vulnerable to allergy.

Sometimes, though, it's hard to determine that dairy is the underlying trigger. Many dairy-sensitive kids paradoxically crave dairy, and therefore eat and drink such quantities of milk products that there is no before and after, only *during*. This is why a trial off of dairy—removing 100 percent of dairy products for one month—can be so helpful. For those who struggle with dairy, temporarily removing it from the diet may offer relief or even resolution of persistent health problems.

You can ask that your doctor request blood or skin tests to look for dairy sensitivity. Even an equivocal (not quite positive) response is enough reason to trial off dairy for one month. But don't rely solely on those results. No available tests—skin prick, scratch, or blood test for IgE, IgG, IgA—are perfect at detecting sensitivity. The best way to determine that your child is sensitive to dairy is to eliminate it for at least a month, and then reintroduce it and look for a return or exacerbation of symptoms. See below to learn how to conduct an elimination diet as well as recommendations for dairy alternatives.

## Take a Trial Period Off a Suspected Offending Food

To truly know whether your child is reactive to a certain food, I recommend this monthlong elimination diet.

- **Stop 100 percent of the allergen.** If you buy processed foods, read labels. If you're stopping milk, look for anything with milk, cheese, butter, sour cream, cream cheese, whey, casein, or lactalbumin. Milk means any milk or milk-based product that comes from animals: cow, goat, sheep, buffalo, you name it. (Dairy does not include eggs.)
- **Really commit.** Sometimes, parents tell me, "Well, we're not sure if it helped, but we were still doing milk in the cereal a few days a week" or "I couldn't take away pizza day at school." Make sure your child is *strictly* free of the suspect food; any food you purchase should be free of that ingredient. If you're going to the trouble of a trial, do it all the way. Don't cloud the picture with incursions.
- **Reintroduce.** After a month without the suspected food, choose a weekend day to reintroduce the food in a significant way (unless, of course, your child's reaction is anaphylaxis). If gluten is in question, a bagel for breakfast, pasta for lunch, and so on. Watch for a return or exacerbation of symptoms during the next 24 to 72 hours. A reaction following reintroduction may look different from what you expect. It may present like a recurrence of the symptoms you've wanted to eliminate or it can look like a cold or flu, chronic nasal congestion, bellyaches, fatigue, insomnia, headache, or totally impossible behavior. My friend called me after a reintroduction of dairy and said that she couldn't tell how her daughter was doing back on milk because she had been sick with a "cold" for the three weeks since she had added it. She stopped dairy again and the

mucus, coughing, and fatigue promptly disappeared. Any symptoms associated with eating the food—whatever they are—mean that the body is unhappy.

- **Keep a journal.** I don't believe in coincidence. From stuffy nose to emotional lability to ear infection to poor sleep, document what being off the food looks like, and what being back on the food looks like. Keep a journal because it's difficult to see patterns unless you objectively record what you see in the moment. Spend no more than ten minutes at the end of each day writing down what your child ate and any symptoms you are rating on a daily basis or that you noticed (it can be helpful to use a scale of 1–10).

- **Reactions, sensitivities, and even allergies need not last forever.** As the body recovers, matures, and heals, physiological shifts can occur. The immune system is constantly changing and learning, which means that under the right circumstances, food reactivity can lessen or disappear. And that means that sometimes problem foods can be reintroduced. Though every child is different, it is possible to try a reintroduction in a small way after six months or one year off of the reactive food. If the allergy is severe, it may take much longer and should be done under the supervision of a physician. But it's more important to know that if your child improves off dairy (or other foods), that doesn't necessarily mean she'll never eat yogurt or ice cream again. To be sure, this may begin at just a teaspoon a week (to eventually become more frequent). But in time, your child may tolerate larger or more frequent exposures.

- **Every child has a different threshold for these foods.** One child's peanut butter sandwich is another's stomachache and another's life-threatening reaction. After the initial period of 100 percent elimination, you learn how strict to be based on your child's tolerance level. It's the difference between removing your child from the same room as that food versus eating ice cream at the occasional birthday party or having one dairy day a week. Beware of the slippery slope, though—it can be easy to become complacent, which can sometimes see a return of problematic symptoms.

- **Look at the whole list of clinical symptoms to measure improvement.** Even though you may be focusing on one target goal, don't forget to celebrate the steps getting there. Perhaps the problematic hyperactivity may take further steps to address, but wow, better sleep and calmer moods are fantastic!

NOTE: Reaction to a food that was removed and then reintroduced can be more obvious or extreme than the symptoms were when the child was eating a lot of that food. Sometimes the immune system is able to more clearly express sensitivities or allergies when not overloaded with a problematic food.

## Stopping Milk

If you've tried an elimination diet and found that your child does better without dairy (which means that he or she can't tolerate foods with the words "milk," "milk powder," "casein," "whey," "butter," "sour cream," or "cream cheese" on the label), then your child should continue avoiding those foods for at least three to six months as you take steps to help her body to heal. Don't panic. I know that it can feel intimidating to navigate meals without a beloved food. But think of it this way: Whether it's eczema, ear infections, hyperactive behavior, acne, seizures, or migraines, your child is living in struggle. Within a few days or weeks, "dairy-free" becomes part of the routine. And many times the resulting improvement is so beneficial that you won't want to go back in a hurry. Here are some great foods to substitute for dairy to help your child not feel deprived.

### Alternatives to Cow's Milk

- **Almond milk:** For kids who tolerate nuts, almond milk—or other nut milks—is my favorite alternative. It is high in protein, healthy fats, and minerals, and it is easy to make from scratch. Make sure to avoid additives like carrageenan.
- **Coconut milk:** Filled with beneficial medium-chain triglycerides, organic coconut milk offers a naturally sweet option to replace cow's milk in smoothies or even cereal. Ideally purchase non- or minimally sweetened, best in glass containers.
- **Rice milk:** Though it's not my favorite milk replacement—it's high in sugar, and rice has been found to contain varying levels of arsenic—using it a couple of times a week is fine.
- **Hemp or flax milk:** The average dairy-reactive child will tolerate hemp or flax milk, which can be enjoyable plain or used in baking.

### Cow Milk Alternatives That May Cross-React with Cow's Milk

- **Goat's milk**: Compared to cow's milk, goat's milk is lower in allergenic casein and more of the (for most people) less allergenic whey. However, many dairy-allergic or sensitive children still don't tolerate it. After a 6- to 12-month period using only dairy-free foods, small amounts (starting with a teaspoon daily) of homemade goat's milk yogurt can be a good way to reintroduce and evaluate tolerance. Do not use goat milk during a trial off of milk!
- **Soy milk:** Soy can cross-react with dairy, so **I don't recommend it as a milk replacement for a dairy-free trial.** Note also that nonorganic soy in the United States almost always is GMO and has been sprayed with pesticides. It also contains phytochemicals that can interfere with thyroid function, and phytoestrogens that in high amounts may impact a child's hormones. Best to avoid it.
- **Raw camel's milk:** I see the shocked expression on your face, but hear me out: This long-traditional food for desert-dwelling

nomads in the Middle East is coming into vogue in the United States. Some Amish farms actually carry it. The fats and antibodies are small in size and are therefore less allergenic and more easily absorbed. Some children with significant digestive problems—and who struggle with dairy—can tolerate and even thrive on camel's milk. In fact, a doctor in Israel published a paper describing cognitive and behavioral improvement in autistic children who drink it, although more research must be done before such a benefit is confirmed. Because the benefits are only observed in raw camel's milk, however, it is essential to find milk certified to be free of brucellosis and other potentially problematic contamination, as with any raw milk. Do not try camel's milk during a dairy-free trial.

Stories like those of my patients who improved physical and neurological illnesses after becoming dairy-free have led some doctors, nutritionists, and activists to claim that milk is not a good food for humans. "Cow's milk is good for baby cows" is commonly repeated by those opposed to drinking milk. Milk detractors point out that we are the only species that drinks milk into adulthood, and the milk we drink is from another species. Ultimately, I don't buy this argument. Drinking milk may not be ideal for certain people and at certain times of life, but humans have consumed dairy for as long as they've herded animals—long before they began to farm during the agricultural age. Milk has played a pivotal role in human survival and health for thousands of years—indeed, in leaner times, humans haven't had the luxury of choosing not to consume dairy. Why, then, does milk seem to be more problematic today than ever before?

The likelihood is that, as with peanuts and soy, a combination of factors makes milk a problem for some people today. As I said earlier, milk itself is not a villain. It's just milk . . . a primal food that has been consumed for millennia, rich with nutrients, fats, immune factors, prebiotics that feed gut bacteria, enzymes, and often a source of beneficial bacteria as well. But agribusinesses invest a great deal of energy into "improving upon nature," otherwise known as making "value-added" products. Processing milk then changes it in ways that our bodies may not be able to handle. **Nature is complex and our understanding limited, so we cannot predict the long-term effects of the changes we make to food.** But clearly, we have created unintended consequences. More on that in Chapter 11.

## Eggs

Eggs are a common food allergy, especially for babies and young children. Leora had sensitive skin as an infant and often broke out in rashes—sometimes hives—for unknown reasons. At a year old, she began to eat scrambled eggs on occasion and often coughed or sneezed repeatedly after breakfast. Sometimes, she also vomited. Her mother suspected that the texture bothered her, but the vomiting worsened. Eventually, her mother took her to an allergist, who diagnosed an egg allergy.

Eggs are a common allergy trigger, especially for babies and very young children. To understand why egg allergies have increased, we should examine how we come by eggs these days. My family's eggs come from our own feathered ladies (as we call our chickens), and I am responsible for what they eat and how much time they get to scratch dirt for bugs and nibble on plants. But most laying hens are factory raised and live in crowded cages with no fresh air, sunlight, exercise, or any of their beloved snacks of bugs and worms. These layers are not very healthy and certainly not happy. They live indoors day and night—under artificial lights to induce them to lay more eggs—and administered antibiotics to keep them from getting sick in less-than-ideal, less-than-natural living conditions. They eat (genetically modified) soy-based feed (including waste like recycled vegetable oil from fryers), and no fresh greens or scraps or forage or bugs. A 1993 US Department of Agriculture (USDA) study found that hens taken off pasture and fed a diet of soy, corn, wheat, or cottonseed meal laid fewer eggs. Fewer of their chicks gestated to term, and the hatched chicks had higher rates of death and illness. If that's what happens to the chicks that grow in the eggs, what might eating the eggs do to us?

Just as our terrain affects our bodies, the hens' terrain affects theirs. The hens' stressful, sedentary, medication-heavy, nutrient-deficient lifestyle changed the quality of the eggs they laid. I simply brush my eggs free of debris and leave them on the counter until scrambling them. Commercial eggs are washed with chemical-heavy detergent, rinsed with warm water plus sanitizer, then dried and coated with mineral oil. This processing inherently changes the egg and ultimately the bodies of those who eat these eggs. An egg laid by a nourished, thriving hen is more nutritious and less allergenic than an egg that's the product of antibiotics, unnatural diet, lack of sunlight and fresh air, and doused in chemical cleansers.

Again, the egg in and of itself—like milk—is not "bad." Good eggs are worth their weight in gold. But not all foods are created equal.

### Gluten

Wheat today is also different from the wheat our grandparents ate. And, like other gluten-containing foods such as spelt, rye, barley, and some oats, it can trigger troubling symptoms in children.[50] The species of wheat planted today differ from those that were a hundred years ago, and they are planted in monocrops covering thousands of acres. Their shallower roots grow in soil that lacks biodiversity; they're sprayed with multiple rounds of the pesticide Roundup; they are milled and further processed differently. Some data suggest that glyphosate—an herbicide found in Roundup—is associated with the skyrocketing numbers of celiac cases as well as increases in cancer, Parkinson's, thyroid disease, and kidney disease.

We're exposed to plenty of Roundup by way of our wheat. At harvesttime, wheat crops are sprayed with Roundup up to six times, to kill it, so that it releases its seed more easily. This increases crop yield, which is good for business, but as a result we are consuming ever-increasing amounts of the toxic herbicide each time we eat wheat-based products. According to the USDA, as of 2012, 99 percent of durum wheat, 97 percent of spring wheat, and 61 percent of winter wheat had been treated with herbicides—a significant increase since

1998.[51] Roundup may well play a role in the increase in food allergies through numerous means, including killing particular gut bacteria,[52] impairing detoxification,[53] depleting nutrients, and improperly triggering the immune system.

Wheat allergy can be difficult enough, but in celiac disease wheat and gluten trigger a full-body autoimmune reaction. Although a child with celiac classically presents with digestive symptoms, skin rashes, and failure to thrive (not gaining weight or growing appropriately), robust data show that these symptoms aren't the only way to detect a reaction. Celiac can present with neurological and other symptoms. According to the scientific literature, ataxia (unsteady gait), ADHD, migraines, worsening autism symptoms, seizures, and tics can all be seen in a child with celiac.[54]

My patient Cheri was a petite five-year-old who was under the fifth percentile for weight and height. She had chronic asthma, for which she had been hospitalized multiple times. She had seen numerous pediatricians, pulmonologists, gastroenterologists, and allergists in her short life. Her parents brought her to me not for the asthma or failure to thrive, but for difficulty focusing in school. After administering a battery of laboratory tests, I found that her celiac antibody levels were off the charts. She underwent further tests with a gastroenterologist and was confirmed to have celiac disease. Off gluten, her asthma has disappeared, she's started to gain weight, and lo and behold, her focus has also improved. Her body was so sick for so long that she is still healing, but even so, she's been weaned off most of her medications and continues to improve.

I believe that **any child with behavioral problems or neurological symptoms—sensory, cognitive, attentional, or otherwise—should have a screening for celiac *and* a gluten-free trial for at least one month.** Not every child with a neurological condition has celiac, nor will every child improve off gluten. But it is worth knowing, especially with the incidence of celiac at 1 in 100 and gluten sensitivity having recently been proposed as a different but important presentation of reactivity.[55]

Billy was three years old and had been developing normally. His distraught mother brought him to me because Billy was standing in the closet in preschool, crying and screaming for hours, "I'm going to kill you!" or "I'm going to kill myself!" His mother had had an array of symptoms that improved when she stopped eating gluten, but she had not tested positive for celiac. Similarly, Billy's celiac testing, both blood and biopsy, was negative. Given the alternative of serious medications with unknown long-term effects on brain development, we removed gluten for one month to see if he shared her sensitivity. Within a week, the screaming stopped completely.

Removing gluten can reduce other symptoms dramatically. Based on both scientific literature and clinical experience, I also suggest that a child trial off of gluten for one to three months if there is a history of seizures. Children with epilepsy have a higher rate of celiac than the rest of the population,[56] and it's been documented that seizures can reduce or even disappear after removing gluten from their diet— particularly if they have brain calcifications on an MRI.[57,58,59] Some children with autism can also improve significantly in sleep, bowel habits, even speech and cognition,[60] though not every child with autism responds equally to such diet changes. Another red flag can be frequent broken bones or problems with teeth, as celiac also affects integration of calcium into the body and brain.[61]

An important caveat: I don't think that "gluten is bad" per se or that children should never eat it so long as they tolerate it well. Many times, the processed gluten-free substitutes are far less wholesome than good-quality, organic wheat that's *freshly ground*—especially nutrient-dense ancient varieties that are higher in protein but lower in gluten, such as spelt, emmer, and einkorn.

### Corn

Corn is ubiquitous in processed food and is often a hidden ingredient. In the United States, conventionally grown corn is frequently GMO and therefore increases your exposure to pesticides. It can also be highly allergenic. If you notice your child demonstrates symptoms after eating corn, remove corn for a trial. This can be challenging because it appears in a lot of products that are not labeled as corn. Cornmeal, corn oil, cornstarch, and corn syrup are obvious, but powdered sugar and baking powder can also contain corn. Vitamin C—including ascorbic acid and citric acid—is often derived from corn. All infant formulas as well as PediaSure contain corn. Believe it or not, the most hypoallergenic infant formulas are derived almost entirely from corn! Many fruits and some vegetables are coated with a corn-containing wax. Even BPA-free lining can be made from corn. Please note that most people are not sensitive to these trace corn derivatives, so start with obvious sources.

## Removing All Grains

Some children with more severe digestive problems—stomach pain, chronic loose stool, severe constipation, painful bloating, especially with other associated symptoms—improve when they eliminate sugar, grains, and legumes for a trial period of a month or more. Clinical studies indicate that a percentage of these children—with conditions from Crohn's to autism—improve dramatically.[62] Some people remain on this diet long term, while others can reintroduce these foods in soaked or sourdough forms after a period of healing. Those who respond and need such a diet long term should be monitored by a health-care professional experienced with these diets. Examples: Specific Carbohydrate Diet (SCD), Gut and Psychology Syndrome Diet (GAPS), Paleolithic diet.

## Removing Carbohydrates

Some children with severe neurological symptoms—notably intractable seizures, but also some children with autism or other neuropsychiatric symptoms—benefit from removing many or most carbohydrates from their diet.[63,64] Studies implementing this diet in almost all kinds of epilepsy show the potential for drastic improvement or resolution of symptoms that can persist even after the diet is stopped. **However, the kinds of proteins and fats used can make or break the success of this diet** (see Chapter 15 for more details on healthy fats). Examples: the Modified Atkins diet and Ketogenic diet.

Children do best with a wide variety of nutrients as they rapidly develop. Unless you have expertise in nutrition, restrictions this severe should be implemented only with the aid of a doctor or nutritionist experienced in monitoring such a diet to ensure that no dangerous deficiencies develop.

## Other Foods

When my middle son was in preschool, he sometimes developed red cheeks and ears for no apparent reason. He also woke frequently in the night, agitated and inconsolable. One day, we noticed his red cheeks after he had had a cup of lemonade at the park. We did a trial off of citrus fruits for one month. Lo and behold, the redness disappeared and his sleep totally normalized.

If you notice that your child looks, feels, or acts differently after eating a certain food, consider removing that food for a trial. Keep a journal to track his or her symptoms and how they change on the trial. Reintroduce the food after a month and watch carefully for the next 48 to 72 hours to see if old symptoms recur or weakened symptoms get more pronounced. Some examples of foods that cause reactions are strawberries, citrus fruit, soy, tree nuts, peanuts, and shellfish.

Here are the steps for following an elimination diet.

### Elimination Diet How-To:

1. First, remove foods that are not food: additives, dyes, processed sweeteners, etc. Sometimes this is all that is necessary to see a huge improvement. More on this in Chapter 6.
2. If you suspect symptoms are connected to a particular food, try eliminating that food for a trial period of one month. Keep a journal and look for improvements. Reintroduce at the end of that time and look for exacerbation.

3. If your child is sick and has still not improved considerably, or you suspect that other foods are involved but you've no idea which ones, you can:

   a) Get blood RAST IgE testing. Any doctor can order this test, not just allergists: Test for casein, whey, soy, egg white, egg yolk, corn, wheat, peanut, tree nuts, lemon, orange, chicken, beef, and other foods that are frequently consumed. A celiac panel can be included.

   b) Some people eliminate the "big allergens" for one month: dairy, gluten, soy, corn, egg, nuts, peanuts, shellfish. If this isn't too difficult for you, go for it. Then reintroduce foods one by one.

   c) Otherwise you may need to play detective. If your child eats a tremendous amount of one food (like dairy or peanut butter), it may be worth removing the food for a trial period of a month.

4. Engage your child. Let him know why you are undertaking this process and what you are hoping to accomplish together. Talk about things that he cares about: getting in trouble at school, having better skin, not having stomachaches, fewer migraines. Build a teamwork mentality rather than being the tyrant who takes away the food he loves.

5. Find replacements for favorite treats—in the long term, the "free-from" products can be just as junky as the allergen-containing processed foods. In the short term, though, using those products occasionally might make the implementation of the elimination diet easier.

6. Look for environmental instigators of allergy. For example, mold in the home or school can be a significant culprit—check for areas of leaks or repeated moisture and remedy them.

# TAKE HOME

1. Traditional allergy tests don't tell the whole story of food reactivity. Neither do tests for IgA, IgG, or others. IgE/IgG blood testing is reasonably useful to evaluate which foods trigger reactions.
2. The best way to determine whether a food contributes to your child's symptoms—whether allergy, sensitivity, or otherwise—is to eliminate it from his or her diet for a month and then reintroduce it to see if the worrisome symptoms recur.
3. It's fine to initiate a one- to three-month trial off a food, but only remove a food from the diet for a longer period if your child objectively improves when you remove the food or objectively worsens when you reintroduce it.
4. If your child must stop one or more foods, consider consulting with a nutritionist to ensure that your child gets the full array of nutrients and doesn't suffer from any significant deficiencies.
5. Food allergies or sensitivities mean that the gut and immune system are disordered, but allergies may not persist for life. Don't simply remove a food and leave it at that. The information in the next chapters will help you heal your child's body so that healthy, whole foods eventually can be reintroduced.

## CHAPTER 6

# Artificial Food: Flavorings, Dyes, Preservatives, and Other Toxic Additives

When I was growing up, my family made strawberry Popsicles in the summer. We'd throw fresh local strawberries in the blender with water, honey, and lemon, pour them into molds in the freezer, and check repeatedly to see if they were fully frozen. Then we'd delight in their vivid red color, heady fragrance, and intense flavor (while getting our daily dose of flavonoids). When I went to my friends' houses, I discovered that food companies made their own mass-produced version, but eliminated fresh fruit entirely, using artificial flavors and colors to approximate color, smell, and flavor.

Instead of investing in real ingredients from fresh food, which impart the flavors, colors, and textures that our bodies crave, industry uses cheaper chemicals to make "food products" that appear to be something they're not. Meanwhile, it spends top dollar on research to determine how chemicals can imitate or "surpass" the flavor and feeling of real food. Since most people don't purposely choose foods filled with chemicals, especially for children, industry experts use labeling to mislead parents who want to buy "natural," "fresh" foods. And they do it to boost their bottom line.

**Food additives are used for one reason: to deceive.** Consider these "foods" to see how far manufacturers have gone to ensure predictability and desirability in their products: Is your child's "Very Berry" juice a beautiful vibrant color and fruity-tasting because it's made from fresh fruit? Is packaged pumpernickel bread brown from the addition of actual pumpernickel flour? And are your pickles bright green as a result of traditional preparation? Nope. The bread is likely dyed with artificial caramel color; the pickles dyed with Yellow

Dye No. 30; and the berry juice probably doesn't contain any fruit at all. When the Center for Science in the Public Interest evaluated a drink called Cherry Berry Blast, it found that, despite the name of the drink, it contained *0 percent* berry and cherry juice. The bright red color comes not from fruit, but artificial dye Red 40. Your carrot cake mix likely has no carrots, but rather "carrot-flavored pieces" processed from corn syrup, flour, corn cereal, partially hydrogenated cottonseed or soybean oil, and artificial colors FD&C Yellow 6 and Red 40.

You might be surprised to discover that nearly every prepared food product currently packaged and sold in the United States contains additives—dyes, preservatives, flavorings, binders, and texturizers—to achieve an approximation of food prepared from nourishing (and real) ingredients. When we eat these lab-made ingredients, we're not just missing out on the healing powers of real food, we're filling our basins with unhealthy substances that make us sick.

In my review of the scientific literature on additives, I found that many of them are used as toxins in laboratory experiments. To cause damage to cells in their labs, researchers use sodium benzoate,[1] MSG,[2] aspartame,[3,4] sodium nitrate, and other common and "safe" food additives. Our children consume these toxins many times a day. I'm not saying that the doses used in experiments are the doses that our children are consuming or that the outcome will be the same as it is for a mouse. But a compound that causes damage to a mouse cell often causes damage to a human cell. Mice and humans are obviously different, but oxidative stress and mitochondrial damage look very similar on a cellular level. That's why we extrapolate from lab animals to humans to learn about health conditions.

I discovered many disturbing papers about the effect of food additives on children's bodies. A landmark double-blind, placebo-controlled study published in the highly respected medical journal *The Lancet* showed that a combination of commonly used food dyes and preservatives increased hyperactivity in two- to three-year-olds and eight-year-olds.[5] In an animal study, combinations of dyes and other additives reduced the detoxification abilities of cells and caused damage to the liver.[6] Yellow dyes—tartrazine and sunset yellow—are xenoestrogens, which disrupt our children's hormones[7] and are implicated in breast cancer and liver disease. Yellow Dye No. 5 also negatively influenced learning behavior in mice—and not just in one generation, but throughout several generations—meaning the dye can affect our brains and our epigenetics.[8] Sodium benzoate increased anxiety and caused motor impairment in animal studies.[9]

It's no wonder that in 2010 the E.U. required warning labels for foods containing artificial colors, stating, "Consumption may have an adverse effect on activity and attention in children." Ultimately, processed foods and their artificial ingredients offer the body no benefits. Even worse, they damage us in ways small and large at a cellular and mitochondrial level.

Avoiding these compounds is your first step in healing. We'll get into much more detail about how to do that in a way that feels manageable, but please read on for an introduction to the major players.

## FOOD DYES: COLOR THEM DANGEROUS

We are drawn to brightly colored foods instinctively because, in nature, bright color equals nutritious phytochemicals. We need phytochemicals to survive, heal, and be well: lycopenes in red tomatoes, carotenes in pumpkins and carrots, ellagic acid and other flavonoids in grapes and blueberries. These beneficial compounds enhance our health on every level: They build our gut flora, help us detoxify, regulate our immune system, strengthen mitochondria, and even make us more intelligent by promoting brain plasticity.

And who are most attracted to brightly colored foods? Kids, of course! Their systems need the intense support of phytochemicals because they are developing so rapidly—physically, mentally, and emotionally. Yet most food dyes are made from petroleum by-products. Yes, petroleum—what we use to fuel our cars and factories (the original food dyes came from toxic coal tar). The food industry taps into children's deep, biological desire to eat gorgeous, bright food with products that mimic food with healthful attributes.

Yet artificial dyes can actually *detract* from health. Is it worth it to feed our kids ingredients that potentially contribute to poor focus, hyperactivity, motor skill issues, allergies, and even cancer?[10]

Another problem with food dyes is the *amount* used. The FDA concluded that **the maximum consumption of food dyes per day shouldn't exceed 30 milligrams.** But a recent study from Purdue University measured the quantity of food dyes in products such as Skittles, M&Ms, Kraft Macaroni & Cheese, and General Mills' Trix cereal and found that they contained more than 30 milligrams per serving.[11] Consider these popular foodstuffs:

| | | |
|---|---|---|
| Trix cereal: 36.4 mg | Fruity Cheerios: 31 mg | Cap'n Crunch Oops! All Berries: 41 mg |
| Target Mini Green Cupcakes: 55.3 mg | Skittles: 33.3 mg | M&M's: 29.5 mg |
| Kraft Macaroni & Cheese: 17.6 mg | Keebler Cheese & Peanut Butter Sandwich Crackers: 14.4 mg | Kraft Creamy French Dressing: 5 mg |

Beverages are the most commonly consumed source of artificial colors in the average U.S. diet. Purdue researchers published another study in 2013 that revealed levels of dye in an 8-ounce serving of many popular drinks:[12]

| | | |
|---|---|---|
| Powerade Orange Sports Drink: 22.1 mg | Crush Orange: 33.6 mg | Sunny D Orange Strawberry: 41.5 mg |
| Kool-Aid Burst Cherry: 52.3 mg | Full Throttle Red Berry Energy Drink: 18.8 mg | |

These numbers illustrate that a child who eats a fairly typical amount of processed food each day could easily take in well more than 100 mg a day, maybe even *double* that. While some of these companies are phasing out synthetic food dyes (without actually adding any real food to improve nutrition), food dyes are still widely used in processed foods.

It turns out that just because the FDA says something is safe doesn't mean it is. Over the years, regulators from the FDA have taken occasional action against some colorings used in the United States that were linked to negative health effects in animal studies. Examples: the banning of Green 1 (liver cancer); Orange 1 and 2 (organ damage); Red 1 (liver cancer); and Sudan 1 (toxic and carcinogenic).

Each of the banned food dyes had been considered "safe"—they'd been used on produce and in spices, candies, and other packaged foods—right up until the ban. They were only removed after researchers demonstrated their devastating impact on health *and* because public outcry demanded it. A host of other dyes are still in use while under investigation. Until these damaging additives are taken out of our food, you should avoid them.

**Where You Find It:** Food dyes are in the obvious products—rainbow-colored candy, fluorescent sodas and energy drinks, and brightly hued cereals—and also often added to foods like yogurt, soup, and even bread.

**Code Words: Any ingredient with a color in its name: red, yellow, green, blue.**

## Rethinking Ingredients

The word "ingredients" usually refers to foods that go into a recipe—eggs, butter, spinach, rice, salt, pepper and so on. Note that most cookbooks aren't calling for two tablespoons of MSG, a dash of aspartame, some BHT, and TBHQ. That's why I object to companies labeling food additives as "ingredients"—they're not natural components of food. Petroleum or coal tar is "natural" in that it comes out of the ground—but it's not what we want to feed kids.

## MSG: SAVORY POISONS

I first became interested in MSG when I noticed that several of my patients had first-time seizures after eating take-out Chinese or Japanese food for a few days in a row. Others had exacerbated migraines or felt agitated after eating foods that contain MSG in high amounts.

Monosodium glutamate, MSG, re-creates a natural flavor called "umami," which is sometimes referred to as the "fifth flavor" (after sweet, sour, salty, and bitter). Umami is savory, meaty, and delicious. It naturally occurs in foods like miso, tamari, umeboshi plums, mushrooms, seaweed, tomatoes, cheese, bone broths—typically long-cooked or fermented foods that are naturally high in glutamate. Ajinomoto Company of Japan found that synthetic umami could cheaply season foods, without the work usually involved in making deeply flavored dishes. Preparing a traditional rich, earthy broth isn't difficult but takes time—roasting bones, simmering them for hours with vegetables and aromatics, straining, and simmering again. That time invested yields tremendous delicious and nourishing benefits. Suddenly, one little MSG-spiked "flavor packet" allowed the home cook to whip up a meal bursting with savory flavor in just a few minutes—but with considerably fewer health benefits. This "magic" ingredient also stimulated the appetite, so manufacturers added it to everything, including hospital meals and even baby food. Why not!? MSG was removed from baby food in the 1970s due to public outcry, but it remains in a large number of processed products.

There's been a lot of debate about the safety of MSG. Some researchers have produced studies saying that it's completely safe to consume, yet many of those studies have been funded by industry or industry front groups. The problem is that MSG is like naturally occurring glutamate in food, but with one small tweak—it contains S-isomers (compounds that are very similar but not exactly the same). However, it doesn't behave in the body as natural L-glutamate isomer does.

Glutamate is an amino acid and a neurotransmitter. Its job in the nervous system is to be "excitatory," meaning it's stimulating. There are several types of receptors in the brain just for glutamate because it's critical for learning and memory. It's so important that the blood-brain barrier (BBB)—the defense system that guards the inner sanctum of the brain and central nervous system from the rest of the body's circulation—selectively admits glutamate, sometimes to the exclusion of other necessary amino acids. Most foods contain small amounts of natural glutamate as part of an array of other amino acids, balanced both by micronutrients like magnesium that confer a relaxing effect, B vitamins that help transform stimulatory glutamate to relaxing GABA, and neuroprotective phytochemicals.

Just as cooking with MSG flavor packets adds fast flavor to meals, eating it adds fast glutamate molecules to your body and brain. Neurons exposed to a flood of free glutamate can be highly stimulated, which results in an overfiring that generates copious free radicals. Though some free radicals are part of the normal metabolic process, large amounts deplete our antioxidants and cause cell damage. This is known as oxidative stress—*not* what you want to happen in your child's brain. And this excitotoxicity, as it's called, also undermines a child's blood-brain-barrier protection by increasing its permeability.[13]

When vulnerable people consume high amounts of MSG-containing foods, neurological struggles can begin: headaches, pain, agitation, insomnia, even seizures (in children who are susceptible).[14] Some families with children on the autism spectrum describe how their children can even be sensitive to foods naturally high in glutamate, and that eating a low-glutamate diet helps tremendously.

If neuronal damage doesn't send you running from Cheez-Its and instant ramen, consider that researchers use MSG to *induce* obesity. Adding MSG to the diet increases food intake, weight gain, and metabolic syndromes in animal studies.[15] In neonatal mouse studies, it damages the hypothalamus, a section of the brain that, among other things, controls appetite.[16] These mice then develop "MSG-induced obesity." Researchers use MSG in newborn mice to target their brains at their "most vulnerable." Do we really want MSG added to our children's food when their brains are most vulnerable?

**Where You Find It:** MSG is found mainly in savory products. Anything that has a flavor packet is a likely culprit (rice mixes, instant soups), as is anything cheesy (Cheez-Its, Goldfish crackers, mac and cheese) or intensely flavored (sour cream and onion chips, ranch dressing, buffalo sauce).

**Code Words (names of ingredients that always contain processed free glutamic acid):** MSG goes by a number of names. No one really *wants* to eat MSG, so manufacturers have gotten tricky. When scanning a label, look for any of these names. Some products even list MSG three or four times using different names.

Ajinomoto
Any "hydrolyzed protein"
Anything "enzyme modified"
Anything "hydrolyzed or autolyzed": soy, vegetable, wheat, yeast proteins
Anything "protein fortified"
Calcium caseinate, sodium caseinate
Gelatin
Glutamate (E 620)
Glutamic acid (E 620)
Magnesium glutamate (E 625)
Monoammonium glutamate (E 624)
Monosodium, monopotassium, or calcium glutamate (E 621, E 622, E 623)
Natrium glutamate
Soy protein, soy protein concentrate, soy protein isolate
Soy sauce, soy sauce extract
Textured protein
Umami[17]
Vetsin
Whey protein, whey protein concentrate, whey protein isolate
Yeast extract, torula yeast, yeast food, yeast nutrient

**Names of ingredients that often contain or produce processed free glutamic acid during processing:**

Any "flavors" or "flavoring"
Anything "ultra-pasteurized"

Barley malt, malted barley
Brewer's yeast
Carrageenan (E 407)
Citric acid, citrate (E 330)
Malt extract
Maltodextrin or oligodextrin
Natural flavor
Pectin (E 440)
Seasonings[18]

## Junk Food at a Glance

- When food producers financially support studies, the results often minimize health concerns associated with their products. According to a JAMA review of hundreds of studies on the health effects of milk, juice, and soda, conclusions favorable to the industry were several times higher among industry-sponsored research than studies that received no industry funding. "If a study is funded by the industry, it may be closer to advertising than science," said one of the reviewers.
- Food companies make big bucks (with our tax dollars) turning government-subsidized corn, wheat, and soybean commodity crops into fast foods, snack foods, and beverages. High-profit products made from subsidized commodity crops are generally high in calories and low in nutritional value.
- Less-processed foods are generally more filling than their highly processed counterparts. Fresh apples have more fiber and nutrients than applesauce. Added sweeteners increase the number of calories without making applesauce more filling. Apple juice has almost no fiber or nutrients. This stripping of nutrients happens to every processed, packaged food.

## PRESERVATIVES AND OTHER ADDITIVES

Traditionally, rural families smoked, cured, preserved, or fermented their food in sugar, salt, or vinegar. **Preserving fruits and vegetables at their peak freshness meant retaining their nutritional value and creating beneficial bacteria.** These benefits built the health of the gut and bolstered the immune system through the challenges of winter.

As food became a commodity, the food industry used equipment and knowledge derived from canning food for U.S. soldiers to offer products to consumers—foods with long shelf lives that eliminated their risk of loss and maximized their profit. Manufacturers scrambled to keep up with demand, packing products with toxic preservatives such as formaldehyde, borax, and sodium benzoate (a derivative of coal tar) in unmonitored amounts. **In short, we went from preserving our foods with healthy bacteria to embalming them with chemicals.**

There was no shortage of toxic additives in this "Wild West" of early food production. The soldering materials used to make cans—lead, copper, zinc—leached into the contents, causing entire families to become extremely ill from heavy metal toxicity. While adulterants were commonly used to give products a "boost" in texture—chalk in flour, hayseeds in jams—industrial canning rendered food unattractive and altered the taste significantly. So industry added bleach to canned corn to make it pearly white, coal-tar dyes to berries that had been bleached white by a reaction with the metal tins, and so on. **Ironically, the more the industry tried to emulate the food in its natural form, the more unnatural the product became.**

In the 1880s and 1890s, some public health officials started worrying about the impact of these additives on human health. Dr. Harvey Wiley of the U.S. Bureau of Chemistry began an investigation into their safety, and in 1902 he formed a group of healthy male volunteers that were dubbed the "Poison Squad," to whom he fed a diet that included preservatives during the course of a year. As the levels of preservatives increased, the men complained of burning throats, pains in the stomach, and dizziness. When the results were made public, people demanded change. Both homemakers and farmers joined forces to fight for unadulterated food. They rallied for the passage of the Pure Food and Drug Act, which managed to pass the House twice but failed in the Senate, crushed by influential manufacturers who didn't want to list additives on their labels. (Sound familiar?) But the publication of Upton Sinclair's now classic *The Jungle*, an exposé of Chicago's horrific meatpacking plants, provided the final impetus to pass the bill. The Pure Food and Drug Act of 1906 became the beginning of the future U.S. Food and Drug Administration.

Unfortunately, more than a hundred years later, we still haven't come very far from bleached veggies and chalk-filled flour. We continue to consume copious additives, from the frightening to the truly disgusting. The toxic flame retardant chemical Brominated Vegetable Oil (BVO), initially used to keep plastics from catching on fire, has been used to prevent artificial flavoring chemicals from separating from liquids. BVO can cause skin lesions, memory loss, and nerve disorders.[19] For decades, the food industry has added BVO to sodas, juices, and sports drinks—Mountain Dew, orange sodas, and some Powerade flavors. (Recently, some large drink manufacturers announced plans to phase out the chemical.) Titanium dioxide, a whitener sometimes contaminated with lead and commonly used in paints and sunscreens, is used to make processed items whiter, including salad dressings, coffee creamers, icings, and hundreds of other products. L-cysteine, used as a dough conditioner in industrially produced bread and baked goods, is derived from human hair and feathers, which can be contaminated with heavy metals—that's just plain disgusting. And then there's castoreum, which contributes to artificial raspberry or vanilla flavoring. It's delicious provenance? The anal glands of beavers.

**Where You Find It:** Most processed foods contain one or more additives for color, flavor, or texture, or to chemically prevent spoilage.

**Code Names:** Things that sound like something you'd use in a chemistry experiment.

## IF WE CAN BUY IT, IT MUST BE SAFE—RIGHT?

Our government agencies must be keeping us safe from toxic foods—aren't they? Not exactly. Once the Pure Food and Drug Act passed, the food industry was subject to a certain amount of oversight. But industry lobbied for—and won—the opportunity to influence policy in favor of its interests. Then and now, the political maneuvering and lobbying money of industry are powerful roadblocks to children's health. And the FDA persists in telling us that additives have no ill effects.

A quick search on its website yielded this statement: "Color additives are very safe when used properly," says Linda Katz, MD, M.P.H., director of the Office of Cosmetics and Colors for the FDA's Center for Food Safety and Applied Nutrition (CFSAN). "There is no such thing as absolute safety of any substance. In the case of a new color additive, FDA determines if there is 'a reasonable certainty of no harm' under the color additive's proposed conditions of use."[20]

With a little more digging on its site—all publicly accessible—I found a document that analyzed several studies on the detrimental effect of food additives on children's behavior. The studies included one in which researchers found that "exposure of this group to various individual provoking food items may result in behavioral changes associated more with irritability, fidgetiness, and sleep problems.... This food intolerance may involve some type of immunologic process possibly involving a non-IgE cellular response to antigen..."[21] Another study included in its review found that hyperactive children reacted to food colors more than "normal" children did, and proposed a possible genetic predisposition for hyperactivity and sensitivity to food colors.[22]

From the FDA document:

*Exposure to food and food components, including artificial coloring and preservatives, may be associated with behavioral changes, not necessarily related to hyperactivity, in certain susceptible children with ADHD and other problem behaviors, and possibly in susceptible children from the general population.*[23]

Translated, the FDA says here that certain vulnerable children—whether with ADHD, problem behaviors, or just in the general population—may experience behavioral changes when consuming artificial colors and preservatives. This means that food additives are not, in fact, safe—at least for a certain population of children.[24]

But the FDA decided that foods containing artificial color should not require warning labels because no causal relationship had been established in the general population. Confused yet? You are forgiven. These contradictions between the FDA's official position and its internal safety evaluation of additives on children's behavior indicate that even the experts at the FDA are "confused."

The European Union, however, doesn't suffer from this confusion and banned all synthetic dyes from foods consumed by babies and small children. In England, the government asked food companies to voluntarily remove artificial dyes in products marketed to children by the end of 2009. All companies—including those from the United States—complied. **In 2011, the U.K. branches of Walmart, Kraft, Coca-Cola, and Mars removed artificial colors, sodium benzoate, and aspartame from their product lines as a result of consumer pressure and government recommendations**. But take note! The very same company that produces cereal without food dyes for European distribution produces the very same cereal with food dyes when it is distributed to children in the United States. Because we Americans want our babies to get that extra kick of toxicity, right?

I know. It's shocking.

The European Union operates with the precautionary principle in mind, which dictates that action should be taken when there is documented risk to health, even before reaching conclusive proof of damage. Unlike its E.U. equivalent, however, the FDA does not require companies to pull products of concern off the market, nor does it require a warning label, nor is it sponsoring further studies for further evaluation. Even in light of the concerns that arise from its own safety evaluation, the FDA rejected recent petitions filed by the Center for Science in the Public Interest to ban eight of the nine currently approved synthetic food dyes. Why is the FDA ignoring the very troubling science of which it clearly is aware? Why isn't the FDA summarizing the science it evaluated so that parents can easily find it and come to their own conclusions? Is it protecting our children or industry?

Are you outraged yet?

Many children right now are getting special services, therapies, or medication for behavioral problems, or trouble focusing, or learning issues. These conditions may be exacerbated because the FDA, our safeguard agency, will not reliably protect our children from known instigators. So we parents, caregivers, teachers, principals, and health-care providers must do it ourselves. And I'm sad to say that schools can be the worst culprits, allowing teachers to distribute junk food in class or providing foods awash with additives in the cafeteria. Many behaviorists even recommend processed "treats" to reinforce desired behaviors in children with autism, who are, if anything, more sensitive to additives than others. In many cases, the "treat" can achieve the exact opposite of the desired outcome, causing children to be more fidgety, hyperactive, and irritable.

This may be hard to hear. It's one thing to want your child to be well, it's quite another to worry that you have to single-handedly take on your kid, your school, and the food industry. I understand your concerns as a parent—that giving up these foods will make your kids feel different or deprived, that your child refuses to eat healthy foods, that he or she will become hysterical, and so on. *But you can change what they eat.* It is not as difficult as you might imagine to find real foods—without chemicals—that your child will eat and enjoy.

We'll review all of the information you'll need to make good choices for your family. It starts with reading the label. Labels allow you to identify (to a great extent) what is in your food, which will help you decide whether you want to eat it or avoid it.

## LEARNING TO LOVE THE LABEL

Labels are the only way we can know anything about the contents of a sealed container of food. And more often than not, if we read the labels at all, we throw the package in our cart without understanding all the mystery words. Most people tend to rely more on the promises on the front of the label marketing descriptions than the ingredients listed, even though the contents go into our children's bodies and brains.

Beginning in the early 1900s, when prepared foods began to change urban eating, food companies had to work hard to convince people to eat what they couldn't see. Consumers were used to going to the outdoor markets, handling their produce, and asking questions about the animals—not opening a can and eating mystery ingredients. People were initially suspicious of meals that could have a "shelf life" and last months without spoiling.

To gain consumer trust, labels became the food industry's tool for projecting a "fresh" image . . . even when they didn't actually reflect a product's contents. At first, labels and images directly related to what people knew: food processes or places of origin. Lard labels depicted a farmer wielding a knife among his happy-looking hogs. Canneries used images of placid lakes, ostensibly filled with their fish. Cereal pictured the tall corn stalks from which it was derived. Even then, though, these appealing pictures belied the contents inside—coal-tar dyes, bleach, and fillers that sickened consumers.

**The food industry and the shopper have entirely different uses for the label.** Industry wants to inspire craving and desire in the shopper, whereas shoppers want to educate themselves about the food inside. Consumer surveys have shown that three out of four shoppers read and act on the nutritional information provided on labels; at least half of those consumers admit to studying labels to avoid various additives—salt, fat, sugar, artificial colors, etc. These same polls show that health concerns are paramount in how consumers choose their food. **Yet since the beginning of processed foods, industry has used labels to conceal instead of reveal.**

Let's look at the ingredients listed on a label of a leading self-described "healthy" cereal:

Corn, Whole Grain Wheat, Sugar, Oat Clusters (Sugar, Toasted Oats [Rolled Oats, Sugar, High Fructose Corn Syrup, Partially

Hydrogenated Soybean Oil, Molasses, Honey], Wheat Flakes, Crisp Rice [Rice, Sugar, Malt, Salt], Corn Syrup, Polydextrose, Honey, Cinnamon, BHT [Preservative], Artificial Vanilla Flavor), High Fructose Corn Syrup, Salt, Honey, Malt Flavoring, Alpha Tocopherol Acetate (Vitamin E), Niacinamide, Zinc Oxide, Reduced Iron, Sodium Ascorbate and Ascorbic Acid (Vitamin C), Calcium Pantothenate, Yellow No. 5, Pyridoxine Hydrochloride (Vitamin B6), Thiamin Hydrochloride (Vitamin B1), BHT (Preservative), Vitamin A Palmitate, Folic Acid, Beta Carotene (a source of Vitamin A), Vitamin B12 and Vitamin D.

*Zzzzzz.* **The desired effect of the "scientification" of label ingredients is for your eyes to glaze over.** Industry knows that the harder a label is to read (either through complexity or the tiniest of typefaces), the less attention a consumer will pay to what's inside. But this list is filled with vital information and tells us that this item is filled with **sugar**, PROCESSED FAT, <u>food additives</u>, and *synthetic vitamins*. (Remember: Any food that is enriched with vitamins essentially means the inherent nutrients have been lost in processing!)

Corn, Whole Grain Wheat, **Sugar**, Oat Clusters (**Sugar,** Toasted Oats [Rolled Oats, **Sugar, High Fructose Corn Syrup**, PARTIALLY HYDROGENATED SOYBEAN OIL, **Molasses, Honey**], Wheat Flakes, Crisp Rice [Rice, **Sugar, Malt,** Salt], **Corn Syrup, Polydextrose, Honey,** Cinnamon, <u>BHT [Preservative],</u> <u>Artificial Vanilla Flavor)</u>, **High Fructose Corn Syrup**, Salt, **Honey, Malt Flavoring,** *Alpha Tocopherol Acetate (Vitamin E), Niacinamide, Zinc Oxide, Reduced Iron, Sodium Ascorbate and Ascorbic Acid (Vitamin C), Calcium Pantothenate,* <u>Yellow No. 5,</u> *Pyridoxine Hydrochloride (Vitamin B6), Thiamin Hydrochloride (Vitamin B1),* <u>BHT</u> <u>(Preservative),</u> *Vitamin A Palmitate, Folic Acid, Beta Carotene (A Source of Vitamin A), Vitamin B12 and Vitamin D.*

And this cereal is billed as "healthy"! Think about the health claims on the front of the cereal box, made in plain English, and usually in easy-to-read typeface. "Less sugar," "More fiber," "Pure," "Natural," etc. Industry is hoping you don't ask any more questions. (Less sugar or more fiber than what? What do "pure" and "natural" really mean?) When we look to the back of the box, where the real information lives, we drown in tiny print and long words from a chemistry textbook. It's so difficult to interpret these confusing labels that we sometimes throw up our hands in defeat and just buy whatever.

**Bad labels are never a mistake. Labels are deceptive** *by design*. The industry works hard to influence regulation regarding what it does and doesn't have to say and what it is allowed to state on labels. More often than not, these are the goals of industry:

1. Try to make you believe the food has attributes that it doesn't have.
2. Try to make you believe the food *doesn't* have attributes that it does have.
3. Conceal troubling properties about ingredients.

Let me give you some examples:

"100% Natural" applesauce. Sounds nice. I'm picturing a sun-dappled apple orchard with large rosy apples that are handpicked and placed lovingly into bushels. I'd assume that no chemicals are added if they're *natural*.

I'd be wrong. "Natural" actually has no standardized meaning in the food world. The same thing goes for "Pure," "Farm-Fresh," and other similar claims. Those apples could be grown with chemical fertilizer, sprayed with pesticides and antibiotics, coated in wax derived from animal products, and drowned in high-fructose corn sugar along with preservatives and artificial dyes and flavors. Yet many people erroneously believe that "All-Natural" means the same or even better than the superior USDA Organic label that actually sets a high standard with significant oversight.

And what happens when the food industry tries to make you believe your food doesn't have attributes that it *does* have? Let's take the example of "No Added Sugar." I wince when I hear my patients' parents say: "We buy juice/jam/etc.—the healthy kind *with no added sugar*." These families have fallen for the trap. As you'll see in the next chapter, sugar is one of the most reliably addictive components of any processed food. But since it has become demonized during the last few decades, industry has found a way around disclosing that it has added it to its products. It adds fructose—concentrated, processed sugar derived from fruit—to the juice, jam, or fruit pops. **Manufacturers are permitted to categorize fructose as "fruit" and not list it as fructose.** Note also that they're not required to list added sugar content separately from total sugar content, so those consumers who read the label assume that juice has vast amounts of sugar *naturally*. When Michelle Obama proposed this change, the backlash from industry was enormous.[25]

**Labels should be simple, understandable, and honest.** The more our labels tell us about the story of our food, the more we can ensure that our children's stories have a happy ending.

## MAKING A PLAN THAT WORKS FOR YOU

Start gradually. People find incredible comfort and well-being in their eating rituals. For some families a sweeping approach can work, but others may find themselves in the midst of a full-blown mutiny. It's okay to put this advice into practice one step at a time. I've outlined these steps so you can make changes in a way that feels comfortable and doesn't create World War Three around food in your house.

### Step One: Just Read the Label

Go through your kitchen and read labels. Do you recognize all the ingredients listed or are there "science-isms" that sound like they belong in a laboratory instead of your breakfast? Is there any MSG? Additives? Food dyes? You might have to squint—that print is tiny for a reason!—but for now, just read.

## Step Two: Make Simple Swaps

Think about easy, parallel swaps. For example, if you were buying flavored rice mixes, consider buying plain white, red, or brown rice and
cooking it yourself with olive oil, broth, and spices. Swap out your
cereal with additives for one with none. Or replace cereal with eggs
and nitrate-free bacon, or unflavored hot cereal with a bit of honey.

## Step Three: Add in New Foods

At this point, you've cleaned out most if not all of the offenders mentioned in this chapter from your pantry. You've mostly transitioned to
foods that are closer to their whole, unprocessed form. You buy and
use glass instead of plastic. It's time to start exploring delicious foods
that will offer even more health benefits, which we'll talk more about
in coming chapters.

## CHAPTER 7
# Sickly Sweet Food: Sugar and Sweeteners

**S**ugar. It is the subject of extreme controversy, and everyone has a different opinion: "Who cares about sugar? Fat is the problem." "Sugar is fine in moderation." "Sugar is the greatest evil." One thing is true. Kids desire sugar like nothing else. While I do encounter an occasional kid who doesn't care for dessert, most children can be convinced to do anything for a sweet treat. Sugar has become ubiquitous in food, and it is marketed like mad to children by the food industry.

It's time to tell the truth about sugar. Let's start with some facts: Our intake of sugar and other sweeteners has exploded during the past decade. In that time, more than half of American adults became overweight, a quarter of them obese.[1] And children, especially teens, are consuming the lion's share, with some adolescents consuming more than 40 percent of their daily calories as sugar. As a result, kids today now suffer from conditions that used to afflict only adults. Triglycerides, a compound in the blood partly related to sugar and carbohydrate intake, have skyrocketed in children.[2] Type 2 diabetes in children, unheard of until a little more than a decade ago, rose 30 percent between 2001 and 2009 alone.[3] And the vast amounts of sugar and processed carbohydrates being consumed have led to an epidemic of fatty liver—think foie gras in children instead of geese—in 10 percent of all adolescents.[4] Once rare, it is now the most common reason for liver transplants.[5,6]

How did we get here? A hundred years ago, it took people five days to consume the amount of sugar that is found in a single can of soda today. And many people are now consuming that same amount *every seven hours*. That adds up to the equivalent of 22 teaspoons of sugar per person, per day. Our intake of drinks in particular—teas, sodas, sport "ades," vitamin waters, and energy drinks—has increased by more than 30 percent during the last three decades[7] and doubled during the past decade to *14 gallons per person per year*.

Besides contributing to fatty liver and type 2 diabetes, diets high in sugary snacks and fast food can increase the risk of ADHD, behavioral issues, anxiety, and sleep problems.[8]

Take Gareth, a six-year-old boy who came in with a diagnosis of bipolar disorder/ADHD. Nicknamed the "Tasmanian Devil," he was in turmoil. In my office, he threw things randomly and also at me, ran his arm along my assistant's desk to push everything to the floor, screamed uncontrollably, and pinched his mother. He was completely out of control. Yet during the course of several visits, I observed that he'd enter my office in a calm state, then the minute he ate a snack—whether something sugary or some cut fruit—these behaviors began. He spent most appointments detained in a therapeutic hug by his mother. But after he stopped eating sugar—even fruit, for a period of time—Gareth became a regular, reasonable kid. I waited for an outburst for an entire appointment, but he simply colored, read a story, and cut out paper hearts for his mother and me. Having apparently identified one part of the issue, we went on to address his gut health and support his body's natural blood sugar regulation—ultimately, we wanted him to be able to eat fruit and the occasional sweet in moderation.

**Our bodies are hard-wired for sweets.** If you've considered kicking sugar from your own diet at any point, you've probably recognized this. Beginning with that first sip of breast milk, which is high in the milk sugar lactose, our bodies learn to crave sweet tastes. It's more than the sweet flavor; the body releases endorphins that induce euphoria and reduce our perception of pain. It's called comfort food for a reason!

## SUGAR ADDICTION: COCAINE, HEROIN, AND . . . SUGAR?

Study after study on sugar shows its highly addictive nature—more highly addictive than cocaine. An astonishing 94 percent of rats that were allowed to choose between sugar water and cocaine-infused water chose sugar.[9] Even rats already addicted to cocaine quickly switched their preference to sugar given the choice. The rats were also more willing to work for sugar than for cocaine. The researchers speculated that the body's receptors for "sweet"—which evolved in ancestral times when the diet was very low in sugar—have not adapted yet to our modern ways of high-sugar consumption. Excessive stimulation of these receptors by our sugar-rich diets generates extreme reward signals in the brain, which can override normal self-control mechanisms and lead to addiction. This research found cross-tolerance and cross-dependence between sugars and addictive drugs. For example, animals with a long history of sugar consumption became tolerant (desensitized) to the pain-relieving effects of morphine.

Here is more research illustrating sugar's addictive qualities:[10,11]

- Sugar stimulates the brain's reward centers via the neurotransmitter dopamine, like other addictive drugs.[12]
- Brain imaging (PET scans) shows that high-sugar and high-fat foods work just like heroin, opium, or morphine in the brain, stimulating release of the brain's own opioids (morphinelike chemicals).
- People (and rats) develop tolerance to sugar—they need more and more of the substance to be satisfied—just as with drugs of abuse like alcohol or heroin.
- A drug called naltrexone—that blocks the brain's receptors for heroin and morphine—also reduces consumption and preference for sweet, high-fat foods in both normal weight and obese binge eaters.
- Many obese individuals continue to eat large amounts of unhealthy foods despite severe social and personal negative consequences, just like addicts.
- Animals and humans experience withdrawal symptoms when suddenly cut off from sugar, just like addicts detoxifying from drugs.[13]

Sugar activates our own internal narcotic system. It's why sugar-containing solutions are used in neonatal intensive care units and newborn nurseries to calm crying babies. Administering a sucrose solution as a pain reliever has been shown to reduce the duration of crying in preterm or term babies undergoing painful procedures.[14] (Interestingly, though, some recent studies find that using such a solution repeatedly may be associated with neurobehavioral effects later on.)[15] Parents of infants know this as well—a baby who has consumed his or her fill of lactose-rich breast milk or formula will often fall into what looks like a drunken stupor, an activation of the endogenous endocannabinoid system—the same response the body has to taking drugs.

Our bodies contain special receptors for detecting sweetness, found in our mouths, stomachs, and pancreas, which line our digestive tract from esophagus to stomach to pancreas. These receptors communicate with the brain from their outposts in the digestive tract through the nervous system, stimulating our centers for appetite, desire, and reward. And foods containing processed sweet and fat are far more addictive than nonprocessed sweet and fat.[16] This makes sense—much of the pleasure that we derive from eating sweet foods begins as soon as sugar hits those receptors. And the less effort needed from our body to convert carbohydrate to sugar, the faster our reward center says "Ahhhhhh." Simple, processed sugar is a faster, more powerful hit than complex sugar from something like fruit.

Eating sweet foods creates cravings for more sweet foods. In other words, feeding kids sugar strongly builds their desire to eat more sugar. Not an "I'm in the mood for something sweet" kind of desire, but something much more powerful. Research from the 1960s showed that rats would overcome their natural instincts to stay near walls and corners if sweet foods were placed in the center of their cage. When given all the sweets they wanted, those same rats would gorge themselves to the point that they overrode any biological signal to stop.[17]

Surprised by this? You may be hearing it for the first time . . . but you can bet that the food industry knows this data inside and out.

## Exploiting a Weakness

The food industry is well aware of how potently children crave sweet. In the 1970s, its studies showed that children were most likely to crave foods that were salty and sweet.[18] Its subsequent research into "bliss point"—the amount of sweetness that makes food and drink maximally appealing—showed that when given the choice, children ages five to ten prefer their food two to three times sweeter than adults do—so industry made its food sweeter.

The industry term for a frequent consumer of its products is "heavy user." As a former Coca-Cola CEO said, "Your heavy-user base is, by definition, very important to the business." Food companies are aggressively targeting kids to become future heavy users. Philip Morris—the tobacco company that marketed cigarettes to children for the very same reason—now owns companies such as Kraft and General Foods. It has converted its child-directed marketing strategies from cigarettes to food by way of kid-friendly packaging, cuddly mascots, and misleading claims such as "all natural" (meaningless) and "fortified" (adding in supplements because the food is depleted of nutrients).

Food manufacturers also dedicate sky-high budgets to scientists who investigate how food can optimally stimulate our pleasure centers and cravings. These food scientists have essentially become specialists in addiction, and their work is used against children to create mini-addicts. Gerber's chairmen summed up their hypocrisy best when asked to comment on why the company was dropping two highly sweetened baby foods from its lineup in response to public outcry: "We never said they were particularly nutritious. We just said they tasted good."[19]

---

**TIP** ———————————————————————————————————

### Calm Kids with Organic Teas

Sugar cravings may be related to anxiety and stress in kids. Adrenal glands are responsible for pumping out stress hormones like cortisol, which can drive sugar (and salt) cravings. Use daily tea blends that include calming nervines like passionflower, linden, lemon balm, and chamomile, as well as adaptogenic, balancing teas made from drinkable herbs like holy basil (tulsi) or astragalus. Throw in rose hips or hibiscus for a huge boost of vitamin C, also in higher demand when the body is under stress. Observe the sugar cravings—and stress—decrease.

## Secret Sugar: It's Hiding in Your Food and Drinks

You might be reading this and thinking, *My kid doesn't eat that much sugar. He doesn't even drink soda.* Great. What if I replaced "soda" with "juice"? Processed juice and soda are in many ways equivalent, both filled with empty calories. **Most juice is no longer made from fruit.**

The food industry understands how deeply parents care about their children's health, and it knows **that successful children's products have the veneer of health.** To convince parents to shell out for their kids, it created "juices": Kool-Aid, then Tang, were made almost entirely of artificial colors and flavors and, of course, sugar. Manufacturers added barely half a teaspoon of real fruit juice per bottle and fortified it with vitamin C so they could market it as "healthy." They pictured fruit on the label and created various artificial fruit flavors and aromas. Parents thought they were cleverly sneaking nutrition into their children with these "fruit drinks." This industry charade even extended to "real" juice, when the food industry doubted that the natural sweetness of apples or grapes was enough to strike the child's bliss point; so it added "fruit sugar" to these products, too—without listing it on the label. Finally, a fruit drink that can sit on a supermarket shelf for weeks, months, or even years without spoiling is not likely to retain many health benefits even if there were actual fruit added.

**Bottom line:** Store-bought juice, Gatorade, and Powerade are hardly better than soda. And let's not forget Vitamin Water, another brilliant conception that's duped many health-conscious parents. It's really just sugar with some synthetic vitamins thrown in.

## Dessert for Breakfast?

Cereal was the brainchild of John Harvey Kellogg, a physician with the best of intentions, who ran a sanitarium in Detroit to help people with digestive issues. In 1894, he created a flaked wheat cereal as well as a corn version to serve his patients. Notably, he banned sugar from the sanitarium, believing it was a primary contributor to the nation's health woes. But in 1908, Kellogg's brother secretly stole the recipe, added copious amounts of sugar, and began marketing Kellogg's Toasted Corn Flakes. Eventually, Post joined in with Grape Nuts. General Mills then charged ahead of the pack by releasing its cereal, Sugar Crisps, which was unabashedly coated in sugar. Not to be outdone, the other companies answered with Sugar Corn Pops, Sugar Frosted Flakes, Sugar Smacks, Sugar Jets, and others. Adding sugar made the cereal taste better, take on a golden-brown color, and stay crisp in milk.

By the 1970s, the cereal market expanded as more women began to work outside the home and needed quick breakfasts for their children. By the 1980s, the cereal market was worth $4.4 billion. Sugar had become a primary ingredient in nearly every cereal on the market and was under scrutiny as a trigger for many illnesses, including diabetes and heart disease. Yet the FDA refused to comment on sugar as a threat to public health or to even require companies to disclose sugar content on their packaging.

More alarmingly, investigation by public health advocates showed that cereals with the highest sugar content—as high as 70.8 percent—were the ones most heavily marketed to children during Saturday-morning cartoons. Sugary cereals were promoted as many as four times per *half hour* on each network. Frequent advertising did, in fact, spur increases in children's consumption of those products, encouraging activists to speak out. One such advocate, Harvard nutritionist Jean Mayer, advocated that cereal be appropriately labeled. "Any cereal containing over 50 percent sugar should be labeled 'imitation cereal' or 'cereal confections,'" he said. "And they should be sold in the candy section rather than the cereal section." Headlines like "Is It Cereal or Candy?" ran around the country. The response? Companies dropped the word "sugar" from their names . . . but not from the cereal itself. Sugar Frosted Flakes became Frosted Flakes, Super Sugar Crisp Cereal became Super Golden Crisp, and so on.

It didn't end there. After adding cinnamon marshmallows to Apple Jacks, Kellogg's aired a commercial that portrayed a sugary cinnamon stick as "sweetly protecting" Apple Jacks' flavor from a surly character named "Bad Apple."[20] And soon after, Kellogg's advertised a study claiming that eating Frosted Mini-Wheats for breakfast increased children's attentiveness by 20 percent. "Keeps 'em full, keeps 'em focused," the ad said. Turned out that Kellogg's had designed and paid for the study, and its report of the findings wasn't quite accurate. Only one in nine children had a boost in attention of 20 percent after eating the cereal, and they were being compared to some kids who hadn't eaten any breakfast at all. When angry parents took Kellogg's to task for false advertising and the Federal Trade Commission issued a complaint,[21] Kellogg's created a $4 million fund to refund products as part of a settlement agreement. While Kellogg's denied any wrongdoing, it agreed to downgrade its claims to say: "Clinical studies have shown that kids who eat a filling breakfast like Frosted Mini-Wheats have 11 percent better attentiveness in school than kids who skip breakfast."[22]

The sugar wars still rage. Now even low-sugar cereals like Cheerios have undergone sugar makeovers like Dulce de Leche Cheerios, Cinnamon Burst Cheerios, and Fruity Cheerios. To this day, sugar content for most cereals remains higher than 50 percent.

## Savory Sugar?

You'll also find sugar in many products that are not considered "sweet," including bread, ketchup, salad dressing, and tomato sauce. Sugar is often the second ingredient in many of these foods. Yogurt, for example, can have as much or more sugar than a can of soda. The food industry loves sugar because we love sugar. It knows that we will buy anything we can't resist—especially if it's affordable (and even when it's not). The industry also depends on sugar to make industrial food profitable and possible—sugar means bread doesn't go stale, cereal looks golden and stays crispy in milk, and donuts stay fluffier. The food industry is as addicted to sugar as we are.

## Stealth Marketing of Sugar

How much sugar we eat is often related to how strongly it's marketed to us.[23]

In "Sugar-Coating Science: How the Food Industry Misleads Consumers on Sugar," the Union of Concerned Scientists (UCS) urges us to beware of:[24]

1. *Sugary foods with a feel-good health claim.* Companies will do whatever it takes to brand sugary food as healthy. Coca-Cola advertised its high-sugar Vitamin Water brand by using buzzwords like "defense," "energy," or "enhanced." General Mills claimed Fruit Roll-Ups were "made with real fruit" when they in fact contain none. Studies find that many products advertised as "whole grain" or high in protein or other valuable nutrients are often more sugary than foods without those claims.
2. *Misleading language like "natural" and "naturally sweetened."* Some companies have removed heavily processed sweeteners like high-fructose corn syrup from their foods and replaced them with an equivalent amount of another processed sugar.
3. *Using brand recognition to market unhealthy alternatives.* Cheerios has 1 gram of sugar per serving, but you've probably seen more ads for the cereal's sweeter versions, Honey Nut (9 grams of sugar) and Apple Cinnamon Cheerios (10 grams). Using an established brand with a healthy reputation gives the veneer of health to sugary variants.

4. *Using "cause marketing" to sell sugary foods.* According to the website for Yoplait, the "Save Lids to Save Lives" campaign has donated more than $34 million to various breast cancer causes. Yet a single cup of Yoplait averages 26 grams of sugar—more than the American Heart Association recommends women consume in an entire day.

## Where Is the Regulation?

For more than three decades, federal officials have exempted sugar from recommended maximum limits that they've set for two other major players in processed foods—fat and salt—even though the data for sugar are more damning. Manufacturers are not obligated to differentiate how much sugar they *add* to their products from natural sugar content—only the total amount in the product. In 2009, the American Heart Association (AHA) took a stand and recommended that adults ingest no more than 5 to 9 teaspoons per day—the equivalent of half a 12-ounce can of Coke, one and a half Fig Newtons, or a half-cup of Jell-O for the *entire day*—with the thought that industry would be pressured to reduce added sugar in its products. But 5 teaspoons is a drop in the bucket when it comes to processed foods. For instance, a half cup of Prego tomato sauce alone has more than *2 teaspoons of sugar*—equal to a tube of Go-Gurt or two Oreo cookies. Industry fought the AHA recommendation quickly and thoroughly. Nothing changed.

## So What Should You Do?

While the medical fury about out-of-control sugar consumption is justified, demonizing all sweeteners is misguided. The problem is not the ingredient itself, but how we've changed it. Unprocessed maple syrup, honey, even the original sugarcane plant have health benefits when consumed in small amounts. We'll focus on them in Chapter 15.

## How to Spot Secret Sugars on the Ingredients List

Use this easy trick to spot secret added sugars on the ingredients list: Anything that ends in "–ose" is sugar, and so is anything with "sugar" or "syrup" after the name. Here are some of the different names for sugar:

| | |
|---|---|
| Agave nectar | Evaporated cane juice |
| Barley malt | Fructose |
| Beet sugar | Fruit juice concentrates |
| Brown rice syrup | Glucose |
| Brown sugar | High-fructose corn syrup |
| Buttered sugar | Honey |
| Cane crystals | Invert sugar |
| Cane juice | Lactose |
| Cane sugar | Maltose |
| Caramel | Malt syrup |
| Carob syrup | Molasses |
| Castor sugar | Muscovado sugar |
| Coconut sugar | Natural sugar |
| Corn sugar | Rice bran syrup |
| Corn sweetener | Rice syrup |
| Corn syrup | Sorghum |
| Corn syrup solids | Sorghum syrup |
| Crystalline fructose | Sucrose |
| Date sugar | Syrup |
| Dextrose | Turbinado sugar |

## SUGAR UNMASKED: A CHEAT SHEET

Here's a list of products where secret sugars are typically found: [25]

- Condiments and sauces such as ketchup, barbecue sauce, teriyaki sauce, plum sauce, or other Asian sauces
- Low-fat or fat-free salad dressings and marinades
- Dips and spreads
- Side dishes from the supermarket deli (macaroni or potato salad, or coleslaw)
- Canned biscuits and pizza dough
- Takeout, especially pizza and Chinese food

### Secret Sugars in the Freezer

- Frozen entrées (low calorie or otherwise)
- Processed meats (sausage, hot dogs)
- Frozen veggies prepared with sauces
- Breakfast sandwiches
- Mini pizza bagels or pizza rolls, or pocket sandwiches
- Frozen bread and rolls
- Potpies

### Secret Sugars in the Pantry

- Pasta sauce
- Rice mixes
- Instant or flavored oatmeal
- Granola or fruit-and-grain bars (whole-grain varieties included)
- Cereal bars
- Sweetened corn bread mix
- Whole-grain cold cereals
- Bread, whole grain/white/pita
- Baked beans
- Trail mix
- Whole-grain crackers
- English muffins
- Tortilla wraps

- Taco shells
- Yogurt, fruity or flavored

## SUGAR'S SIDEKICKS:
## HIGH-FRUCTOSE CORN SYRUP AND ASPARTAME

The food industry is constantly in search of "magical" ingredients—inexpensive substances that are "too good to be true." High-fructose corn syrup (HFCS) and aspartame are the reigning king and queen of this category—HFCS delivers super-sweetness cheaply and efficiently, and aspartame packs intense sugary flavor without calories. Both of these substances exploit our preprogrammed love for all things sweet, hooking even the savviest of us.

### High-Fructose Corn Syrup

High-fructose corn syrup is literally liquid sugar: easy to add to all sorts of products and *cheap*. Manufacturers use vast amounts of it for mere pennies in all kinds of food products: cereal, breakfast bars, breads, lunch meats, yogurts, soups, and condiments. All of this sugar wreaks havoc on our bodies.

In the way that MSG packs a punch with free glutamate, HFCS consists of unbound molecules of fructose and glucose, which allows them to be rapidly absorbed by the liver all at once. Glucose triggers big spikes in insulin—the body's major sugar regulating, fat-storing hormone—increasing inflammation that can lead to weight gain, diabetes, heart disease, cancer, dementia, and fatty liver. Normally, increased insulin levels modify our food intake by inhibiting appetite with leptin release, which tells us we're full.[26,27,28,29,30] Meals high in high-fructose corn syrup, however, can reduce circulating insulin and leptin levels,[31] contributing to increased hunger and weight gain. Fructose intake does not generally result in the degree of satiety that you would feel with an equally caloric meal that contains glucose or sucrose.

Unlike naturally occurring fructose that is part of fruit, free fructose from HFCS demands high energy to be absorbed by the gut and depletes the body's energy stores of ATP. As a result, mitochondria are under greater stress to produce the energy necessary to maintain the integrity of the intestinal lining. Normally each intestinal cell membrane has a tight junction with its neighbors, which prevents food, toxins, bacteria, and the like from "leaking" across the intestinal membrane and triggering body-wide inflammation. But high doses of free fructose can punch holes in the intestinal lining, allowing undesirable substances into our bloodstream.[32] This is part of what triggers an inflammatory response that promotes conditions like asthma, seizures, autism, ADHD, obesity, diabetes, and cancer.

High-fructose corn syrup also contains measurable amounts of mercury due to contamination from processing. In 2009, almost half of the tested samples of commercial HFCS contained mercury, detected also in nearly a third of 55 popular brand-name food and beverage products where HFCS is the first- or second-highest labeled ingredient.[33] Worse, the government was aware of the contamination and attempted to cover it up.

In 2004, Renee Dufault, an environmental health researcher at the FDA, stumbled upon an obscure Environmental Protection Agency report on chemical plants' mercury emissions. Some chemical companies, she learned, make lye by pumping salt through large vats of mercury. Since lye is a key ingredient in making HFCS (it's used to separate corn starch from the kernel), Dufault wondered if mercury might be contaminating the ubiquitous sweetener that makes up one of every ten calories Americans eat. Dufault sent HFCS samples from three manufacturers that used lye to labs at the University of California–Davis and the National Institute of Standards and Technology. The labs found mercury in most of the samples, and the UC Davis scientists believe it is likely organic mercury—the most neurotoxic form.

In September 2005, Dufault presented her findings to the FDA's Center for Food Safety and was shocked by what happened next: "I was instructed not to do any more investigation," she recalls. The FDA claimed its decision against further investigation was because it wasn't convinced "that there was any evidence of a risk."[34] It subsequently removed her from fieldwork. No risk, except that individuals could be ingesting up to 200 micrograms of a neurotoxin per week—three times more than the amount the FDA deems safe for children, women who are or plan to become pregnant, and nursing mothers. Of course, the Corn Refiners Association disputed the study, stating it had used mercury-free versions of hydrochloric acid and caustic soda for years. Then it hired ChemRisk—the consulting firm whose scientists testified on behalf of a polluting utility in the lawsuit portrayed in *Erin Brockovich*—to attack Dufault's report. It worked.

We may never know exactly why these peer-reviewed studies detected mercury because the production process remains top secret. But at a minimum, four plants in the United States and hundreds of plants abroad still use the chloralkali process that requires mercury. Industry continues to use HFCS with no obligation to disclose how it is produced.

High-fructose corn syrup isn't just wreaking havoc on our bodies' internal terrain. It's also hurting the external terrain of our environment. HFCS is derived from industrially raised corn, grown in a way that depletes soil, requires high pesticide use, and burns fossil fuel energy to truck it to where it can be processed. The kicker? You're paying for it, thanks to the Farm Bill, which heavily subsidizes our country's overplanting of crops like corn, wheat, and soy. Your tax dollars are subsidizing cheap, often GMO corn to be made into sugar that damages your family's health. As long as the government incentivizes this practice by footing the bill and refusing to ask questions, industry will continue pumping these foods into the market.

My advice: Read labels and **avoid HFCS.**

Aspartame (also known as NutraSweet, produced at one time by Monsanto) is an artificial sweetener used in more than six thousand products, including soft drinks, chewing gum, candy, desserts, and yogurt, as well as in more than five hundred pharmaceutical products, including syrups and antibiotics for children.

Aspartate, a major component of aspartame, acts similarly to glutamate as an excitotoxin. Animal studies show that it crosses the blood-brain barrier straight into the sanctuary of the brain and even alters frontal-lobe activity in measurable ways.[35] Aspartame breaks down to aspartate, phenylalanine, methanol, and diketopiperazine, a known carcinogen that converts to neurotoxic formaldehyde in the cell.[36] Like glutamate, phenylalanine competes with many necessary amino acids for transport into the central nervous system, which can limit the brain's access to other building blocks.[37] Rats fed 5 percent aspartame in their diets for only two hours had significantly lower brain levels of serotonin—which modulates well-being, anxiety, and sleep—when compared with controls.[38] Phenylalanine and aspartate both can promote cancer,[39] as can prenatal exposure to aspartame.[40]

Human studies also demonstrate health problems from aspartame. Drinking artificial sugar does not keep us thin. "Non-nutritive sweeteners" like aspartame replicate the very same cravings and addictive behaviors as sugar[41] and drive weight gain. A two-year study involving 166 schoolchildren found that the more diet soda they drank, *the more weight they gained*.[42] The Growing Up Today Study, involving 11,654 children ages 9 to 14, also reported that boys drinking diet soda gained weight. For each daily serving of diet beverage, their BMIs increased.[43] Another study of almost one thousand children found diet soda drinkers had significantly elevated BMI and waist circumference.[44] Worse, a 2014 study on artificial sweeteners including aspartame, Splenda, and saccharine showed that they all induced glucose intolerance by altering gut microbiome.[45] Our guts and flora play a critical role in modulating diabetes.[46] Yet diet sodas and foods filled with aspartame are frequently recommended as good replacements for sugary foods for diabetic kids—even though these foods may worsen their issues.

Clinically, several studies have linked aspartame consumption with disrupted electrical activity in the brain as well as other health issues including headaches and various kinds of cancer including brain.[47,48,49] One study in *Neurology* showed that ten children newly diagnosed with epilepsy spent 40 percent more time in spike-wave activity after a dose of aspartame than one of sucrose.[50] Some studies in adults had similar results.[51,52,53] Aspartame also has been shown to be a migraine trigger in susceptible people.[54,55,56,57]

And if that isn't bad enough, when NutraSweet is flushed out of the body and down the toilet, data show that water-treatment plants don't remove chemical sugars from sewage effectively—so now they pollute our waterways.[58]

My advice: **Avoid all artificial sweeteners,** and never look back.

# TAKE HOME

1. Children are eating massive amounts of sugar in many forms from treats and sweets to "healthy" foods like bread, yogurt, and sauce.
2. Sugar can be listed under many names in processed foods—or not listed at all—so it can be hidden in plain sight. Avoid high-fructose corn syrup and all "corn-based sugars."
3. Beware of high-sugar foods with a veneer of health: cereal bars (or power or protein bars) are particular offenders, as are "healthy" drinks like Vitamin Water or Snapple. Claims like "no added sugar" are a ruse.
4. Compare carbohydrate and sugar content in any processed foods you buy to get a sense of the playing field—tomato sauce, bread, yogurt, even ice cream. Organic brands may or may not add less sugar.
5. Cooking for yourself with the basic ingredients means you control much of what's in your food. This doesn't mean you need to can your own tomatoes—you can buy tomatoes canned in glass jars (free of BPA!), add olive oil, garlic, and spices, and simmer your sauce while you prepare the rest of the meal.
6. Diet sugars are not the answer either; quite the opposite. Instead, try to minimize your need for sweeteners altogether, especially in beverages.
7. Even standard white sugar is best avoided. I don't keep any in my cupboard. When you need sweet, always go for the natural ones: raw honey, real maple sugar, date sugar, stevia leaf, and blackstrap molasses. They will satisfy!
8. If your kid craves sugar, helping your child's body to feel nourished and relaxed will help relieve those cravings and make the transition off sugar easier. Try calming teas, plenty of foods high in vitamin C, more sleep, and other activities that promote relaxation and joy.

# PART III

—

## STEP TWO: Nourish

*Of all the paths you take in life, make sure a few of them are dirt.*
—JOHN MUIR

A couple of generations ago, our food was diverse, we ate what was growing in season, and we prepared it ourselves. Protein, carbohydrates, and fat were not yet known entities. Multivitamins didn't exist, in concept or in practice. The word "vitamine" was coined only in 1912; during the next 30 years, chemists discovered these compounds and how to manufacture them.

## EAT WHOLE FOODS FROM NATURE

Our scientific understanding of nutritional compounds has led us to regard food as a chemical amalgam of compounds that exists solely for our benefit. **Yet food is complex, derived from living entities that do not exist exclusively for us.** Indeed, this complexity is exactly what makes it so beneficial for us. Nourishment is more than protein, carbohydrates, and fat; it's more than vitamins and minerals and even phytonutrients (plant compounds that confer color, flavor, and health benefits). We are as nourished by food's vitality and complexity as by any one of its components.

Food nourishes us on a physical, emotional, and spiritual level. It establishes and maintains the health of our terrains. Water, minerals, and other eternal bits of the natural world travel through us for a short time to do their work, and then reenter the natural world again. Food is not simply fuel nor is food mere medicine—food is an ally that promotes resilience through sacred partnership with the natural world.

Food is the most intimate conversation we have with the natural world as we ingest it, daily. Food—real food—is the embodiment of all the healing properties of nature: rich soil, warm sunshine, fresh air, living water, and diverse microbes. Real food connects our inner terrain to the outer terrain, and aligns them. This alignment makes us well and keeps our bodies resilient.

The next step in your child's healing journey—after eliminating foods and substances that can actively hurt the body—is exploring foods that actively nourish. And your child's nourishment starts with soil. That's right, *dirt*.

The benefits of fruit, vegetables, grains, high-quality meat, milk, and eggs come from the vitamins and minerals, fiber and phytonutrients ... but everything we eat derives benefits from interactions with soil and its many components. Dirt is much more than what we spend our time cleaning. Fertile soil is a repository of microbes and nutrients critical to our children's guts and microbiomes, their immune systems and brains—even, as you'll see, their emotions. When we plant, grow, and harvest our own food, traces get onto our skin and into our mouths and nostrils. In turn, these soil traces transmit diverse flora into our bodies in ways that trigger chemical reactions to produce compounds like serotonin and endorphins. These allow our bodies and minds to run optimally and make us feel wonderful. The health of the soil is directly connected not just to the health of our food, but also to our children's health.

Plants are nourished from the soil. We eat plants, and the animals we eat also eat plants. **We are what we eat eats.** We are actively nourished by the contents of soil; we integrate it into our bodies. Healthy soil has favorable tilth, which means it's well aerated, drains water well, and has good consistency. When soil has good tilth and is dense with nutrients, bacteria, and other microorganisms—then our bodies will be healthy and balanced, too. Conversely, depleted soil produces sicker plants and animals. To find the best possible food for our bodies, we must provide the best possible food for our food.

Along with air, water, and sunshine, soil is the terrain of plants, animals, and humans, as well as the microbiome that lives within and on us. Ninety percent of all organisms live underground. In addition to bacteria and fungi, the soil is filled with protozoa, nematodes, mites, and microarthropods—as many as ten to fifty thousand species in less than a *teaspoon* of soil. **That same teaspoon of soil holds more microbes than the Earth holds people.**

Soil bacteria and fungi are part of a healthy soil terrain. Soil nutrients and microorganisms nourish and protect plants and give them the "grit" to survive dramatic changes from drought, floods, and climate swings. They also serve as "intestines" of plants by forming symbiotic relationships with plants' roots to procure and assimilate nutrients that the plant needs.

Let's look at one example: mycorrhizae, fungi that live on the roots of plants—particularly legumes—channel the nitrogen that the plants need from the atmosphere, which they otherwise can't access.[1] These mycorrhizae facilitate the release of necessary minerals from rocks for plants to access. They also channel nutrients from deep in the soil: Their filaments extend the reach of plant roots more than *one hundredfold*, transmitting nutrients to the plant and allowing plants to communicate and set up defense systems. These healthier plants are hardier and more nutritious for us.

Like our own microbiome, mycorrhizae not only aid "digestion," but also regulate the plants' immune system. A broad bean plant attacked by aphids transmits a signal through the mycorrhizal filaments to other, healthy bean plants nearby, triggering those plants to produce defensive chemicals that repel aphids and attract wasps, a natural aphid predator. Diseased tomato plants also use the underground network to signal healthy tomato plants to activate their defenses to prevent being attacked. Those defense chemicals are phytonutrients— the stuff of "superfoods." Produced when plants are under stress and transferred to us when we eat them, phytochemicals regulate our digestion, immune system, nervous system, mitochondria, and DNA, which strengthens the resilience of our internal terrain.

As if that weren't enough, mycorrhizae are "basin" cleaners extraordinaire, detoxifying our soil and plants by removing pollutants. They "eat" toxins so we don't have to! These super-microorganisms also keep the earth cool—they sequester carbon for hundreds of millions of years in amazing mycorrhizal filaments. This is just one of the amazing microbial communities that contribute to the perfect terrain that includes us and is—or should be—in our soil.

Farmers know that soil tilth and fertility are key. Indeed, many farmers taste their soil to determine if its components are in balance. The smell of soil is called "geosmin," and chefs honor the flavor it imparts on beets and carrots. When our soil flourishes, our food flourishes and we flourish. We know proteins, vitamins, and minerals are nutrients. In a very real sense, dirt is a nutrient, too.

The diversity found in healthy soil facilitates an array of necessary reactions in the body. Microbial diversity alone influences our immune health, affecting conditions such as weight gain and the development of allergies and autoimmune disease. Newer probiotics, which are what we call beneficial bacteria we intentionally ingest, are being developed to include SBOs (soil-based organisms): bacteria from the soil. Eating actual dirt? Yes! And it's straight from the scientific literature. The common soil organism *Clostridium sporogenes* has been shown to help kill cancer cells and protect healthy cells during chemotherapy.[2] Another soil bacterium, *Mycobacterium vaccae,* improved both long-term survival and quality of life for cancer patients with malignant melanoma.[3,4] Soil organisms can also powerfully affect mood and cognition: treatment of mice with *M. vaccae* boosted serotonin levels and improved mood in ways comparable to that of antidepressant drugs.[5] Anxiety dropped and cognitive performance improved.[6] Researchers likewise discovered that exposure to farm dust causes the lining of the respiratory tract to react less severely to allergens because of a protein known as A20, which is produced by our bodies when we're in contact with farm dust. This makes us less likely to develop asthma.[7] All that . . . from dirt!

We are an integral part of our terrain, and our terrain—with all of its living components—is an integral part of us. Yet we no longer actively engage in that connection. Instead, we have outsourced the growing of our food to industry that has little interest in our internal or surrounding terrain. As a result, soil of commercial agricultural lands has been largely neglected and depleted. Just as we have unwittingly destroyed vital microbes in the human gut through overuse of medications like antibiotics and by eating highly processed foods, we have devastated soil microbiota through overuse of chemical fertilizers, fungicides, herbicides, pesticides, heavy tilling, and planting countless acres of monocrops with no diversity or rotation. Microbes are unable to do what they have done for millions of years—conserve and cycle nutrients and water into plants, sequester toxins, and regulate the climate. We've sacrificed the abundant biodiversity in soil, microbes, and plants that ensures our health.

**You can change this loss of diversity in ways large and small.** Begin by simply understanding the importance of terrain. Buy foods that are grown and raised responsibly, or even grow food responsibly yourself. Compost food and yard waste and feed it to your soil instead of sending it to a landfill.

Acting as custodian of the ecology around you naturally leads to a healthy inner ecology for you and your child. A healthy inner ecology translates to a child who is resilient and healthy. **What we do to soil, we do to ourselves.**

## CHAPTER 8
# Soil Power: Organic Fruits, Vegetables, and Plants

**W**e evolved with plants. Our bodies recognize them. Plants were our main source of medicine less than one hundred years ago, and they remain a source of inspiration and information for pharmaceutical development today. Unlike pharmaceuticals, however, plants are complex and contain countless compounds that are in constant conversation with our cells. From their aromas and flavors to their vibrant colors, plants insinuate themselves into every nook and cranny of our physiology by way of antioxidants, enzymes, pheromones, stem cells, and phytonutrients that influence our bodies to be strong and resilient.

Fruits and vegetables are more than a vehicle for delivering vitamins, minerals, and fiber into your body. A wealth of impressive studies show plants' curative powers in all manner of conditions. A meta-analysis of 34 studies found that high consumption of fruits and vegetables reduces asthma symptoms in children and adults.[1] In 2011, a Phase I trial at Ohio State University showed that consuming 60 grams of black raspberry powder—a variety of raspberry exceptionally high in phytonutrients—slowed the growth rate of colorectal cancer cells and the blood vessels that supply them in just two to four weeks.[2] Black raspberry also showed powerful benefits in preserving intestinal tissue in models of ulcerative colitis.[3] Capsaicin, found in hot peppers, combined with diindolylmethane (DIM) in kale and other cruciferous vegetables, has powerful anticancer properties.[4]

I also see these benefits firsthand in my practice. Cranberries— ideally unsweetened—effectively prevent *H. pylori* and urinary tract infections (UTIs) by discouraging adhesion of bacteria to the bladder or gut wall[5] and they reduce recurrent infection almost as effectively as antibiotics.[6] When I've given cranberry juice or extract in pill form to children suffering from chronic UTIs—including those with chronic illness requiring catheterization—they've no longer required frequent rounds of antibiotics for prevention or treatment. After reading a compelling study that beet juice boosts physical performance,[7] I began to recommend one to two cups daily of freshly juiced beets to fatigued teens struggling to recover from severe illnesses—and not just the teens but their families *and* teachers indeed noticed a big difference in areas like school attendance, homework completion, and return to sports.

Garlic has been used as an antimicrobial for everything from impetigo, staph, clostridia, pseudomonas, and other chronic or resistant infections. It helps to dissolve biofilm, a slimy substance secreted by bacteria trying to evade antibiotics or our immune systems. Garlic is effective alone or as an adjunct with antibiotics.[8] Scientists were amazed when a thousand-year-old Anglo-Saxon "Eye Salve" recipe—made from garlic, onions or leeks, wine, and oxbile—decimated MRSA, a superbug resistant to our most powerful antibiotics.[9] Hearty doses of chopped fresh garlic mixed with pastured butter, ghee, or olive oil, spread on sourdough bread or steamed veggies, act as an effective treatment for severe sore throats. Even picky kids find it helps to relieve their symptoms.

Elderberries prevent proliferation of different strains of influenza virus.[10] Every season, I hear from parents that my patients on regular elderberry were the "lucky ones" in their family to avoid flu. I've seen it with my own family: the elderberry bushes we planted as part of my "food forest" now provide a bumper crop of elderberries each summer from which I make syrup. When my children drink a teaspoon every day—more frequently at the first signs of sickness—our winter is free of the illnesses everyone else gets. They *ask for* homemade elderberry syrup—with added star anise and cinnamon—because it's delicious. But it also makes them feel better. It also happens to deactivate bronchial viruses and act against methicillin-resistant staph aureus (MRSA),[11] reduce inflammation in the brain,[12] and improve mood.[13]

Fruits and vegetables aren't just medicine for when you're sick. Plants help maintain balance in the body, with benefits that are ongoing and cumulative. Eating plants regularly balances your gastrointestinal, endocrine, immune, and neurological terrain so that you don't become acutely or chronically sick. Their phytonutrients and other components kick up our immune function while simultaneously absorbing inflammation and free radicals created by the immune response.

Though most of us make cancer cells occasionally, healthy immune systems eliminate them before they proliferate. Studies show that alliums such as garlic, onions, and leeks,[14] cruciferous vegetables such as cabbage and kale,[15] and berries,[16,17]—just to name a few—reduce our risk of developing many conditions including cancer. We often can't easily detect why a child's immune and detoxification systems go awry, as both genetics and "invisible" exposures also play roles—with or without healthy food. But we can empower children's immune systems simply by feeding them diverse, seasonal produce every day. This way, their terrain becomes considerably less hospitable to severe infection, unbridled inflammation, and cancer cell proliferation.

Eating diverse plants is the closest thing we have to a "magic bullet." Your mission—should you choose to accept it—is to offer plants in all forms as the biggest part of your meals, starting today. Pay the farmer instead of the doctor.

## PHYTONUTRIENTS

Like us, healthy plants benefit from some stressors. Phytonutrients are the immune system of plants; they increase a plant's ability to survive and overcome hardships—insects, microorganisms, UV rays, drought, and nutrient deprivation. Why do the brightest, best apples grow at the top of the tree? They're most stressed by UV radiation and predators, and produce copious phytonutrients to compensate. Phytonutrients provide flavor (the bite of the onion), fragrance (citrus), and vivid color (berries). When plants want to attract pollinators (humans included!), they present an appealing phytococktail of color, fragrance, and flavor. Phytonutrients can also repel predators by creating a bitter taste, rancid smell, or even unpleasant pheromone release. **Contact with plants that have a healthy internal terrain enhances our own internal terrain.**

Take Brussels sprouts. It turns out Grandma was right when she forced you to eat those green minicabbages. That's because all brassicas—Brussels, cabbage, kale, collards, cauliflower, broccoli, and watercress, to name a few—contain a powerful phytocompound called sulforaphane, which powers up gene transcription factors like Nrf2 that act to protect our cells: they prevent brain, breast, ovarian, and testicular cancer;[18,19,20,21] enhance learning and memory;[22] aid in better recovery from concussions or brain injury;[23,24] decrease inflammation;[25,26,27,28] encourage better detoxification; and complete a nourished microbiome. A 2012 study reported that eating just a few grams of broccoli sprouts a day reduced insulin levels and insulin resistance within four weeks' time.[29] Sulforaphane can help shut down the neuroinflammatory response,[30] which can target the neuroinflammation and microglial activation that exacerbate neurological disorders like seizures, migraines, tics, and ADHD.

Broccoli got another huge gold star when a 2014 Harvard study found that sulforaphane may effectively treat some physiological abnormalities in children with autism.[31] All fruits and vegetables have phytochemicals that demonstrate not just one but many such benefits. **When children eat their fruits and veggies, they change the present and future health of their bodies and brains.**

## Is My Produce Really Fresh?

If you've ever eaten fresh-picked fruits or vegetables, you know that they taste entirely different from what you buy from the store. The taste and texture reflect high amounts of phytonutrients and antioxidants that naturally preserve freshness, but begin to deplete the moment the produce is picked. Most store-bought produce was picked long ago, shipped from afar, stored in a warehouse, then placed on shelves in the grocery store for you to buy and eat. Most plants are bred to maintain good looks, but not to retain taste and fragrance.

Enhance your phytonutrient boost by buying fresh carrots and radishes with tops still attached (greens go bad long before most roots, which last for months), cauliflower with no brown spots, and cherries or apples with sturdy stems still on. If you buy from farmer's markets (or grow your own), be prepared for a transformative produce experience!

## Why Bitter Is Better

Most of us are drawn to sweet flavors in produce, which we've evolved to love. Sweet sends a message to our brain that says, "This food is calorie dense! Load up, so you'll have energy to get through another day." A bitter taste, on the other hand, alerts us to the possibility of poison. Yet bitter foods confer enormous health benefits.

Bitter receptors extend far beyond our mouths. They line the digestive tract—esophagus, stomach, intestines, liver, pancreas, and gallbladder—and even our nasal and respiratory tracts. When activated they stimulate the immune system to prevent infection (sugar receptors do the opposite). They've even been found in breast, testicular, and brain tissue.

**An important way that plants benefit us is by stressing us.** When cells in the body perceive bitter phytonutrients—which they interpret as potential poison—they kick into action, especially those in the immune system and detoxification machinery of the liver. The "kick" is an example of *hormesis*, a beneficial health effect that results from a low-dose exposure to an agent that may be toxic at higher doses. As discussed, our cells respond to teensy challenges—in this case bitter compounds, accompanied by antioxidants and dense nutrients—which prepare us for the many, truly nasty poisons that will inevitably come our way. Think of hormesis as a military drill. Eating most bitter plants primes the liver and other cells—especially our mitochondria—to jump into action in case of adversity. Then they are prepared to prevent accumulation and damage when real dangers like heavy metals, pesticides, plastics, and industrial chemicals come their way. **Bitters improve the drainage of our basins and help maintain homeostasis on all levels, while simultaneously nourishing us with nutrients.** *This is a big deal.*

When manufacturing industries are under fire for causing toxic exposure, they like to throw around hormesis as a last-ditch argument against taking responsibility: *We didn't poison your children with lead; we're actually helping them!* Please don't fall for that. Every person has a different threshold between hormesis and being poisoned. Heavy metals and industrial waste are toxic.

The importance of bitters, however, has been recognized for thousands of years in traditional Chinese medicine and Ayurveda. Bitters stimulate the T2R receptor, which in turn impacts every organ system in the body. As usual, everything begins in the gut. Bitters promote gastrointestinal balance from motility to digestion to absorption to immunity.

The skins and peels of fruits and vegetables tend to hold the highest concentration of bitter elements, so we're often throwing away the most concentrated areas of these phytonutrients! Dried orange peel, for instance, is a bitter that modulates hunger,[32] improves digestion and absorption of nutrients, and speeds up the metabolism.[33] It reduces gas, heartburn, and burping, relieves nausea, and promotes normal liver function. Bitters are also known to regulate appetite both for those who eat too much or too little.

Bitter compounds have powerful metabolic function in the body, affecting fat storage,[34] insulin release,[35] blood sugar levels, and wound healing, even in diabetics.[36] In my practice, I've used bitter melon as an adjunct treatment for children with types 1 or 2 diabetes. The result? Their blood glucose levels and need for insulin dropped noticeably.[37]

All bitters increase the gut's nonspecific immune system response, which prevents gastrointestinal infections.[38] The immunity extends beyond the gut; nasal fluids that contain bitter compounds protect us from infection in the sinuses, while nasal fluids higher in sugar content (as in diabetics) actually suppress the important immune response in the ear, nose, and throat, which can lead to more colds, coughs, and sore throats. Bitter receptors that line our nasal passageways and respiratory tracts powerfully stimulate our immune system, which dissolves phlegm, reduces coughs, and alleviates asthma.[39] In my practice, many children who had asthma unresponsive to medications improved only after they incorporated bitters—culinary and medicinal—into their regimen. Eating bitter is like insurance against infections for your family.

Avoid too much sweet and add some bitter to your family's regimen for better digestion, detoxification, and immune function. You might even say that a spoonful of bitter helps the sugar go down.

By introducing bitter (and reducing sweet) in the diet, your child can have

1. balanced appetite,
2. better digestion, including less reflux, burping, gas, and bloating with more regular bowel movements,
3. stronger immune response,
4. better absorption of nutrients due to increased release of stomach acid and bile, which improves protein breakdown and healthy fats,
5. reduced risk of food allergies due to better breakdown of proteins from stomach acid,
6. more balanced blood sugar levels by modulating insulin, helping to reduce inflammation and obesity, and
7. better detoxification.

And all this is just what we know so far in one category of plant compounds! What were we saying before about plants being the magic bullet?

Even so, you may be thinking, "Bitters? No way!" Allow me to introduce you to two very popular bitter plant tonics enjoyed by many—if not most—adults around the world: coffee and beer. The bitter compounds of coffee can confer impressive health benefits, reducing risk of conditions like Parkinson's disease and type 2 diabetes.[40,41] No, I'm not recommending that children drink coffee—though organic roasted dandelion root tea tastes somewhat similar and is truly wonderful for kids—just keep in mind that bitter is an acquired taste. Even whole-grain bread has a mildly bitter flavor (manufacturers add high-fructose corn syrup to disguise it), as do peels of apples and carrots. And for children, with their sensitive palates, a little can go a long way. Kids need less bitter flavor than adults to achieve the same physiological benefits. Taming bitter vegetables so they're appealing to your family can be as simple as cooking them with a little fat, salt, and some umami. More on that in Chapter 15.

## MORE FRUIT, LESS FRUIT, OR NO FRUIT?

Most people take for granted that fruit is healthy and, for the most part, it is. For a healthy child, some organic fruit in the diet is ideal. Fruits that are smaller and naturally less sweet (i.e., crabapples, currants) tend to be higher in phytonutrients, because a plant that budgets energy toward making carbohydrates has less to "spend" on producing phytonutrients. Wild fruit is inherently higher in phytonutrients than their grocery store cousins, because no one is looking out for their well-being—pulling off bugs, spraying them with herbicides and pesticides, or fencing out deer.

Don't give your children fruit-*flavored* products because they usually have lots of sugar without the benefits of the real plant. The food industry has surmised that the word "fruit" means "healthy" to many parents and uses terms like "enriched fruit juice," "sweetened applesauce," "fruit leather," and "fruit roll-ups" to sell essentially high-fructose corn syrup with artificial dye and fruit flavor thrown in.

Some diets demonize fruit as "sugar" and recommend avoiding it. On the one hand, it is nonsense to equate eating fruit with consuming high-fructose corn syrup or processed sugar. Isolated chemical structures can be similar, but neither food nor children are just a bundle of isolated chemical structures! Fruit contains vitamins, minerals, insulin-stabilizing fiber, and powerful phytonutrients. Extracting and using only the fructose removes those healthy benefits. On the other hand, fruit becomes a problem when children consume vast quantities to feed their sweet tooth, to the exclusion of vegetables and other foods. Such craving can both reflect and feed dysregulated gut flora.

NOTE: Some phenol-sensitive children have sulfur-related polymorphisms that can trigger symptoms in response to fruit's colorful phytonutrients. Remember that phytonutrients can act as tiny poisons. Some children simply don't yet have the reserve and resilience to come back stronger. These children can present with symptoms that include frequent red ears and cheeks, hyperactivity or tantrums, bloated belly or loose stool, dark circles under the eyes, headaches, difficulty falling/staying asleep at night—which can crop up immediately after having certain fruits. These include but are not limited to reds and purples (including tomato—yes, it's a fruit!). If you recognize these symptoms in your child, stick with pears, mangoes, papayas, and pineapples for one month and look for improvement.

## Juice Is Not Fruit

Fresh juice can pack a punch of produce all in one go. By fresh, I mean juicing whole fruits or veggies with a juicer and promptly drinking it—right away or within 24 hours if it's well sealed and refrigerated. Most people, however, aren't drinking juice that's fresh. Once juice has been pasteurized or stabilized to sit indefinitely on a shelf in a container at room temperature, the benefits decrease significantly.

Almost all "fresh-squeezed" orange juice has undergone a deoxygenation process to "maintain freshness." Your fresh OJ can sit in storage for *more than a year* before you buy it (losing much of its inherent nutrition—especially vitamin C—in the process)! To add back flavor, fragrance, and appeal, manufacturers add extracts from pesticide-laden orange peels, "natural flavorings," and GMO-derived enzymes that break down nutrient-dense pulp. The frozen juice concentrate so popular in the 1970s actually contains more phytonutrients than the big-name so-called fresh-squeezed

OJ of today. And if you want to "drink" apples as a treat, very cloudy, unfiltered cider contains four times the nutrients of commercial apple juice—just stick with organic.

Remember how "no sugar added" juices can have undeclared fruit sugar added? Well, even if you juice yourself, it takes many fruits (four to five apples) to make one cup of juice. The high natural sugars in fruits mean even the freshest fruit juice should be a treat rather than a many-times-a-day beverage.

In general, unless you juiced it yourself, watched it be juiced, or know the people who juiced it: AVOID IT.

This leads me to . . . My "Food How-Tos." Here's a simple guide to enjoying fruits and vegetables to get the most benefit from them:

1. **Use all parts of plants, from root to leaves to flowers, flesh to seeds.**

    Different parts of plants are optimally nutritious at different points in the season. Early in the season, sprouts are tremendously nutrient-dense and are a great way to get a powerful punch of nutrients in a small package. Leaves or stems tend to be most nutritious during the spring, before the plant flowers. When the flowers blossom, the plant focuses on producing a delightful flower—making it most nutritious. The flowers from arugula plants taste deliciously peppery and a touch bitter, just like arugula—same with those of broccoli, mint, ginger, and other flowers that you might not have thought you could eat. As the season continues, ripe fruits and vegetables are the most nutritious, followed by edible seeds (sunflower, pumpkin, squash) as the plant goes to seed, which are wildly nutrient-dense and tasty. Edible roots—potatoes, carrots, parsnips, beets, for example—are most nutritious in the autumn/winter, when the plant is storing nutrients to survive the cold weather.

2. **Eat fruit, with a side of peel.**

   The peel tends to be the most nutritious and gorgeous part of our produce—apples are rosy red or golden, nectarines a blushing pink, and grapes a deep purple or vibrant green. The color comes from being "sun-kissed," which means that UV radiation from the sun stressed the fruit enough to boost colorful phytonutrients. Birds know that fruit at the top of the tree is far more nutrient-dense than lower-hanging fruit. The slightly bitter taste of the peel means that it's doing a body good, in many cases even more so than the flesh of the fruit. I leave stripes of peel intact if I peel a carrot. You can add organic lemon or orange zest to veggies, fruit dishes, soups, smoothies, and desserts to enhance flavor and nutrient content.

3. **When it comes to fruit, bigger is not always better.**

   Hybridization created bigger fruit with fewer phytonutrients. Almost every modern fruit started out as a smaller breed with more phytonutrients. It makes sense—the energy a plant has is finite. Plants that budget less energy to grow have more energy to produce phytonutrients. Apricots have more phytonutrients than peaches or nectarines. Crabapples have many times higher nutrients than regular apples; currants have more than raisins. Even smaller cherries and grapes have higher nutrient content, which also often means more intense flavor.

4. **Choose an array of fruits and vegetables, including the "ugly" ones.**

   Eat an array of the most fragrant, brightest, and freshest-looking produce. Sometimes the nose knows better than our eyes how to detect hybrids bred to look nice but taste bland. Take a chance on the "uglier" options, too; especially produce with mouth-watering aromas. Rougher, green, or even brown-skinned fruits of heirloom varieties may be far more delicious than the more common commercial options. Don't always look for the perfect specimen, either. While wilted produce connotes spoilage, imperfect apples sporting a little bug hole or bruise may have undergone more stress and therefore actually may have a higher phytonutrient count—and more unique flavor—as a result of mounting a "pest defense." By eating an array of produce choices, you're getting tens of thousands of biodiverse phytonutrients.

5. **Go wild for wild.**

Wild plants have grit—they have to look out for themselves and produce their own kick-ass defense system. From stray dandelions to surprise apple/pear/plum trees, less hybridized plants hold a treasure trove of flavor and nutrition. Many wild foods enhance liver cell function and promote detoxification of the very toxins kids' bodies need to flush—including pesticides like Roundup and atrazine, endocrine-disrupting plastic chemicals like BPA, and industrial contaminants like carbon tetrachloride.[42] You can forage these goods yourselves (many kids adore that—just avoid pesticide-laden areas such as those bordering conventional agriculture fields or golf courses), or find them at a farmer's market, which is a great place to find prized foraged foods. At our market in New York, we get seasonal feasts of fiddlehead ferns, morels and chanterelles, garlic ramps, and lion's mane mushrooms. Yum!

When we consume plants like dandelion, burdock, yellow dock, goldenrod, elderberry, barberry, and even wild radish, we derive not only nutrients but physiological protection. And wild food doesn't have to mean exotic: A cup of pine needle/bark tea is an exceptional source of vitamin C (five times that of a lemon and ten times that of orange juice!), vitamin A, and many other phytonutrients that boost your immune system and protect against disease. In fact, white pine needles are a source of shikimic acid, the compound used in the conventional flu treatment Tamiflu. (Avoid consuming yew, Norfolk Island, or Ponderosas, however, as these can be toxic.) Wild blueberries have been shown to boost cognition and memory, and they generally promote optimal health—even as juice (when 100 percent juice). You can make jams, syrups, and preserves using natural sugars to enjoy these concentrated phytonutrients long after harvest.

6. **Enjoy fruits and vegetables in season.**

Buy or pick in season whenever possible. Out of season, root vegetables, winter squash, apples, and pears maintain their nutrients for longer than other produce. You can store them in cold cellars, attics, garages, or your refrigerator. Freeze or dehydrate produce that doesn't store well, or preserve them by pickling, fermenting, or making jams or sauces.

## THE REAL DIRT ON EATING ORGANIC

**USDA Organic is one of the few meaningful certifications on labels today.** It exists because many people do not want to expose themselves and their families to synthetic pesticides and chemicals. Children's rapidly developing nervous systems are particularly vulnerable to pesticides. A study of more than a thousand U.S. children showed that those with higher organophosphate pesticide traces in their urine were twice as likely to have an ADHD diagnosis as those with lower levels.[43] A meta-analysis of several studies concluded that exposure to pesticides around the time of birth (in or out of the womb) disrupts the baby's thyroid and neurotransmitter function and is associated with ADHD and autism spectrum disorder.[44] Many pesticides are also endocrine disruptors that elicit premature puberty, polycystic ovarian syndrome (PCOS), miscarriages, or infertility; hypo- or hyperthyroidism; obesity or growth delay; as well as neurodevelopmental problems.[45]

Pesticide exposure may be contributing to a "silent pandemic" of developmental neurotoxicity[46] by crippling mitochondria and reducing liver enzyme activity necessary for detoxification.[47] These chemicals affect different people differently, depending on genes, epigenetics, and previous exposures. The problem is that we don't know how much pesticide exposure will push a given child past his or her tipping point.

A growing body of research shows that pesticides affect children before they're even born. In a study of eight hundred women with prenatal exposure to common organochlorine pesticides like DDE or PCBs, their children, ages zero to eight, had a significant increase in the occurrence of ADHD, depending on pesticide exposure and amount.[48] Prenatal pesticide exposure increases the risk for neurological problems including autism spectrum disorder by 24 months.[49]

**Even when exposed mothers had no apparent adverse health effects from exposure, their children's development was adversely affected in long-lasting ways.**

Pesticide exposure during childhood affects children's health as well, and it has been linked to obesity, asthma, cancer, the increasing incidence of food allergies,[50,51,52] and delayed or abnormal development. The famous Guillette study showed that the children exposed to pesticides in a Mexican community demonstrated significant developmental delays that nonexposed children didn't.[53]

Does eating organic make a difference? Children who eat conventionally grown food excrete higher levels of organophosphate pesticide metabolites than those who eat organic foods,[54] metabolites associated with a six-times higher risk of ADHD.[55] The good news is that those metabolites drop within days of switching to an organic diet.[56,57] **Whatever has happened before today, changes that you make right now can affect your children's health from this moment forward.**

## FARMING, THEN AND NOW:
## WHY LEAD AND ARSENIC ARE IN FOOD

For most of human history, farming was more sustainable than it is today. Our ancestors rotated selections of crops (instead of season after season of a single crop) and occasionally allowed land to remain fallow, which naturally discouraged pests, kept the soil nutrient-rich, and also preserved its health. For pests, families developed their own remedies of black walnut hulls, tobacco, or lye. They knew that the real defense mechanism of crops was in healthy soil, facilitated by compost and plant clippings.

The driving force behind new "technologies" in pesticides conveniently came from industries that were no longer permitted to dump their toxic waste in rivers and lakes. They saw farmland as a receptacle of hundreds of thousands of acres. Industry figured that by convincing farmers to buy toxic waste as a "product," it could reduce illegal dumping and make a profit to boot. Companies advertised in agricultural journals, remaking lead and arsenic into pesticides like Paris Green and

London Purple (both pigments used in paints and fabric dyes), touted as the latest and best in fighting mold and insects.

Many farmers, experts, doctors, and the population at large were reluctant, as they already knew that these substances were toxic and could accumulate in the soil and in animals and people.[58] Even in the nineteenth century, toxicologists warned the USDA and Bureau of Chemistry that arsenic would cause health problems. The Bureau, fearful of political repercussions, meekly asked farmers to spray less. But there was no going back, because pests had become resistant as quickly as farmers ramped up pesticides.

Fast forward a few decades' worth of events: physicians detected clear cases of arsenic poisoning in people throughout the United States; the British embargoed American fruit because of high arsenic levels; and an article in the *Journal of the American Medical Association* linked cases of pediatric eczema to arsenic in breast milk (in the 1930s!). Yet the U.S. government and industry insisted all the while that use of these poisons was safe.

When arsenic no longer had any effect on newly resistant pests, producers added lead, which helped the arsenic stick better to leaves. Lead arsenate is a particularly dangerous poison for children.[59] By the 1950s, the arsenic and lead combo predictably had become utterly ineffective against pests, and was mostly (though not entirely) retired as a pesticide. Something new and sinister was available: DDT.

Thanks to a surplus of nerve gas after World War II and a great advertising campaign designed by Theodor Geisel (aka Dr. Seuss), nerve poisons like organochlorines and organophosphates used in warfare were reconfigured as pesticides. These wreaked havoc on plant, animal, and human health. After decades of damage, Rachel Carson's 1969 book *Silent Spring*, which described the devastation caused by DDT on birds, butterflies, amphibians, and beneficial insects, helped end the use of DDT in the United States. But close behind was yet another wartime chemical, 2,4-D, aka Agent Orange, used to kill huge swaths of Vietnam jungle and, in the process, poison half a million U.S. serviceman and a generation of Vietnamese people. Roundup (glyphosate) was next in line—more on that in Chapter 9 when we discuss genetically modified organisms. In October 2014, the U.S. EPA approved adding the pesticide Agent Orange to Roundup on non-organic crops that we will feed our children. **Unfortunately, industry and government have historically colluded to minimize and—when possible—conceal the impact of pesticides on public health rather than protect individuals.** And so these poisons continue to be used extensively in our food supply.

When you read headlines like "Arsenic in Apple Juice: How Much Is Too Much?" or "Rice Linked to Arsenic Poisoning" (and more alarmingly, "More Than Half of Popular Rice Cereals Exceed Limits for Arsenic"[60]), you are witnessing the result of our country's past reliance on arsenic-based pesticides. Though some arsenic formation occurs naturally and can contaminate groundwater, inorganic arsenic didn't just happen to be in our soil. It's there because we put it on our crops! And that's how much of it got into our drinking water, too. Even California, which has some of the strictest regulations for pesticide use, still uses hundreds of thousands of pounds of arsenic in agriculture every year. It's used also for cottonseed, which is not regulated as a food, even though 80 percent of it is fed to dairy cows (and occasionally to us in the form of cottonseed oil). Yikes.

Testing by numerous reputable sources has shown that certain apple juice and rice products—including cereal bars, rice pasta, and organic nondairy *baby formula*—have arsenic levels far exceeding the "safe level" set by the EPA.[61] Further, the amount of inorganic arsenic in rice according to 2013 FDA data was significantly higher than in 2012. Regular exposure to even small amounts of arsenic can increase the risk of bladder, lung, and skin cancer, as well as heart disease and type 2 diabetes. A baby exposed to arsenic in utero may have a compromised immune system. Yet there's still no federal limit for arsenic in rice and rice products.[62]

TIP ————————————————————————————

Systemic pesticide administration, a common process by which pesticides are injected into the plant, means that a careful washing of our food is not an effective way to eliminate our exposure. Buying or growing food organically or biodynamically offers the safest and most optimal choice.

---

While reducing toxin exposure is benefit enough, growing data also show that organic produce is more nutrient-dense. Studies not funded by industry (or its front men) show that organically raised vegetables develop much higher levels of vitamin C, antioxidants, carotenoids, and polyphenols.[63,64] Not surprisingly, these plants are also better at surviving stressful conditions like drought. Phytonutrients at your service!

**Plants grown organically are healthier, and enable us to be healthier.**

## FERTILIZERS: A FORMULA FOR NUTRIENT DEPLETION

For the past 70 years, the most widely used chemical fertilizers have been made from a simplistic, man-made combination of nitrogen, phosphorus, and potassium. During that time, chronic disease has increased. Some scientists see a connection. The late, great soil scientist Dr. William Albrecht conducted studies on this topic for almost 50 years: he demonstrated that chemical fertilizers create nutrient imbalances in soil and increase growing plants' vulnerability to attack. He noted that a less fertile soil also results in malnutrition and health problems in animal and human populations. Sound familiar? Albrecht also correlated soil infertility with tooth decay (people in areas with better soil fertility have less tooth decay) and fitness for the army (men from areas with the worst soil fertility were more often found physically unfit to serve).

Albrecht noted that red clover, often used in feed for animals, is a magnesium-rich plant. Yet as soil fertility—and as a result, soil magnesium levels—dropped, red clover became increasingly difficult to grow and thus increasingly expensive. Chemical fertilizers decrease magnesium in plants by flooding soil with potassium, which competes with magnesium uptake. As plants have become magnesium-deficient, so, too, have animals who eat those plants. And in turn, so have we.

Magnesium is a critical nutrient for neurological and overall health, yet many of us suffer from symptoms of magnesium deficiency. Normally, it acts as a neurorelaxant, calming the brain from overstimulation of excitatory neurotransmitter function of glutamate. Children who are deficient can suffer from constipation, asthma, anxiety, ADHD, migraines, tics, and seizures. Adults can have similar symptoms, as well as hypertension, muscle cramps, and preterm contractions during pregnancy. In many cases, administering a daily magnesium glycinate or threonate supplement in sufficient quantity (up to 400 mg) can ameliorate symptoms relatively promptly. But synthetic vitamin supplementation, taken from somewhere else that needs its minerals, is not a sustainable answer in the long run. Ultimately, we should be getting this and other minerals from the plants and animals living off our own rich soil that we nourish by giving back to it.

The complex minerals we need come from rocks—yes, rocks—that release potassium, calcium, phosphorus, magnesium, and many other necessary elements for our metabolism. Healthy plants obtain minerals from rocks with the help of mycorrhizae by secreting mild acids and enzymes that extract nutrients from rock particles, atom by atom. And a healthy ecosystem holds on to these minerals, recycling them. Falling leaves or dying plants in a forest ecosystem, for example, recycle 98 percent of calcium and magnesium again and again. In contrast, chemically fertilized land retains only about 40 to 50 percent annually.

We need to reject this outdated, harmful, and simplistic practice of chemically fertilizing our soil. Composting is a better option, which creates complex, nutrient-dense fertilizer from waste that nourishes soil. This, in turn, liberates precious minerals and organic waste that would otherwise sit forever in plastic bags in landfills. Win-win.

## Synthetic Nitrogen Degrades Soil, Water, and Plants

- Degraded soil lacks nutrients that make food nutritious.
- Plants in poor soil have weak root systems, are vulnerable

to drought and disease, and require increased irrigation and application of pesticides.

- Increased erosion promotes rapid runoff into our water supply, causing surface algae bloom that results in dead zones where no aquatic life can survive.
- Nitrates from fertilizers cause tumors in laboratory animals and are linked to reproductive problems, urinary and kidney disorders, and bladder and ovarian cancer.
- Nitrates in drinking water used for infant formula can cause potentially fatal blue-baby syndrome.
- Nitrates contribute to smog, greenhouse gases, and acid rain, while destroying protective ozone.

Changing your child's food can change your child's health. Ultimately, eating organically guarantees that you're reducing your exposure to food and animals grown with pesticides, synthetic fertilizers, irradiation, GMO, hormones, sewage sludge, and antibiotics. That's serious benefit! To ensure you're feeding your family the best possible produce, keep the following in mind:

## GUIDE TO BUYING QUALITY FRUITS AND VEGETABLES

1. **Eat fresh.** The sooner you consume just-picked produce, the more phytonutrients you get—which means superior texture, taste, and health benefit.
2. **Eat organic and biodynamic whenever possible.** Buying organic food is healthier and supports organic growers, which minimizes the impact of pesticides that affect your family and children everywhere. Biodynamic has even higher standards than organic and specifically nourishes soil in ways that nourish us.
3. **Eat diverse plants.** We're learning that no food is 100 percent "toxin-free"—especially because plants act to clean the soil by internalizing toxins like arsenic, lead, or thallium. But this need not

cause despair. The healthier the soil—replete with microorganisms and nutrients—the lower in toxins the plants will be. Eating diverse plants is key, both for the full array of nutrients that support effective detoxification and for a lower exposure to any unwanted compound as well. Well-nourished bodies are effective at detoxifying.

4. **Avoid the "Dirty Dozen Plus."** If you can't afford to buy all organic or don't have access to a variety of organic produce, at least you can avoid what the Environmental Working Group has dubbed the "Dirty Dozen Plus," conventional foods that consistently test high for pesticide residue. Their list currently includes:[65]

Apples
Strawberries
Grapes
Celery
Peaches
Spinach
Sweet bell peppers
Cucumbers
Cherry tomatoes
Snap peas (imported)
Potatoes
Hot peppers
Kale/collard greens

Conversely, you could buy the "Clean Fifteen," the conventionally raised fruits and vegetables that test lowest for pesticide residue. Check the Environmental Working Group's website for the most recent list:[66]

Avocados
Sweet corn
Pineapples
Cabbage
Sweet peas (frozen)
Onions
Asparagus
Mangoes

Kiwi
Eggplant
Grapefruit
Cantaloupe
Cauliflower
Sweet potatoes

5. **Support local farmers who grow organically and who care about soil.** By supporting these farmers through farmer's markets, Community Supported Agriculture (CSAs), or buying directly from them, you are investing in small-scale agriculture that allows for careful farming from soil to seed to plant to plate. Farmers who use biodynamic or permaculture methods see themselves as custodians of soil. Let your conventionally growing farmers know that minimizing pesticide application is important to you and that they will have your support as they shift their practices. And consider growing some food yourself, even fresh herbs in a sunny corner of an apartment.

## Pickle Me! Fermenting for a Healthy Microbiome

Fermenting foods at peak season means you can enjoy them long after harvest time while also boosting your gut, immune system, and brain. Cabbage, cucumbers, and even watermelon rind taste delicious after sitting submerged in brine for six weeks. I pickle organic Meyer lemons in sea salt and their own juice; the rind is a tangy addition to meat and veggie dishes. Pickled veggies are easy to make from scratch with pickling salt and spices. Try it! If you're intimidated by the process, get your feet wet this way: Save brine from your jar of full sour pickles, then add cut-up kohlrabi, beets, turnips, or carrots, keeping veggies fully submerged. Let the jar sit on the counter with the lid loosely on for up to a week. Bubbles mean fermenting bacteria have shown up. Store them in the fridge and enjoy for a week or two. Be warned, they'll go fast!!

1. Eat all parts of plants, from seeds and sprouts to stems, leaves, flowers, and fruit. Eat all colors—make a rainbow on your plate. In rare instances, certain parts of edible plants, like rhubarb leaves, are not safe for consumption. Double-check for safety before you experiment too wildly.

2. Buy food seasonally, preferably locally. The sooner you eat food from when it's harvested, the higher the phytonutrient content. Get your fix out of season by eating preserved forms: jams; flash-frozen products; and pickled, dehydrated, or dried options. DIY options are higher in phytonutrients than what you can buy from the supermarket.

3. Look for organic and especially biodynamic, permaculture, or "beyond organic" produce, grown by farmers who cultivate superior soil. Flavor, aroma, and nutritional content will be superior as a result. For more information on biodynamic growing: http://www.demeter-usa.org

4. Avoid power-washed vegetables, though it's fine to rinse your veggies before eating. Just keep in mind that a teeny film of soil and the microbes therein are good for you.

5. Shop at farmer's markets. Join a CSA or a community garden. Grow your own food and swap with other people who grow their own.

6. Forage. Wild foods are free and delicious, and kids love gathering and eating them. Learn how to identify what you're looking for and avoid foraging in heavily sprayed or toxic areas.

## CHAPTER 9
# Unlocking Seeds: Nutritional Powerhouses

*The creation of a thousand forests is in one acorn.*
—RALPH WALDO EMERSON

S eeds are available year-round, throughout the seasons. They are compact, powerful packets of energy that can lie dormant for years, decades, even centuries. Seeds beget new food, and more seeds. As the first—and last—step in the life cycle of most plants, seeds complete the circle of life. It's why many cultures throw seeds like rice at weddings.

Seeds have played a pivotal role in human history. The pharaoh of Egypt consolidated power by forcing farmers to pay taxes partly in seeds; when famine struck, Egypt's amassed seed bank allowed it to control food supply for surrounding lands. Captured African women on slave ships hid seeds in their hair to ensure a continued supply of food and medicine. During the Nazi's nine-hundred-day siege of Leningrad in World War II, 12 Russian scientists in the Pavlovsk agricultural station chose to starve to death rather than eat the unique collection of seeds and plants they were protecting for humanity, which Hitler aimed to seize. Grain shortage can precede civil unrest, from the French Revolution to the Arab Spring. Seeds remain the object of struggle for commercial power today.

The word "ingrained" means "in the seeds." Seeds—including grains, nuts, and beans—are our history and our future, continuity between our ancestors and future generations. They safeguard biodiversity, which allows for abundance. Above all, they produce plants that are vital to our very survival.

## LEGUMES

There is evidence that our ancestors gathered tiny wild legumes more than twenty thousand years ago, likely because they remained edible long after being harvested. Legumes like beans and lentils are high in protein, but lack an essential amino acid called methionine. This is why legumes are commonly eaten with methionine-rich grains, which together provide a "complete protein." Generally, legumes that are colorful—red, purple, black—have the highest levels of phytonutrients. Their soluble fiber can slow digestion and keep you fuller longer.

Soybeans, when grown and prepared properly, are also legumes. Soy isn't always bad, just as it isn't always good. Processed soy found in packaged products in U.S. groceries is almost always genetically modified, which means it's heavily sprayed with Roundup or other pesticides. Soy also has high phytoestrogen levels; this impact on our health is controversial. But some organic, fermented soy seems to be fine for those who don't react to soy. Fermenting helps release soy's beneficial compounds and mitigates many negative ones. Fermented soy includes miso, tofu, tempeh, soy sauce, and tamari. Eat them in small to moderate amounts and minimize exposure to processed soy products and the ubiquitous soybean oil used in nearly every restaurant (If you don't believe me, just ask!).

### Nuts

Nuts are dry, single-seeded fruits with high oil content enclosed in a tough outer layer. Many seeds also fall into this category (such as sunflower and safflower). Some nuts, like peanuts, fit more than one description (legume and seed). Historians hypothesize that ancient societies about ten thousand years ago likely centered on the harvesting of nuts, which may then have fostered agriculture. They're nutrient-dense with generous amounts of calories, fats, complex carbohydrates, protein, vitamins, minerals, and fiber. And they're good sources of minerals like magnesium, zinc, and selenium, which are often underconsumed in today's largely processed Western diet.

Nuts and seeds protect against disease. They're rich in phytochemicals and plant sterols, which help keep cholesterol levels in balance and reduce cancer risk. People in countries that eat lots of nuts have lower incidence of cardiovascular diseases than those in countries where few eat nuts. In a study of more than 34,000 Seventh-Day Adventists, those who consumed nuts at least five times a week halve their rate of heart attack compared to those who rarely ate them; eating nuts once a week still lowered risk by 25 percent compared to nut avoiders.[1] The Nurses' Health Study, involving more than 86,000 women, reported lower rates of heart disease among frequent nut consumers than nut avoiders,[2] and the Physician's Health Study of over 20,000 men found lower rates of mortality from all causes in those who consume nuts.[3,4]

Despite their reputation as a high-calorie, fat-filled snack, nuts and seeds may actually enhance weight loss and maintenance. Nuts promote satiety, which can reduce consumption of other foods.[5] Of 65 people on a weight-reduction program, those who ate a diet rich in almonds lost more weight and maintained their weight loss compared with those who ate a diet rich in complex carbohydrates.[6] In another study, participants who ate 3 ounces of peanuts daily reduced their intake of other foods because they felt satiated, which helped them control their weight.[7]

Consuming nuts may even play a role in diabetes prevention and glucose control. Nut consumption can lower risk of type 2 diabetes in women. Eating almonds helps avoid spikes in blood glucose from foods that are known to raise blood sugar levels.[8] Nuts and seeds in general, with their low glycemic index and dense nutrient profile, can play a role in preventing or controlling diabetes.

The nutrients and other bioactive components in nuts and seeds benefit the brain and cognition. Walnuts in particular protect the hippocampus, our memory center, from oxidative stress and other damage.[9] (They also look like little brains!) Regular nut consumption—ideally soaked, then roasted—may prevent and help reverse brain dysfunction.[10]

Over the last several years, obtaining unprocessed nuts has become increasingly difficult. Industry pools almonds from hundreds of farmers, which amplifies the risk of contamination. A contaminated batch from one farm causes limited problems because we can trace it back to the source, but when that batch is combined with thousands of other batches from other sources it has led to massive recalls mostly due to salmonella or listeria.[11] As a result, many nuts sold in the United States—and all almonds—are irradiated, which can cause nutrient losses due to formation of highly reactive free radicals that degrade the structure and activity of vitamins.[12] Formation of radiolytes and radioactivity in the food itself pose their own health (and environmental) hazards. No labeling exists at this time that allows consumers to identify which foods are irradiated, though it's worth knowing that typically Italian and Spanish almonds are not irradiated. They can be obtained from several Internet-based nut companies.

### "Antinutrients"

In order to protect themselves from being destroyed before germinating, beans, seeds, nuts, and grains have several defenses, which some call "antinutrients," that allow them to survive insects, mold, fungus, and the digestive tract of animals. After all, a primary way that seeds spread is because animals deposit seeds in their scat. An example of an antinutrient is phytic acid, which binds minerals, making them unusable by your body.[13] A diet that includes too many phytates means that calcium, iron, and zinc may bind to phytic acid to form insoluble complexes, resulting in reduction of these minerals in your body.[14] Phytic acid can also exhaust phosphorus supplies. In populations where cereal grains provide a major source of calories, rickets and osteoporosis are more common.[15] Nuts' phytic acid content can particularly block absorption of iron.[16] And eating straight bran or high-fiber foods with bran can contribute to bone loss and intestinal problems.[17] Given their high demand for minerals, growing children can run into problems when eating a phytate-rich diet, due to lower calcium, phosphorus, zinc, and iron.[18]

You shouldn't fear eating grains, beans, seeds, or nuts. Simply source and prepare these foods properly and eat them in moderation. Phytates in small amounts have antioxidant-building and toxin-binding properties—and may even have anticancer properties.[19] Listen to your body. And as always, balance is key.

The way to dissolve phytic acid is with its counterenzyme: phytase. We humans do not produce much phytase, in contrast to cows and other ruminants, but probiotic lactobacillus and our healthy human digestive microflora do.[20] Studies show that the body can adapt to the effects of some phytates in the diet, likely through the microbiome. Subjects who consumed high levels of whole wheat at first excreted more calcium than they took in, but after several weeks, they stopped excreting excess calcium. It seems our flora can adjust somewhat to our phytate input. Similarly, a combination of sprouting/soaking/fermenting/cooking—which benefits our bodies in other ways as well—activates the seeds' innate phytase before even entering our digestive tract, which reduces phytates while boosting nutrients.[21] Similarly, food combinations can make a difference with phytates. For instance, consumption of meat or vitamin C–containing foods increases our absorption of iron.[22] Adding onion or garlic to rice or beans also enhances the amount of iron and zinc you absorb from them.[23] The sulfur-containing phytonutrients that give onions and garlic their pungent smell also "unlock" certain minerals to be better absorbed. Daily consumption might consist of a slice or so of genuine sourdough bread; a handful of soaked, sprouted, and roasted nuts; and one to two servings of properly prepared oatmeal, pancakes, rice, or beans. In a nutrient-dense diet rich in vitamins, minerals, healthy fats, and lacto-fermented foods, most people tolerate up to four to five servings daily.

Problems arise when grains or legumes become the foundation of every meal, especially in children who eat a limited array of foods.[24] This is one reason that children who are raised vegan and even vegetarian can be at a significant disadvantage nutritionally—they're not eating nutrient-dense animal proteins and fats, while they're consuming foods that contain large amounts of antinutrients that bind minerals they need.[25] Children under age six, pregnant women, and anyone with serious illness should be careful to consume a diet lower in phytic acids because their bodies have such a high demand for these minerals.[26] This means preparing phytate-rich foods by sprouting and cooking, and restricting consumption to two to three servings daily. Chronically ill children or those with numerous cavities or bone fractures may benefit from a trial off grains and legumes altogether for one to three months under careful medical supervision and monitoring for improvement. We all benefit from minimizing unfermented soy products, extruded whole-grain cereals, rice cakes, unsprouted granola, raw muesli, and other high-phytate foods, but this group should avoid them.

## GRAINS: THE GOOD, THE BAD, AND THE GLUTEN

Whole grains prepared in traditional ways have clear health benefits, although reactivity to wheat—gluten in particular—has become a significant issue for an unprecedented number of children, as discussed in Chapter 4. Reasons for this reactivity may include poor soil fertility, hybridized wheat strains with shallower roots that can't absorb nutrients from the soil, and residues of the Roundup that are repeatedly sprayed on the wheat. Almost all white flour in the United States—which is designed to last on the shelf but not to be nutritious and flavorful—is treated with chlorine bleach (azodicarbonamide), then sprayed with fungal amylase (which slows down the growth of mold) and potassium bromate. These compounds are associated with kidney and nervous system disorders as well as cancer. Banned in many countries, they're legal in the United States. One old study showed that animals fed white flour suffered from infertility significantly more than those fed freshly stone-ground wheat.[27] Fertility is a window to overall health.

But these are all problems that *we caused*. Traditional grains—both with and without gluten—carry health benefits. Buckwheat, used in an eastern European dish called kasha, contains D-fagomine, a compound that effectively reduces blood glucose[28] and insulin release.[29] It inhibits intestinal adhesion of several kinds of potentially harmful bacteria, such as types of *Escherichia coli* and salmonella, and promotes adhesion of beneficial bacteria like lactobacillus, balancing intestinal microbiota.[30] Quinoa, a grainlike berry, is high in protein and has the high-antioxidant characteristic of berries.[31]

Wheat and its sister grains like spelt and rye have gotten a bad rap despite their nutritional benefits. But that's mostly because we don't go to the best sources and prepare it traditionally. For instance, sprouting wheat increases vitamins A, B$_{12}$, C, and promotes enzymes that facilitate digestion of starches and proteins. Some studies suggest that fermenting or sprouting wheat can reduce the gluten content significantly.[32,33] Sprouting also destroys flatulence-promoting oligosaccharides along with phytates and trypsin inhibitors (which bind nutrients and prevent protein breakdown).[34] Sourdough bread (made using traditional fermentation methods) breaks down phytates by fermentation, which increases mineral availability and digestibility and decreases rate of spoilage. Fermenting gluten-free grains into sourdough has been shown to heal and balance gut microbiome after celiac diagnosis.[35] These preparations also regulate rises in glucose to prevent a subsequent damaging spike in insulin that can lead to inflammation in the body and brain.[36]

Traditional preparation enhances other grains as well. When corn is traditionally prepared by nixtamalization—soaking, cooking in alkaline solution (like limewater), then hulled—it becomes the nutritionally superior masa harina. It's more easily ground, the flavor and aroma are improved, mycotoxins are reduced, and nutrients are more accessible. This process also enhances the availability of niacin, which prevents the deficiency syndrome pellagra—still a widespread problem in the world.

Bob's Red Mill and Gold Mine are a few companies that offer cornmeal prepared as traditional masa harina. Brands like Lundberg, TruRoots, and Now Foods offer sprouted organic rice. In the New York area, Cayuga Organics offers freshly ground wheat, and Biodynamics and To Your Health Sprouted Flour Co. offer sprouted grains more widely.

## A Guide to Eating Seeds

- Choose organic, preferably biodynamic whole grains over processed ones, i.e., brown rice versus white, and steel-cut oats versus rolled.

- Opt for ancient varieties such as kamut, emmer, amaranth, millet, quinoa, or einkorn. These are much less likely to be monocrops, which are depleted of nutrients and excessively sprayed with pesticides.
- If you want to eat corn, try buying (or growing) an heirloom variety, such as the antioxidant-rich blue corn from companies like Anson Mills. Pop your own corn from these beautiful varieties. Avoid microwave popcorn and its chemical-infused packaging, trans fats, and GMO or monocropped kernels. Foods made with properly prepared cornmeal, called masa harina, offer optimal nutrition and flavor.
- Sprout and ferment (sourdough) your grains or flours to aid digestibility and nutrient absorption and to boost the microbiome.
- Find freshly milled flour locally if possible—often a farmer's market is the first place to explore. If you're feeling adventurous, you can obtain and grind your own wheatberries or other grains in a Vitamix blender or a flourmill to experience the fresh, living flour. Yes, fresh flour is more delicious and nutritious in everything from cakes to breads—and you probably won't want to go back to the old stuff for baking.
- Choose sourdough or sprouted breads, gluten-free or not, as tolerated.
- Sprouted nuts taste exceptionally better than the regular kind most of us eat. Many companies offer them sprouted, including Living Intentions.
- Add chia, flax, and hemp seeds to everything from salads to smoothies to homemade cracker recipes. No soaking necessary.
- To reduce the gassiness of beans and increase their nutrient availability, soak them for 24 to 48 hours with a postage stamp–size piece of kombu. Drain and add fresh water before cooking.

TIP ━━━━━━━━━━━━━━━━━━━━━━━━━━━━━━━━━━━━━━━━━━━

### Wild Milky Oats (WMO)

Grains can have medicinal benefits. One week of every year, wild oat plants—which grow in all parts of the country—exude a milky substance. During that week, these harvested oats possess special properties of calm (but without sedation). As a gentle antidepressant and restorative, WMO reduce the stress response; revive the nervous system and adrenal glands; help to restore minerals the body needs; aid sleep; and bestow a feeling of general well-being. WMO makes a relaxing, nutritive tea or tincture (infused in a very small amount of alcohol) that lifts mood and can reduce social anxiety while being gentle enough to be a daily tonic even for young children to "take the edge off." Parents like it, too!

━━━━━━━━━━━━━━━━━━━━━━━━━━━━━━━━━━━━━━━

## DEMONIZING MACRONUTRIENTS

*When we try to pick out anything by itself,*
*we find it hitched to everything else in the Universe.*
—JOHN MUIR

Since macronutrients—fats, proteins, and carbohydrates—were identified, they've taken turns at being considered "bad." Fat of any kind was the fall guy for a long time. Protein and fat from animals are perpetual villains. These days, though, the bad guys are gluten and "carbs."

But as we're learning, foods are more than macronutrients or micronutrients. Equating milk with calcium, or eggs with cholesterol, reduces food to one element and ignores its complexity. Too often, we focus on the "what" of our foods (whether one element is "good" or "bad") and not enough on the when (when was it harvested), how (what kind of soil, how was it grown, processed, and cooked), why (why do we grow and prepare food in this way), and who (who benefits or suffers).

It's true that we're eating more carbohydrates than ever before. A study of general caloric intake between 1909 and 1997 found that people have been eating significantly more calories, and that carbohydrate consumption accounted for *80 percent of those calories.*[37] A 2004 study conducted by the Center for Disease Control and Prevention (CDC)'s National Center for Health Statistics found that carbohydrate intake was at the root of an increase in calorie consumption during the past 30 years (a 22 percent climb for women, 7 percent for men).[38] The real problem, though, may be that these carbohydrates came primarily from processed foods and sugar.

Sometimes eliminating carbohydrates can be absolutely appropriate as a medical treatment, as with children with refractory epilepsy or chronic GI disorders. Indeed, the ketogenic or modified Atkins diets can control seizures better than many epilepsy medications and may improve some cases of bipolar disease.[39,40] Specific carbohydrate diets appear quite promising for Crohn's disease.[41] (Whenever possible, such diets should consist of real food, even blended, over carb-free formulas. Either way, be sure to engage the help of a nutritional expert.)

Yet gluten, carbohydrates, or even sweeteners are not villains in and of themselves. **The whole of the plant is always greater than the sum of its parts.** The fats and phytonutrients of living grains can actually modulate blood sugar and prevent a spike in insulin.[42,43] Moreover, only in times of plenty do we have such choices about what we should eat—cutting out entire food categories isn't sustainable in the long run. Rather than villainizing entire food groups in this reductionist way, I recommend sourcing and preparing them well and eating them in moderation, if tolerated.

## Vegetarian Kids

Though strict vegan or vegetarian diets can be healing at times in adults, I tend not to recommend them in children. While some kids may thrive eating vegetarian or occasionally vegan diets, children's rapid development means they need an even broader array of foods and nutrients than adults. In our current food system, keeping these children optimally nourished and healthy takes exceptional care. Of special concern are vegetarian kids—or as I call them, carb-etarians—who consume diets largely free of vegetables! Although meat is not a must for everyone, pastured animal products like eggs and milk can help restore health, veggies must be copious, and diverse fats (not just olive oil, for example, but pastured butter, ghee, coconut oil, sesame, flax hemp, and more) are critical. Chronic illness may merit a trial of animal protein for vegetarians, just as it can mean the opposite for meat eaters.

## THE REAL DIRT ON GMO: POWER OVER SEEDS

*Our entire much-praised technological progress,*
*and civilization generally, could be compared to*
*an axe in the hand of a pathological criminal.*
—ALBERT EINSTEIN

Genetically modified organisms (GMOs) have become the next chapter in the history of seeds and attempts to control food production. The biotech and food industries say that GMO foods are safe and will "feed the world." The FDA claims that these crops are "exactly the same" as conventionally grown food. Some senators have introduced bills in Congress to allow GMO products to be labeled 100 percent natural.[44] Anyone who disagrees is labeled "anti-science" (industry's term for those who disagree with its spin on science). Meanwhile, 26 foreign markets ban GMOs and 62—and counting—restrict them.

Crops from GMO seeds comprise nearly 100 percent of soybean crops and at least 50 percent of corn, as well as canola, squash (zucchini and yellow), Hawaiian papaya, sugarbeets (another sugar source aside from corn), alfalfa, and cotton. This may not sound like much until you consider that soy, corn, and sugarbeets make up a tremendous portion of every processed food—including institutional and restaurant foods, where industrial products like soybean oil are almost universally used. And you likely consume meat, eggs, or milk from animals that consume alfalfa (or vegetables that are fertilized by the manure from animals that eat genetically modified alfalfa) and cottonseed. GMOs are also commonly used in processed food additives that we've already discussed.[45] Wheat, rice, and flax—considered "high risk"—are not GMO but have genetically modified cousins that can cross-pollinate with them. Indeed, the USDA detected GMO wheat—currently not approved in the United States—in Oregon in 2013 and again in Montana in 2014. These findings caused Asian markets to ban U.S.–grown wheat for a period. After the second finding, Monsanto—the creator of GMO wheat—was fined.

A genetically modified organism has had foreign genes—from a different kind of plant, an animal, even a bacterium or virus—added to its DNA to improve crop yield, resist drought, or evade predators. The problem is that in nature every functional gene—plant, animal, or human—has corresponding regulator genes that determine whether and when to turn genes on and off. Removing a fragment of a gene without its regulator genes means that the transplanted gene can act in untethered ways in its new home in our food's DNA. An even bigger problem arises when these unregulated ("promiscuous") genes enter our bodies. They can lead to unexpected food allergies, toxicity, tumors, and other health problems. **Promiscuous genes—deposited in soil from GM plants or in our own gut—can produce new, foreign proteins that affect our food and our health.**

GMOs currently cover millions of acres of farmland—or should I say pharmland?—across the United States. Here's why that affects you:

The most common GMO seed named Roundup Ready was designed to grow crops resistant to pests. Monsanto creates Roundup Ready crops by injecting a fragment of DNA into a seed to render the plant resistant to the Monsanto-made herbicide Roundup—of which glyphosate is a major ingredient. Roundup Ready plants withstand vast quantities of Roundup without dying, as toxic glyphosate kills "nondesirable plants" or weeds. Yet the "war on weeds" never works for very long, because the weeds develop resistance to an herbicide and become "superweeds"[46,47] that come back stronger than before.[48] In response, farmers apply higher doses of Roundup more frequently.

The amount of glyphosate used since GMOs were introduced in 1996 has increased fivefold (to 880 million pounds a year). All of that glyphosate soaks into the soil, and according to a 2014 study, it is ubiquitous in more than *75 percent of air and rain samples.*[49] So much glyphosate applied repeatedly to crops binds minerals in the soil, preventing them from entering plants.[50] As such, those plants become less nutritious and more vulnerable to pests. Plants need bacteria and mycorrhizal fungi to feed them and build their immune systems, but glyphosate acts as an antibiotic, which further weakens the plant by limiting exposure to diverse microbes that both support them and stress them into producing more phytonutrients. Glyphosate accumulates in the growth points of the plants—seeds, root tips, and shoot tips—which also happen to be the most edible parts of the plant. So both we—and the animals we eat—accumulate glyphosate in our tissues.[51]

Even at very low doses of exposure, glyphosate kills placental, embryonic, and umbilical cells.[52] Glyphosate is associated with genetic damage (mutations), including chromosomal aberrations, *even at doses below those recognized as "safe."*[53,54] The herbicide acts as a potent endocrine disruptor, which can affect future reproductive health of young boys and girls.[55] Glyphosate was even implicated recently in the development of autism, neurobehavioral problems in children, and other neurological diseases, including Parkinson's and Alzheimer's.[56,57] Glyphosate—and other components inherent to using GMOs—are linked to conditions such as increased intestinal permeability (leaky gut), imbalanced gut bacteria, immune activation, food allergies, impaired digestion, and damage to the intestinal wall.[58] Eating GMO crops impairs fertility in livestock.

Above all, glyphosate impairs detoxification[59] and was called out by the World Health Organization (WHO) as possibly causing cancer. A 2014 study from MIT researcher Stephanie Seneff convincingly correlated the precipitous increase in chronic conditions—celiac, thyroid disease, kidney disease, and others—with the increased use of glyphosate. Urinary levels of glyphosate in chronically ill subjects were

significantly higher than healthy individuals.[60] Glyphosate residues are
neither removed by washing nor broken down by cooking. The herbicide residue remains on food for more than a year, even if processed,
dried, or frozen. Bt toxin, also a pesticide (derived from a spore-
forming bacteria), has now been genetically added to GM corn. When
insects ate crops sprayed with Bt, it attacked their gut walls and killed
them—but then was washed off. Now GM corn produces Bt toxin,
which we consume, and which may similarly damage our own guts.[61]
GMOs have spread worldwide, to the dismay of many countries.

Some of the earliest GMO literature described a spike in anaphylactic reactions in the United Kingdom after GM soybeans combined
with Brazil nut genes were introduced from the United States.[62] The
United Kingdom is one of the few countries that annually evaluates
food allergies. In March 1999, researchers were alarmed to discover
that "soy" allergy had skyrocketed by 50 percent since the previous
year. The Brazil nut gene had somehow expressed itself in the GM
soy, which had now become genetically contaminated with hidden
tree-nut allergen and triggered anaphylaxis.

**When industry patches genetic material from one plant or
animal into another, genetic and epigenetic complexity can lead to
unanticipated outcomes in our bodies and the environment.**

In the case of GMO, however, we are not given a choice as to
whether it is something we want our bodies, our food, or our environment to be exposed to: wind and water carry GMO seeds that grow
in one field to other farmers' fields, where they take root and grow.
And because GMO-containing foods in the United States are not required to be labeled, we as consumers cannot choose whether we want
to expose ourselves to this technology.

## Myth: GMOs Are Proven to Be Safe Because They Are FDA Approved

You might imagine that the FDA established safety based on extensive examination of GMOs, using peer-reviewed soil, plant, and
human health studies. Nope. **The FDA has never conducted safety**

**studies on GMOs.** In the 1990s, the FDA classified food from GM seed as generally recognized as safe (GRAS), as if it were like any other food. The FDA justified the GRAS based on the assumption that nutritional components—proteins, fats, carbohydrates—of a GM plant are "the same as or substantially similar" to those found in non-GM foods.[63] Maybe, but aren't we more interested in the differences? In 1996, the FDA first allowed GM foods into world markets, *even as its own scientists warned that genetic engineering differs fundamentally from conventional breeding and poses special risks, specifically production of new toxins or allergens.*[64,65,66,67,68] **The FDA did not use data to approve GM food as safe. The FDA didn't and does not commission independent safety tests on these foods.**

Indeed, the FDA has no mandatory GM food safety assessment process—only a *voluntary* program for premarket review of GM foods, with no legal requirement for companies to participate. Because of a U.S. government decision to "foster" the growth of the GM industry,[69] the FDA does not exercise oversight. Agritech companies may release any GMO product into the market *without even notifying the FDA.* **The only safety testing done is by the very companies that stand to profit from selling their own GM seeds as well as the accompanying chemicals.**

Needless to say, many of the safety studies are flawed or biased. For instance, a 2015 study found that standard laboratory animal feed tested positive for GMO and glyphosate.[70] If both the exposed and nonexposed animals consumed GMO feed, the safety data are invalid, as no group was "GMO-free." Skepticism grew when the *New York Times* revealed that the biotech industry "has published dozens of articles, under the names of prominent academics, that in some cases were drafted by industry consultants" and they'd given scientists unrestricted grants.[71]

David Schubert, professor and head of the cellular neurobiology laboratory at the Salk Institute, stated in a peer-reviewed study: "One thing that surprised us is that U.S. regulators rely almost exclusively on information provided by the biotech crop developer, and those data are not published in journals or subjected to peer review.... *The picture that emerges from our study of U.S. regulation of GM foods is a rubber–stamp 'approval process' designed to increase public confidence in, but not ensure the safety of, genetically engineered foods."* [72] **In other words, our government is staking our children's health on the word of bio-technology companies.**

Our government has been filled with ex-Monsanto executives, lobbyists, attorneys, and board members, from the well-known—Supreme Court justice Clarence Thomas, former secretary of defense Donald Rumsfeld, various members of Congress, even former secretary of state Hillary Clinton worked as an attorney for a law firm that represented Monsanto—to the lesser-known Monsanto employees who attained high positions in the FDA and USDA.[73] Conversely, FDA and USDA officials also have gotten top positions in Monsanto and its subsidiaries after leaving public service.[74] Current FDA deputy commissioner of policy Michael Taylor, for example, orchestrated the FDA's approach to GM foods in 1991.[75] Prior to joining the FDA, Taylor worked at a law firm that represented Monsanto. In 1998, Taylor became Monsanto's vice president for public policy.[76] In 2010, Taylor returned to the FDA as deputy commissioner for foods.[77]

**Simply put, the fox is guarding the henhouse.** While the Hungarian government destroyed all of Monsanto's genetically engineered cornfields within its borders, the U.S. government has never denied a single application from Monsanto for new genetically engineered crops. Not one, ever. According to the *New York Times*, "It was an outcome that would be repeated, again and again, through three administrations. What Monsanto wished for from Washington, Monsanto—and, by extension, the biotechnology industry—got. If the company's strategy demanded regulations, rules favored by the industry were adopted. And when the company abruptly decided that it needed to throw off the regulations and speed its foods to market, the White House quickly ushered through an unusually generous policy of self-policing. Even longtime Washington hands said that the control this nascent industry exerted over its own regulatory destiny—through the Environmental Protection Agency, the Agriculture Department, and ultimately the Food and Drug Administration—was astonishing."[78]

## Myth: GMO Is Just as Nutritious as Conventionally Grown Crops

Glyphosate was first patented as a chelator and antibiotic. Chelators bind nutrients in the soil, reducing what's available for the plant (and us). In addition, glyphosate attacks microbes and mycorrhizae that facilitate nutrient uptake into plants and strengthen plant connections.[79] While glyphosate may help kill some weeds, the weeds inevitably evolve to become resistant. Ultimately, the remaining (or subsequent) crops have fewer mycorrhizae, earthworms,[80] nutrients,[81] and phytonutrients,[82] which impacts soil, plant, animal, and human health.

## Myth: GMO Increases Crop Yields

Biotech companies claim that GM foods will solve world hunger problems by increasing yields and resistance to pests. No studies to date show that genetically modified food can actually increase crop yield. Recent events suggest that it's quite the opposite. In India, the government banned conventional cottonseed in favor of GM to please Monsanto and as a way to receive contingent International Monetary Fund loans to help its economy. Indian farmers were convinced to spend what was often one thousand times the cost of conventional seed on Monsanto's "magic seeds." Yet the crops were often destroyed by bollworms and other kinds of crop failure,[83] demanding costly pesticides and herbicides. The GM crops also required twice the water of conventional cotton to grow—but water in that quantity was not available, so many crops died. Farmers, who subsisted by saving seeds from year to year, discovered they'd have to purchase new seeds every year. To families already in insurmountable debt, this was the final blow. More than 270,000 Indian farmers have committed suicide since 1995, which some claim was in part a response to the monstrous debt incurred as a result of their agreement to use Monsanto's GMOs.[84]

## Myth: GMOs Will Feed the World

GMOs create dangerous monoculture. Biodiversity of crops means some plants will survive and thrive when challenges arise. One hundred percent of soybeans might be Roundup Ready, but the inevitable Roundup-resistant pest or fungus could then decimate 100 percent of soybeans. Drought-resistant crops may survive drought, but not wet weather. **Biodiversity, not GM technology, ensures resilience.**

As for "feeding the world," there is no evidence to date that GMOs can achieve this goal. Moreover, our world doesn't suffer from a shortage of food. The USDA recently published a study stating that Americans throw away 133 billion pounds of food annually, or about 30 percent of the world's available food. It's widely agreed that the world has enough food, but it's not getting to people who need it. Our global food problem is one of distribution, not scarcity. To argue otherwise is a scare tactic meant to manipulate. And GMO-based monoculture is likely a far greater threat to food security, anyway. As Mark Twain said, "A lie can travel half-way around the world while the truth is putting on its shoes."

## GMO: The Hidden Ingredient

Currently, no legislation requires food manufacturers to disclose GM ingredients. But surveys show that more than 90 percent of American consumers want to know whether products are made from genetically modified seeds. At least 62 other countries mandate labeling of these products so that consumers can make an educated choice. Yet the U.S. food industry has invested billions of dollars in a huge battle against legislation that supports consumers' right to know. This isn't about banning GMOs, mind you—they refuse to simply label them so that consumers can make an educated choice. **Industry says, "Food grown from genetically modified seeds is no different from other food so there is no need to label it." Yet simultaneously manufacturers applied for—and** won—patents on these seeds because they consider them fundamentally *different from* regular seeds. **How can they have it both ways?** Another argument that industry makes is, "Americans aren't sophisticated enough to understand how to interpret information about GM food. They will become overwhelmed." Citizens of 62 other countries have managed to navigate such labels, but simpleminded Americans cannot?[85]

## HOW DO I AVOID FEEDING MY CHILDREN GM FOODS?

Shockingly, more than 80 percent of food in North America contains GMOs, much of which is marketed to children—cereals, snack bars, snack boxes, cookies, processed lunch meat, and crackers. Because manufacturers are not obligated to label products containing GM foods, the only way to avoid them is by shopping organic. The use of GMOs is prohibited in certified organic products. This means an organic farmer can't plant GMO seeds, an organic cow can't eat GMO alfalfa or corn, and organic bread can't be made with any GMO ingredients.

## CONCLUSION

GMO seeds may one day have the potential to offer benefit to society. So far, however, GMO technology has been used almost exclusively as a way to allow application or integration of vastly more pesticides to crops. The extensive rigorous, peer-reviewed safety testing we expect simply hasn't been conducted in animals or humans, and the science we do have is highly alarming. At a minimum, consumers deserve transparency as to whether the food they purchase contains GMO.

# TAKE HOME

1. Seeds—grains, beans, nuts, etc.—are nutrient-dense, delicious, and long-lasting. You should buy organic—or even biodynamic—and non-GMO. See if you can find local growers to get the freshest products. Some high-quality producers even believe that grains and rice should be refrigerated from the moment after harvest to maintain the aromatics and other phytonutrients that confer flavor and health.

2. Most grains and beans, and some nuts and seeds, should be soaked, sprouted, then slow-cooked or roasted for full nutritional benefits. More and more companies are offering consumers sprouted options as demand increases for traditionally prepared, nutrient-dense foods.

3. Check resources like *Consumer Reports* for testing on different brands of rice for arsenic and other contaminants.

4. Beware of anything fortified. For instance, fortified grains mean the most nutrient-dense parts of the plant are gone and packagers added, at most, a few vitamins and minerals, which creates a veneer of healthfulness. Synthetic vitamins cannot achieve what nutritious whole foods can. In this case, freshly ground whole grains provide the complex array of nutrients your child needs.

5. Ditch cereal. Feeding your kids fortified cereal is like giving them cookies and milk for breakfast with a few added synthetic vitamins. Actually, many cookies are healthier! Instead, try soaking your oatmeal or eating sprouted granola, good-quality sourdough bread, or warm quinoa or amaranth, with delicious additions like sprouted nuts, cinnamon, ginger, and cardamom; blueberries, maple syrup, and raw honey; extra-dark maple syrup or black-strap molasses. Or forgo grains and eat eggs or soup for breakfast.

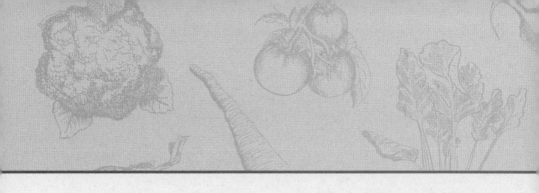

Source grains from companies that offer presprouted options for maximum nutrient availability.

6. Demand GMO labeling and transparency, and rigorous, independent testing for safety for food ingredients, from industry as well as local, state, or federal lawmakers.

# CHAPTER 10
# Meet Your Meat

M any kids think meat comes "from the supermarket," partly because many adults don't want to acknowledge that steaks or burgers come from living animals. Yet every single aspect of an animal's life before it reaches your plate—from the soil that grew its food, to what it ate, to where and how it lived, and even how it died— changes its taste and its impact on your health in tremendous ways. Our relationship with animals that we eat starts long before they reach our plates, and continues long after the meal is done.

Meat is not just meat. When animals eat nutrient-rich plants and live well, they become nourishing food for us. Meat that comes from healthy, responsibly raised animals helps us to fight disease and keep all our parts running the way they should. Grass-fed meat has higher levels of omega-3—the anti-inflammatory fatty acids essential to your skin, gut, immune system, and brain health—than many fish. Cows raised on well-kept pastures contain more micronutrients—like vitamin D and others critical to your health—than grain-fed cows.[1] Grass-fed beef is chock-full of B vitamins, carnitine, and minerals like calcium, magnesium, and potassium; grass-fed lamb delivers additional highly absorbable vitamin E; pastured pork boosts selenium, too.

Not every cow, chicken, sheep, or pig is blessed with these healing properties. Just as farming practices affect soil and plant health, animal husbandry affects the nutritional status of animals. So if you're buying any old chicken or steak, you're likely not optimally benefiting from these foods. In fact, most of the animal products served and sold in this country are actually unhealthy. Not healthy for us to consume directly, and not healthy for the natural world.

When I learned as a teenager how animals are raised for meat, I became a vegetarian until well into my 20s. Eventually I returned to eating meat when pregnant with my first because my body screamed for it—but in the following years, I had to find a way for me, my children, and my patients to eat meat from healthy animals who had died in as humane a way as possible. Finding pastured, conscientiously raised meat (because I only eat kosher meat) turned out to be nearly impossible. I called growers, businesses, and food-to-farm nonprofits, and ultimately I organized a "mindful meat" co-op. I spent hours driving to meet producers who cared for livestock humanely and slaughtered them compassionately. I visited slaughterhouses and observed when the animals were butchered. It was an unexpected crash course in the tough business of raising animals for meat.

Though I no longer run my co-op, I've saved the coveralls I wore while standing on the kill floor. It was an intense and oddly paradoxical experience. As a physician, my life's work is to support life; the entire purpose of the kill floor is to end it. The first time I watched an animal turn from "cattle" to "meat," I couldn't imagine eating it. In the end, I did. As it turned out, eating that meat was unlike any other meal I'd eaten. The steer and I had formed a sacred connection—he had given his life to sustain mine, and I was able to deeply honor his sacrifice and feel gratitude because I had been present for the process. But I also ate less meat as a result of my experience. It became more precious.

It's important to know more about the animals you eat for your own sake and your child's sake. As you will see, it matters—ethically, nutritionally, environmentally, and experientially (i.e., it tastes better). Asking questions before you buy—"Where does the chicken come from?" "What did the pig eat?" "How was the cow slaughtered?"—can be the difference between eating food that nourishes us on all levels and food that damages our bodies, planet, and collective consciousness.

## HEALTHY ANIMALS, HEALTHY HUMANS

Eating animals can be healthy if the animal is raised in a healthy way. Ideally, a pregnant cow births her calf and nurses him for the better part of a year. During that time, the calf will supplement his diet with a grass salad bar—clover, alfalfa, and other diverse native grasses—rotating through a series of pastures to get the most nutrient-dense food possible. Cows that pace the same paddock day after day are not getting the diverse nutrition that they need. Rotating pastures for grazing allows the manure to fertilize the soil, allows the soil to recover, and recharges nutrients and microbes, which enable more diverse grasses and plants to grow. In such a system, the grazed pasture is greener and lusher. And all those vibrant grasses steeped in rich, microbial soil are supercharged with nutrients for that cow, her calf, her milk, and, in turn, us. Moreover, cows' sensory systems help them find what their bodies need. For instance, an animal that has a high demand for sulfur is more likely to eat mustard plants or plants with yellow flowers, which tend to be high in sulfur.[2] That's the innate brilliance of animals and nature!

How can a calf gain well over a thousand pounds just on grasses? Cows (also sheep, buffalo, and goats) are ruminants equipped with multipart stomachs that break down grass with the help of dense populations of microorganisms. Just as with soil—and our own guts—this cow microbiome is critical for turning food into calories and nutrients. Optimally, the ruminant subsists on grass and very little grain. In the winter when grass is scarce, a calf might eat mostly hay (often fermented for improved digestibility and increased sugar availability) with daily treats of grain to help him grow. But on an all-grain diet, the calf's beneficial microbes wane, while not-so-healthy ones thrive.

In simplest terms, animals that eat grass are healthier, which ultimately makes their meat and even fat deeply nourishing for us. I call this the **Rumpelstiltskin Effect,** or **"How Pastured Animals Spin 'Straw' into Gold."** More specifically, grass-fed meats:

- **Have a lower fat content.**[3] They can have the same amount of fat as skinless chicken breast, wild deer, or elk. Lean beef actually lowers so-called bad LDL cholesterol levels. One USDA study compared grass-fed lambs with feedlot lambs fed grain, and found that pastured lambs had 14 percent less fat and 8 percent more protein. (The researchers also mentioned that pastured sheep will "benefit our economy by reducing reliance upon expensive grain supplements.")

- **Have more beneficial fats.** Cattle that eat grass have more omega-3 fatty acids than their grain-fed counterparts in spite of lower overall fat content. And people who eat grass-fed beef have higher levels of omega-3 fatty acids than those who don't. One study in the *British Journal of Nutrition* showed that eating moderate amounts of grass-fed meat for only four weeks boosted levels of omega-3 fatty acids and decreased levels of pro-inflammatory omega-6s. Meanwhile, those who consumed conventional, grain-fed meat ended up with *the opposite ratio*, promoting a pro-inflammatory state.[4] In the appropriate ratio with other essential fats, omega-3 fatty acids lower risks of ADHD, cancer, learning disabilities, and mental illness.
- **Have higher levels of natural trans fats.** Robust science shows that industrial trans fats are absolutely damaging to our health, but natural trans fats from ruminants—like conjugated linolenic acid (CLA) and vaccenic acid (VA)—are actually beneficial.[5] Indeed, CLA is a potent defense against cancer. In laboratory animals, a very small percentage of CLA—a mere 0.1 percent of total calories—greatly reduced tumor growth.[6] Switching from grain-fed to grass-fed meat and dairy products lowered women's risk for breast cancer by *60 percent* compared to those with the lowest level of CLA.[7] You may be able to lower your risk of cancer simply by eating three servings of pastured products daily: an egg; whole-fat milk, yogurt, or cheese; meat or meat fat. You'd have to eat five times that amount of grain-fed meat and dairy products to get the same protection.[8]
- **Have significantly more micronutrients.** Because pastured cows have eaten high amounts of phytochemicals from pasture,[9] they pass along those benefits to us. Necessary nutrients—even fat-soluble vitamins A and E—are uniformly higher in pastured cows than grain-fed, in spite of their lower fat content. The meat from pastured cattle had four times the amount of vitamin E than the meat from feedlot cattle—and almost twice as much as feedlot cows given a vitamin E supplement. Sheep that consumed grass had twice as much lutein—a highly absorbable form of vitamin

E—in their meat than their grain-fed counterparts.[10] Pigs raised on pasture, too, have higher vitamin E and selenium compared with feedlot pigs supplemented with synthetic vitamins.[11]

## THE REAL DIRT ON MEAT

The meat industry has devoted itself to shortening the time from calf to burger, piglet to pork chop, and egg to drumstick to increase profit. Instead of raising animals well, they force us to sacrifice our physical health, environmental health, and compassion in favor of their financial health.

By six months of age, a calf born into a concentrated animal feeding operation (CAFO)—where more than 50 billion food animals are raised and slaughtered each year[12]—joins the one hundred thousand steer crammed into tiny stalls with open sewers and a stench that travels for miles. A calf has 14 months to reach 1,300 pounds, the ideal weight for slaughter. That's not much time—and not even close to how nature works—so he needs help. He's primarily fed corn, which is compact, portable, has a long shelf life, and is one of our country's largest subsidized crops (our tax dollars go to help big agriculture grow corn; it's now cheaper to buy corn than it is to grow it). Corn (usually GMO) is also calorie-dense, but growing it uses a lot of energy because it uses tons of fertilizers, pesticides, and 1.2 gallons of oil for every bushel. Cattle are also fed gallons of liquefied fat (sourced from slaughterhouse refuse, including other cattle) and protein supplements in cattle-feed "milkshakes," delivered by tanker trucks, along with liquid vitamins, synthetic estrogen, corn "enhanced" with protein (usually GMO soy), and drugs (including regular doses of antibiotics and growth hormones). A calf may receive some dried alfalfa and hay for roughage, "feather meal"—ground-up chickens, bones, feathers, and all, including some manure—and old bakery goods, candy, and chewing gum with the wrappers still on. If you don't believe me, check out the study showing that chewing gum could comprise *30 percent* of a cow's diet "without obvious ill effects."[13] After all, sugar is just sugar and all carbohydrates are created equal, right?

There's just one problem: Cows aren't built to eat corn or grain or chewing gum. Though consumers have grown to like and even expect the fat marbling of corn-fed meat, the result is an unhealthy animal, and in turn, an unhealthy human. Research suggests that many of the health problems associated with eating meat are really problems associated with eating sick animals fed corn and other grains. Most studies investigating the impact of red meat on our health use grain-fed, CAFO-raised meat. Just as ruminants have not evolved to eat grain, humans have not adapted to eating grain-fed animals.

## GMOs: Bad for Animals?

For three years, a Danish pig farmer fed his pigs ordinary, non–genetically modified soy. When he ran out, he bought the less expensive GM soy. His herdsmen didn't know anything had changed, but they immediately noticed that the pigs lost their appetites and the piglets developed diarrhea. Worse, more and more pigs began to be born with birth defects—one missing an ear, one with a large hole in its skull, a female born with testes. To understand why this was happening, the farmer euthanized 38 of the deformed pigs and had them tested for glyphosate, the herbicide used in Roundup. The samples of lung, liver, kidney, brain, gut wall, heart, and muscle all tested highly positive.[14] This is just the story of one farmer. Other such stories exist, as does a growing body of concerning research.[15,16,17,18,19] Further rigorous research must be done to evaluate the impact of GMOs and toxic contaminants on livestock health, and how that translates to human health.

Cows fed too much grain or corn develop illnesses like "feedlot bloat." The rumen—which in a healthy animal is filled with microbes to ferment grasses—usually produces copious amounts of gas, normally expelled by belching. But a diet with too much starch and too little roughage traps gas. The rumen inflates like a balloon, pressing against the animal's lungs. Unless a worker relieves the pressure (usually by forcing a hose down the animal's esophagus), the cow suffocates.

Corn-fed cattle can also develop an unnaturally acidic—rather than pH neutral—rumen. Though this condition can be fatal, the cow more commonly experiences diarrhea, ulcers, bloat, liver disease, and weakened immunity, leaving the animal vulnerable to diseases ranging from pneumonia to feedlot polio. As acids eat away at the rumen wall, bacteria enter the bloodstream and collect in the liver, which becomes abscessed. Many feedlot cattle have abscessed livers at slaughter.

The major reason that feedlot animals don't die under these conditions is because they are given copious doses of antibiotics. *More than two thirds of all antibiotics sold in America are used in animal feed.* This practice has led directly to the evolution of antibiotic-resistant "superbugs." As a pediatrician, I was taught to scold parents who asked to treat their children's viruses with antibiotics, warning them of antibiotic-resistant bacteria. Yet livestock ingest 80 percent of the antibiotics sold in the United States to preempt illness, without a word from the powers that be.

As a result, nearly half the meat and poultry sold in the United States is likely to be contaminated by highly dangerous microbes of our own making. A recent study estimated that 47 percent of meat and poultry on U.S. supermarket shelves contains the bacteria *Staphylococcus aureus*, which is not one of the four bacteria—*Salmonella, Campylobacter, E. coli,* and *Enterococcus*—the U.S. government routinely tests for in meat.[20] In 136 samples from 80 brands of beef, pork, chicken, and turkey purchased from 26 grocery stores in five major U.S. cities, DNA tests from staph-infected samples suggest that the farm animals themselves were the major source of contamination. The report states that "densely stocked industrial farms, where food animals are steadily fed low doses of antibiotics . . . [are] ideal breeding grounds for drug-resistant bacteria that move from animals to humans." These bacteria are linked to a number of human diseases and are also resistant to at least three classes of antibiotics. Indeed, a 2013 report by the CDC found that more than two million Americans a year develop bacterial infections resistant to antibiotics, which kill at least 23,000 annually.[21]

These drugs are also linked to the obesity epidemic and obesity-related diseases. Within seven weeks, mice regularly subjected to low doses of antibiotics—like cows, pigs, and chickens on CAFOs—had shifted microbial composition in their guts and had gained 10 to 15 percent more fat mass than controls.[22] Antibiotics administered to livestock—and passed on to us—target bacteria that digest carbohydrates that we otherwise couldn't digest. (Carb sensitivity, anyone?)

The newly acidic digestive tract of feedlot cows has fostered acid-resistant strains of *E. coli* (like the deadly 0157) that survive our stomach acids—and can kill us. By acidifying a cow's gut with corn, we've disrupted one of our food chain's major barriers to infection. One study showed that one of three cattle is contaminated with these acid-resistant *E. coli*, but grass-fed animals had so few acid-resistant bacteria that the number didn't even register. Simply switching a cow's diet from corn to hay in the days before slaughter could reduce the *E. coli* 0157 in manure by as much as 70 percent, but most CAFOs won't voluntarily risk their bottom line in this way just to improve public health.

The industry instead focuses on *disinfecting* the manure that will inevitably find its way into meat, rather than altering the animals' diet, preventing them from standing day and night in their own contaminated waste or even slowing the rapid speed of the industrial kill floor to prevent that waste from splashing the meat. Instead, the industry uses irradiation (or as they say "cold pasteurization") that passes carcasses through a hot steam cabinet and finally sprays them with an antimicrobial solution before they're hung in a cooler.

The same goes for chicken. The European Union takes issue with the standard U.S. practice of washing poultry carcasses in chlorinated water to kill bacteria. It has banned the import of all U.S. poultry since 1997 because it's not convinced that it's safe to ingest the chlorine that remains on the meat, not to mention concerns that it masks unclean processing of animals. E.U. agriculture ministers repeatedly have voted to continue the ban despite aggressive pressure from the United States, concluding it would "threaten the community's entire set of food production standards."[23]

And as recently as 2013, chickens, turkeys, and pigs were administered arsenic-containing drugs to prevent disease and promote growth.[24] The FDA finally tested one hundred chickens who had been administered the drug and found arsenic levels in all of their livers. Their arsenic-laced manure subsequently was used as fertilizer, which contaminated other food, like rice and apples! After decades of data showing that arsenic is toxic, the FDA finally banned three out of four of these commonly used drugs. (The last, Nitarsone, is still used in turkeys.)

Lastly, consider that growth hormones are also administered to factory-farmed animals in the United States. Each calf receives a synthetic estrogen implant behind its ear to enhance growth by 40 to 50 extra pounds. This is banned in the European Union, but American regulatory agencies permit hormone implants because "no risk to human health has been proven yet," even though they admit measurable residues do turn up in the meat (especially the fat) we eat.[25] Pigs, too, may receive hormones—not for growth, but to regulate fertility and sometimes induce abortion.[26] These contribute to the buildup of estrogenic compounds in the environment, which some scientists believe contributes to falling sperm counts in boys and premature maturation in girls. Industry and regulatory agencies say that many of these hormones are naturally found in our bodies. However, the relationship between our bodies and sex hormones we ourselves produce is tightly orchestrated; minute differences in these levels can have a tremendous health impact—especially during fetal development, childhood, and adolescence. Moreover, recent studies have found persistent levels of synthetic growth hormones in feedlot waste, which eventually wind up in the waterways downstream of feedlots where fish exhibit abnormal sex characteristics.

## A Happy Meal

Aside from the ethical dilemmas of eating mistreated animals, meat from stressed or sick animals doesn't taste as good as humanely raised meat. When cattle go to slaughter, they may have a long, cramped ride from the farm and may be kept for days in an uncomfortable lot with stressful sounds, sights, and smells, without food or drink. Their trip to the slaughter floor may be frightening. Even industry knows a deeply stressed animal will have tough "dark meat" due to surges of adrenaline and cortisol in its system. We eat these elevated stress hormones from slaughter when we eat its meat, literally ingesting its stress.[27]

Humans inhabit the same hormonal, microbial, and spiritual terrain as the animals we eat. What we do to them, we do to ourselves. What they become, we become. Whether we consciously know it, what happens to them also happens to us. We incorporate our ethics into our bodies and our children's bodies. When an animal lives and dies horribly, we taste it. When it lives and dies peacefully, we taste that, too. By restricting yourself to eating animals that have been raised humanely and treated well from the beginning to the end of life, you are supporting not just a compassionate and healthier system for animals, but healthier children.

It doesn't have to be this way. We can reduce this pressure on our fellow creatures, our planet, and our consciousness. We can put a stop to an industrialized, fossil fuel–driven method of raising animals and return them to their natural place. Ruminants need little more to survive and thrive than mineral-dense wild forage in rich soil; clean, fresh water; sunshine; and protection in extreme weather. It's the ultimate solar-powered system. Animals transport themselves to the tastiest, best grass. They don't need super-size GMO smoothies or antibiotics. Healthy ruminant manure *is* the ideal fertilizer, resulting in naturally enriched soil that grows healthy, nutrient-dense plants. Everything they need is right at their feet (or hooves).

## Meat: A Buyer's Guide

Because almost all ruminants start on grass, anyone can label meat "grass-fed." Words like "natural," "free-range," "grass-fed," or "fresh" are used to mislead consumers. CAFO producers are always hoping to grab part of the market of people looking for healthy, ethically raised meat, so their misleading labels are designed to gloss over the other 99 percent of the picture. The healthiest cows, lambs, or goats have been fed minimal or no grain, as in less than 10 percent during winter months. But ruminants should eat minimal wheat, corn, soy, barley, and absolutely no animal by-products. To learn more about different certification standards, check out *Consumer Reports*'s www.greener choices.org/eco-labels.

Here are the kinds of words to look for on labels:

**100% grass-fed**
**Grass-fed and finished**
**100% pastured**
**Pasture-fed and finished**

Ultimately, look for the meaningful **FoodAlliance.org** certification, which ascertains that the producer raises animals to the health and humane standards outlined here.

NOTE: Chicken and pigs are omnivores. While they may eat a variety of other foods, they should spend time foraging in pasture and dirt—so knowing they are pastured is just as important, along with USDA organic certification for their feed.

## Certified Humane

The Certified Humane label means that the farms raising the animals for meat, eggs, or dairy met the Humane Farm Animal Care program's standards, which aim to improve humane living conditions and humane treatment during transportation and slaughter. Certified Humane standards also require prudent antibiotic use and prohibit artificial growth hormones and animal by-products in animal feed. They do permit beak trimming and filing the teeth of piglets. Also, the label does not mean that chickens and pigs go outdoors, or that beef cattle and dairy cows have continuous access to pasture for grazing.

## Organic

One hundred percent grass-finished animals may not need an organic certification if they consume only forage, aren't treated with antibiotics, and the fields are not treated with herbicides or chemical fertilizers. On the other hand, "organic" does *not* mean that the animal lived outside or on pasture, or that it had an opportunity to forage. It does not mean that the animals lived in a herd and were able to have natural social interactions, and it does not mean that the animals weren't unduly stressed. But it does mean that its feed was free of pesticides, chemicals, hormones, and antibiotics. Sometimes pigs or chickens given opportunities to forage may not earn an organic label because the farmer couldn't afford to meet all the requirements of organic. Demeter Biodynamic is among the highest standards of certification, including organic, humane treatment, and soil and land stewardship.

Your best bet is to know your producer. Ask questions—don't assume that images of pastured animals mean that the animals don't spend the last few months of their lives in feedlots eating GM feed. In all cases, misleading labels become less relevant when you're certifying the meat yourself! Buying in bulk—and stashing extra in the freezer—minimizes trips to the farm/market and usually means you pay less by eliminating the middleman. Some farms offer a CSA meat share, and sometimes people share a large animal, splitting a pig, lamb, or cow two, four, or more ways. I strongly encourage taking at least one trip to visit your producer's farm (arrange it in advance—don't just show up and interrupt farmers' busy routines!).

## A Note on Cost

There's no denying it: Industrial meat is cheaper than grass-fed meat. But this is largely because the U.S. government subsidizes this system with our tax dollars. Moreover, what is at face value less expensive comes at a huge cost to individual health and public health. The price doesn't account for food poisoning by *E. coli,* antibiotic resistance, environmental costs of industrial farming, or chronic illnesses that result from grain-fed meats or their pesticide and hormonal residues. In the end, it's not less expensive. **We only pay a small part of the real price of this meat at the store; we pay the rest through our taxes and sick care.**

There is an old saying, **"Pay the farmer now, or pay the doctor later."** You get a lot more for your money with grass-fed beef. Not only are you voting with your wallet for ethical and humane practices, but you are better nourished by every part of the animal, from meat to fat to bone, putting money in your body's proverbial bank account. And grass-fed beef has lower water content than factory-farmed meat, therefore it shrinks less when cooked and browns more deeply and flavorfully. Many people find that it actually takes less grass-fed meat to satisfy their appetite.

Another way to lower cost is through "meatless Mondays." This movement aims to lower meat consumption overall *and* to get us off of the destructive treadmill of industrial meat. I support eating less meat, as a way to eliminate both the demand for CAFO meat and the resulting health and environmental impact. To that end, remember meat need not be the centerpiece of every nighttime meal—try reimagining dinners with vegetables as the centerpiece and meat on the side. It can still be filling and exceptionally delicious. Less is more.

## YOU Make a Difference

Antibiotic-free beef, pork, and chicken accounted for only 5 percent of the meat sold in the United States five years ago, but that's been quickly changing. In 2013, sales of antibiotic-free chicken alone rose 34 percent, for example, and producers took notice. In response to consumer demand, some of the largest producers have begun amending their practices. Companies like Tyson, Perdue, and Cargill are phasing out the use of antibiotics and cramped "gestation stalls" for pregnant sows (albeit slowly). **Are they doing it because the FDA demanded they stop? No! It's because people like you are sending a strong message: with dollars and cents.**

# TAKE HOME

1. The animals you eat should graze outdoors on pasture (except in coldest winter), with sources of shade in the summer, in places where land is cared for, and should be fed non-GMO, organic feed when needed.

2. Meat that's certified organic or biodynamic and 100 percent pasture-raised reduces your child's exposure to hormones, antibiotics, pesticides, arsenic, and other additives used in factory farming. NOTE: Organic alone doesn't always mean pasture-fed or that animals are treated humanely.

3. Use all parts of pastured animals for food: meat, fat, cartilage, and bones for broth, and in some animals, skin. Eating organ meats like liver and pancreas (or giblets in chicken) offer the densest nutrition of any part of the animal. Baking chicken skin renders fat for future use, and leaves a crispy snack that kids love. Nose-to-tail cooking, as it's called, is more economical and sustainable as well as delicious and healthy. To me, it also honors the animal's sacrifice to use every part so nothing is wasted.

4. Cook grass-fed steaks or burgers at high temperature only *briefly* so they won't dry out. A tenderizing tool can help. Note that high-heat cooking and charring of meat (or fish) lead to the production of heterocyclic amines (HCAs) that can cause cancer. Quickly grill or broil thinner cuts to remain bright pink/red on the inside, but keep it as a treat.

5. Slow cooking larger roasts and tougher cuts at low temperatures renders them tender and flavorful *and* is the healthiest way to eat meat.

6. Consider Meatless Mondays: Eat less meat each week in exchange for making the meat you eat the highest quality.

## CHAPTER II
# Milk: Pasture-ization over Pasteurization

A mong my friends, I am notorious for imposing travel adventures upon my family that involve finding foods typically unavailable to city dwellers. My quest for raw milk ranks high on that list. Over the course of my journeys, I was startled to discover that many dairy farmers don't drink pasteurized milk from the supermarket, even when the commercial milk includes their own product. Almost uniformly, the farmers I've met prefer their milk fresh and raw. One farmer told me that milk from the store "just doesn't taste good." Another said that she can only tolerate fresh milk from her goats or she experiences severe digestive symptoms.

Farmers sell what the market demands so that they can support themselves—a challenge even in fat times. But farmers have one dependable luxury that city and suburban dwellers alike lack: They can eat all the fresh food they like, exactly as they like it.

I visited a grassy dairy farm in Vermont right after raw milk became legal there in 2014. When I asked to buy pastured raw milk, the farmer explained that all of their milk went to a cooperative that pasteurized it to make ice cream. She was afraid to sell her milk raw. "*One* bad batch anywhere," she said, "means that *all* Vermont milk will get a bad rap and we lose business." I asked her whether she boiled her own milk. She looked at me like I was crazy. "Of course not," she answered. "We drink it raw."

After some serious searching, I tracked down raw milk sold by a certified farm in upstate New York. Certified, in this case, means that New York State requires frequent microbiology checks for various bacteria. If the milk is free of measurable amounts, the farm's milk remains certified. Even with certification, however, state law made it illegal to sell this raw milk anywhere but on the premises of the farm itself. This wrinkle required us to drive more than two hours to obtain the milk.

At the farm store, we bought milk plus cream and plenty of butter. I immediately noticed the deep yellow cast of the creamline milk. That thrilling, golden color reflects rich fats derived from feeding on pasture, as if the cows capture the very sunlight in their milk. Unlike most doctors, I value the fat in pastured milk, both for the taste and the many health benefits. The creamy texture and rich flavor of this milk were heavenly and sated everyone's appetite for hours more than usual. Despite what I'd heard about raw milk staying fresh for less time compared to pasteurized, our unopened half gallons stayed delicious for at least two weeks. One thing was for certain: This milk was far more interesting than the bland stuff I had grown up drinking.

My delight in this new yet ancient food led me to look more deeply into its long and fraught history. Though my intentions were innocent, my trip upstate had not been merely a foodie journey, but a political act. Worry over bacterial contamination had made drinking raw milk controversial. As a result, it's regulated state-by-state. Even so, the dairy industry's lobbying has made raw milk illegal in some states, with only a few states that allow stores to sell even certified raw milk. Raw milk can't cross state lines. You'd think for all the regulations that this liquid was far more illicit than milk.

## FERMENTED MILK: A TRADITIONAL FOOD TEEMING WITH BACTERIA

The debate about bacteria in milk is a modern phenomenon. Before the 1800s, children breast-fed for several years and then consumed milk fermented by bacteria, soured into a yogurtlike beverage called clabbered milk—referred to simply as "milk." The "fresh" milk that we now consider an essential staple for every child was available mainly to those on farms. Along with butter and fresh cheeses, most Americans consumed milk in cultured form, whether clabbered milk, buttermilk, cheeses, or yogurt. Traditional cultures from North Africa to Asia to Europe have long drunk fermented milk in the form of kefir and yogurt, whether from cows, goats, sheep, water buffalo, mares, llamas, reindeer, yaks, camels, or other animals. Drinking fermented milk is highly practical; cultured products are less perishable, highly digestible, and incredibly nutritious. Yogurt and soft cheeses lasted weeks at cellar temperatures, and cultured butter and hard cheeses could last months. Milk products from high-yield, warmer seasons could be enjoyed when production dropped during the colder months; they teemed with bacteria as well as beneficial fats to promote immunity.

Unaltered milk directly from the cow naturally contains diverse bacteria, fats, and enzymes that enable fermentation. Microbial life feeds off lactose and produces lactic acid as a fermentation by-product, causing sweet milk to become sour. While unaltered milk sours with time, pasteurized milk putrefies. The former is delicious and chock-full of health benefits; the latter not so much. The souring of milk gives it a yogurtlike consistency which then separates into semisolid curd and liquid whey. And the lactic acid produced as milk sours naturally inhibits putrefying bacteria and simultaneously facilitates growth of diverse health-promoting bacteria. These bacteria continue beneficial work begun by similar components found in breast milk.

Fermented foods like yogurt, kefir, and cultured butter maintain our microbiome by constantly boosting healthy bacteria. Indeed, fermented dairy has been shown to prevent illnesses in everyone from children to the elderly.[1] In 1908, Nobel Prize winner Ilya Metchnikoff described the longevity of the people living in Bulgaria, ascribing it to the regular consumption of fermented dairy products containing the Bulgarian strain of bacteria (including *Streptococcus bulgaricus*). In fact, three cultures with populations that regularly live into extreme old age—Hunza in the Himalayas, Vilcabamba in Ecuador, and Caucasian Georgia—all depend upon a diet of fermented dairy derived from pasture-fed animals. Moreover, those lush pastures are themselves fed by mineral-rich water from glacier runoff in all three cases. This incredible synchronicity between water, soil, plants, animals, microbes, and humans is what truly makes these people so healthy. Everything that we eat must be rich with nutrients and minerals—all the way down to the water sources that feed the soil that grow the grass that feed the cows that give the milk that we drink. Healthy outer terrain begets healthy inner terrain.

## THE REAL DIRT ON MODERN MILK

Sadly, most dairy cows in the United States live in a manner far less idyllic. They are confined to cramped pens so small they can't even turn around, without sun or fresh air, and fed everything but the pasture they're meant to eat—much like their hamburger-bound brethren. Not surprisingly, these cows tend to be sick. Their milk production is lower and they die more readily, not to mention sick cows are more likely to produce contaminated milk. Because all of this is bad for business, confinement cows are fed daily rations of prophylactic antibiotics. The daily antibiotics further destroy the microbacteria in their already ravaged digestive systems, so their health only worsens.

The milk we drink is supposed to be free of antibiotics, but testers disclose (quietly) that milk that routinely fails is still given a passing grade . . . which is bad news for our microbiome.

This overcrowded way of raising dairy cows—which began around the Industrial Revolution—brought about the introduction of pasteurization. As rural families moved to cities in the 1800s, demand for the fresh milk they'd been drinking on their farms increased. Dairy cows were moved to cities, but were kept in abhorrent conditions—fed whiskey by-products, tied to one spot for their entire, short lives, mired in their own excrement. The sick cows made sick milk, which in turn led to a tremendous number of deaths of babies and children. Infant mortality skyrocketed as distillery dairies became widely established.[2]

Rather than shut down these profitable "swill dairies," which were owned by influential men, public health advocates were forced to allow continued production of this sick, nutritionally deficient milk—with a caveat. Department store magnate and philanthropist Nathan Strauss promoted Louis Pasteur's new discovery based in germ theory: pasteurizing or heating milk to kill any and all bacteria. Nobody yet recognized that bacteria could be beneficial and was not all harmful. So pasteurization was implemented widely, decimating both bacteria resulting from the filth of swill dairies along with the necessary spectrum of diverse bacteria innately found in milk.

Public health advocates subjected certified "country milk" (i.e., unpasteurized milk from pasture) to far stricter standards than industrial milk, with so-called medical milk commissions regulating the number of bacteria allowed in milk. But doctors, especially pediatricians, argued passionately that certified farm milk offered health benefits and should continue to be available. Despite ongoing demand, many small- and medium-size raw milk dairy farmers went out of business. It was either get big or get out: Dairy farms were growing larger and required expensive equipment—electric milking machines, sterile bottling machines, refrigerated bulk tanks—to ship to cities.

As scientists learned that newly identified microscopic bacteria could lead to deadly infections, public health officials and physicians began to believe that fermented foods eaten for centuries, like kefir and sourdough bread, were forms of dangerous bacterial contamination. Bacteria were "bad" and sterile was "best," and the practice of pasteurization endured.

Even as our knowledge of microbes becomes more complex and nuanced, surprisingly little has changed. Still today, the practice of pasteurization remains "necessary" as a way to mask the large numbers of sick cows kept in overcrowded conditions, subject to illness and infections like bovine tuberculosis.[3] The larger the dairy is, the higher the risk. But the question is, do we really want to drink that milk in the first place? Even "discard milk" taken from cows sick with infection, is pasteurized and used as an "economical alternative" to milk replacer for calves at dairy farms.[4] **Pasteurization doesn't improve the quality of the milk; it masks how sick the milk really is.**

Pasteurization is like yanking out your gorgeous flower garden to get rid of the bees. Pasteurizing milk enables inhumane and unhealthy practices in animal husbandry while decimating microbial content, altering proteins, and inactivating necessary enzyme activity. While it's true that in rare cases, milk even from healthy cows can contain bacteria that may render some vulnerable people ill, producers can test for the presence of such microbes on a batch-by-batch basis to prevent consumer exposure to potentially problematic strains. And certified raw milk will always be tested regularly. **Paradoxically, the presence of diverse bacteria and active enzymes from raw milk—rather than their absence—protects milk from overgrowth of nasty bacterial strains.** When in balance, most so-called germs actually bolster our health.

Science verifies the value of raw milk, not just for its microbial content but its whey protein structure when unaltered by pasteurization. A 2011 article published in the *Journal of Allergy and Clinical Immunology* reported that children who drank raw farm milk had fewer cases of asthma, allergies, and hay fever.[5] A 2015 study that followed almost one thousand mothers and infants who drank "unboiled" milk over their first year of life showed they had a 30 percent lower prevalence of fever, ear infections, and respiratory infections, as well as lower blood inflammatory markers.[6,7] In their unaltered forms, milk's diverse microbes, fats, and proteins like whey changed these children's gene expression of innate immunity[8] to produce protective effects that staved off the development of childhood allergies or severe infections.[9] You read that correctly—raw milk transformed the children's epigenetics. NOTE: No children were harmed in the making of these studies.

The health of the cow and its living conditions indisputably play significant roles in the quality of the resulting milk. Yet the FDA has long taken the stance that regardless of the source, raw milk is inherently unsafe. Further, its website, entitled "The Dangers of Raw Milk," states (with no scientific references cited) that "research shows no meaningful difference in the nutritional values of pasteurized and unpasteurized milk."[10] This claim, however, is misleading. If its measure of "nutritional values" includes only protein, fat, and carbohydrate content, perhaps there is no meaningful nutritional difference. But as you now know, nutrition is far more complex than the quantity of macronutrients. It includes the quality: structure of proteins, activity level of enzymes, and diversity of beneficial bacteria, which is unquestionably less in pasteurized milk. Consider that both the American Academy of Pediatrics and the Centers for Disease Control and Prevention advise that excessive heating of breast milk detracts from its nutrition, and they recommend against it.[11] **Would human breast milk confer its many robust health benefits if we insisted that it be boiled before babies drank it? From all we're learning about raw milk, the answer is likely no.**

Unsurprisingly, pasteurization has led to other unanticipated problems. While raw or low-heat milk has a thick, creamy layer that rises to the top, ultrapasteurized milk is far thinner. So the dairy industry adds guar gum, carrageenan, polysorbate 80, and mono- and diglycerides, some of which have been implicated as risk factors for obesity, metabolic syndrome, or inflammatory bowel disease.[12] **The artificial chemicals are only necessary to poorly imitate something that was perfect beforehand.** But industry can't come close to approximating raw milk's health benefits; indeed, its version damages our health.

Ultrapasteurized milk can't even be used to produce cheese. Cheesemakers find that ultrapasteurization renders useless the endogenous enzymes in milk essential to the cheese-making process. If it cannot be used to make cheese, what else is different about that milk? When traditional techniques of food preparation used for millennia are no longer possible because of human intervention, it implies that our interventions have changed food in "meaningful" ways.

You might well ask the FDA where to find its webpage entitled "The Risks of Industrialized Milk," which could explain how pasteurized, homogenized milk from CAFO-raised cows is processed with additives, hormones, traces of antibiotics, pesticides, herbicides, and other contaminants. It also could explain how such milk plays a role in triggering or exacerbating many chronic illnesses children endure: eczema, inflammatory bowel disease, chronic ear infections, asthma, seizures, ADHD, and others.[13,14,15,16] Consider dropping them a note.

> ### There's a Nanoparticle in My Milk
>
> With the rapid emergence of nanotechnology—i.e., the ability to break down common substances into tiny particles and add them to things like textiles (like nano-size silver added to socks for odor control)—agribusiness is adding these tiny particles to our food. Disturbingly, large dairy producers use nano-size titanium dioxide to whiten products like yogurt and soy milk. The FDA acknowledges that these particles may pose big risks but has done nothing to curtail their use in the food supply.[17]

## DOES MILK REALLY DO A BODY GOOD?

Let's debunk a few longstanding myths about milk:

- **Industrial milk is not a natural source of vast amounts of fat-soluble vitamin D.** Our government mandates that milk be fortified with synthetic vitamin D to prevent rickets. Beware of anything fortified! It means that synthetic, often low-quality and less bioavailable vitamins have been added to your food. Commercial milk is almost always fortified with vitamin $D_2$, which may actually inhibit activation of the vitamin D receptor and limit potential health benefits.[18] In order for milk to naturally provide quality vitamin D, the cows would need to live outdoors in sunshine, consume pasture, and retain their full fat (since vitamin D is found in milk fat). Look for full-fat milk, cream, or butter from 100 percent pasture-fed cows.
- **Milk is far from the only source of calcium.** A cow's milk is only as mineral dense as the terrain she grazed, from water to soil to plants. If not fed high-quality pasture, most cows don't consume balanced and diverse minerals. Foods like sardines, some nuts and seeds, bone broths, sesame seeds and tahini, blackstrap molasses, kale, collards, spinach, and turnip or mustard greens all provide greater calcium content per serving

than conventional cow's milk. And when children eat smaller amounts of different nutrient-dense foods, they need not rely on any one food as their only source of a nutrient.

- **Don't fear the fat in your pastured milk.** Many of the beneficial compounds—and delicious flavor—in milk reside primarily in the pastured milk fat and cream along with fat-soluble vitamin A and D. Cows that live outdoors and graze on pasture produce milk rich with healthy fats including CLAs,[19] which paradoxically reduce risk of obesity, diabetes, cancer, and inflammatory bowel disease,[20] and enhance gut, immune, and brain health.[21] Fats actually curb your appetite by triggering the release of the hormone cholecystokinin, which causes fullness. Fats also slow the release of sugar into your bloodstream, ultimately reducing the amount that's stored as fat. In other words, the more fat in your milk, the less fat around your middle.

  Low-fat milk, on the other hand, might actually make you fatter than if you drank whole. A large study from the Harvard School of Public Health observed weight and milk consumption of 12,829 kids ages 9 to 14 across the country. "Contrary to our hypothesis," they reported, "skim and 1 percent milk were associated with weight gain, but dairy fat was not."[22]

- **Drinking skim and low-fat milk may not be as good for cholesterol levels as you think.** Most people don't regard skim or low-fat milk as a processed food, but consider: To standardize fat content, all fat is first removed. The resulting bluish, chalky "skim milk" is then fortified with powdered milk to appear white and add back the desired "percent milk fat." Powdered milk (also added to organic low-fat milks and baby formula) results from spraying the liquid under heat and high pressure. This oxidizes cholesterol,[23] which triggers a host of biological changes, from plaque formation in arteries to heart disease to an increased risk of developing cancer and genetic mutations.[24] Though oxidized cholesterol levels vary, it's impossible to say how much could be harmful to any given child.

- **Even whole milk is not whole.** "Whole milk," too, often has fat removed and replaced, as it's a regulation 3.5 percent, rather than roughly 8.5 percent milk fat found naturally in "udder milk." The rest goes to more lucrative butter, ice cream, and other value-added products. Unhomogenized milk bought directly from farmers will offer full health benefits—and is worth the effort.

Ultimately, real milk is a whole food. Cows do not produce skim and low-fat milks; such products are man-made, aided by machines that remove the cream with all of its nutritional benefits, and add it back in standardized amounts to create nonfat, reduced-fat, or "whole" milk.

## rBGH

Industrial dairy cows live in confinement facilities and their calves are taken away at birth. These mothers, after being separated from their babies, exhibit depressed, anxious behaviors that discourage milk production. So they're given ongoing doses of hormones like Monsanto's rBGH (recombinant bovine growth hormone) to maintain milk production. The hormones fed to these cows end up in the milk we drink.

The safety of rBGH has been controversial. Onset of puberty has gotten so much earlier during the last two decades—as many as two years earlier—that the American Academy of Pediatrics actually adjusted the lower limit of "normal" for puberty to seven for girls and nine for boys.[25] And if the child is African-American, it's considered "within normal limits" to enter puberty a year earlier than that. Yes, it's officially okay for an African-American girl to develop breasts and pubic hair at *six years old*. This problem has become so widespread that we've actually created a new normal.

What might be behind this extreme change? One reason floated is *better nutrition*. Yes, really. I take issue with the idea that childhood nutrition—pumped up on processed foods as it is—is better now than it was 30 years ago. Moreover, nourished children's bodies still shouldn't prepare to make babies at six years of age. Increased obesity also has been investigated as a cause, as have plastics and increased consumption of soy phytoestrogens (because of the high amounts of soy not only in processed and restaurant foods but also in animal feed).[26]

A very worrisome—and likely—contributor is that rBGH, a synthetic estrogenic hormone that has become ubiquitous in our milk supply. Milk naturally contains estrogenic hormones—another reason why drinking more than one to two glasses a day is inadvisable, particularly during puberty, when hormones rage. Yet industry justifies adding synthetic hormones to milk (and yogurt, ice cream, and other dairy products) as being "no more than that which is naturally in milk." Synthetic hormones behave differently in our bodies than endogenous ones. And even if true, then they've *doubled* the estrogenic hormones!

The revolving door between our government and Monsanto allowed rBGH to happen. For the FDA to determine whether Monsanto's rBGH was safe, Monsanto was required to submit a scientific report. Margaret Miller, one of Monsanto's researchers, assembled the report. Shortly before the report was submitted, Miller left Monsanto and was hired by the FDA. Her first job for the FDA was to determine whether to approve the report she herself wrote for Monsanto. In a sense, Monsanto approved its own report. Deciding whether rBGH-derived milk must be labeled fell under the jurisdiction of another FDA official, Michael Taylor, who previously worked as a lawyer for a firm representing Monsanto. No labeling was required. "Monsanto should not have to vouchsafe the safety of biotech food. Our interest is in selling as much of it as possible. Assuring its safety is the FDA's job," said Phil Angell, Monsanto's director of corporate communications, without any hint of irony.[27]

### How Should You Drink Milk, if You Drink Milk?

Milk may not be for everybody. I see many children who are sicker when consuming commercial dairy products than when not. I don't recommend you consume industrially produced milk—ever—but unaltered milk products can have powerful health benefits for those who tolerate dairy. Many of the health problems we face today are iatrogenic, that is, man-made. Data suggest that these problems have more to do with what has been done to "improve" milk rather than the milk itself.

Milk that's good for you comes from cows that consume foods

that nature intended, in the environment that nature intended: grazing on choice pasture outdoors, with perhaps a treat of GMO-free grain. Healthy animals make healthy milk, and the milk you drink should be as close to "udder milk" as possible. In short, **I promote "PASTURE-IZATION" OVER PASTEURIZATION.**

You can't just expect milk to be healthy, delicious, and safe—you must demand it. If large dairies can't provide unaltered, nourishing milk, you must seek and support small dairies that will. If necessary, simply stop drinking milk. As consumers, your voice, vote, and food dollars create change.

## Does Breed of Cow Matter?

Cow's milk contains six proteins, one of which, A2 beta-casein, underwent a natural mutation in European dairy herds that changed the type of beta-casein in their milk. European breeds like Holsteins and Friesians began producing an A1 version, which is found in most milk in northern Europe and America. Unlike A2, A1 beta-casein tends to be digested in our bodies into an opiate fragment called BCM7, which can trigger significant inflammation in vulnerable individuals and is associated with an increased risk of developing autoimmune disease, heart disease, diabetes, autism, and even schizophrenia. New Zealand milk has converted almost entirely to A2 milk for this reason, and this milk is now becoming available in the United States. Jerseys, Guernseys, and Normandes, as well as African and Asian breeds, produce the more desirable A2 milk.[28]

Here's what to seek in milk:

1. **Pastured:** Check the label for "100% grass-fed" or "pasture-raised." A humane certification is ideal, too.
2. **Full fat:** Fat in milk from pastured cows is healthy in moderate amounts. The cream contains conjugated linolenic acids, immune

factors, and fat-soluble vitamins. It's a case of something delicious actually being good for you!

3. **Unhomogenized:** It's widely available; just look for the cream-line. Skim the cream from the top or gently shake the bottle, depending on whether you prefer milk creamier or slightly less so. Don't forget to eat the skimmed cream with fruit or in oatmeal, or use it to make butter, crème fraîche, or other delicious options.

4. **Unpasteurized:** Enjoy the flavor and health benefits of *certified* raw milk that you're missing in pasteurized milk. Find a certified farm near you, or on www.realmilk.com. Or raise your own goat or dwarf cow. It's way easier than you might imagine! Never drink ultrapasteurized or ultraheat treatment (UHT) milk.

5. **Fermented:** Yogurt, kefir, fermented sour cream, crème fraîche, and other traditional foods feed your gut, boost immunity, and are associated with longevity. Fermented proteins are easier to digest because their bacteria do much of the work for us. You may tolerate fermented dairy even if fresh milk bothers you.

## Milk at a Glance

*Certified organic milk*

This milk does not contain pesticides. The cows must consume only organic, non-GMO feed and cannot be treated with antibiotics or hormones. However, cows that produce certified organic milk may or may not live in humane conditions or be raised outdoors on pasture. Confirm by reading labels carefully, calling the company directly, and looking for certification from Food Alliance or American Grassfed.

*Certified raw milk*

This milk is not pasteurized and is typically unhomogenized. It contains unaltered protein plus healthy fats, immune factors, enzymes, and diverse bacteria unaltered by heat. Some people briefly heat their milk to a very low boil to make traditional treats. Can be used to make kefir, yogurt, cheeses, and sour creams. In most states, raw milk is not permitted to be sold in stores and must be purchased directly from the farm or as part of a farm share. **Raw milk should always be independently certified to ensure its safety.**

*Kefir*

The "champagne" of milk; a slightly bubbly, fermented milk drink low in sugar, easily digestible, and filled with beneficial bacteria critical for health. Made from cow, goat, and other milk.

*Ghee*

A clarified butter product popular in India. When from grass-fed animals, it's very high in omega-3s, CLA, and other healthy fats. Unlike butter, ghee lacks milk sugars or proteins and therefore may be better tolerated than butter by allergic or sensitive individuals.

**A guide to "supermarket milk"**

*Homogenized milk*

This milk's fat has been removed, then added back in standardized amounts. In order to prevent a creamline from developing again (where the cream naturally rises to the top of the milk), the fat particles are processed into smaller particles that will more easily remain immersed. This leads to increased spoilage of the fat and may have detrimental health effects as well. Unhomogenized cow's milk will have a visible creamline—and the thicker the creamline, the better the milk's quality. Goat's milk may not have a creamline, as the fat globules are naturally smaller and do not separate from the remainder of the liquid as naturally.

*Skim milk, nonfat milk, fat-free milk*

These products contains casein (milk protein), whey, and lactose with no milk fat to be found, and they are fortified with fat-soluble vitamins A and D (because the original nutrients are removed with the milk fat and require fat to be well absorbed). The amount of milk fat in milk is inversely proportional to lactose, so skim contains proportionately more milk sugar. Because fat comprises much of milk's flavor, industrially produced nonfat milk is also exceptionally bland. Most contain added powdered milk solids (rarely listed on the label) that further boost lactose levels and contain problematic oxidized fats and cholesterol. Not very tasty, not very good for you, and always homogenized.

### Reduced-fat milk

Creating 1 percent and 2 percent milks involves using a nonfat milk base, then adding powdered milk solids and fats to the liquid in standardized amounts, depending on the desired fat percentage. Fat-free milk is combined with powdered milk to 0.5 percent milk fat (low-fat milk), 1 percent milk fat, or 2 percent milk fat. Always homogenized.

### "Whole milk"

Deceptively named, most whole milk is not whole. It, too, has been homogenized and pasteurized. Milk and milk fat are separated by centrifuge and recombined to an arbitrary standard of 3.25 percent milk fat content. Powdered milk is rarely added to the "whole milk" product because the higher cream content provides sufficient body and taste.

### Half-and-half/light cream

A vaguely defined product that contains varying combinations of milk and cream by volume, with milk fat content ranging from 10.5 to 18 percent. Light cream is similar to half-and-half in that it contains varying combinations of milk and cream.

*Heavy cream*
Contains at least 36 percent milk fat. If pasteurized or ultrapasteurized, it may contain numerous additives and thickeners that are best avoided. Raw heavy cream is nourishing, nutrient-dense, filling, with minimal milk protein and milk sugar levels, and thus is less likely to cause dairy sensitivity.

*Reduced-lactose milk*
Intended for those with lactose intolerance, its milk sugar is reduced. Milk proteins like casein and whey are still present, so most dairy-allergic or -sensitive individuals still cannot tolerate it. Typically pasteurized, homogenized, and not raised on pasture.

# TAKE HOME

1. In moderation, milk can do the body good—when it comes from a certified farm, pastured but unpasteurized. Ideally, the farms are biodynamic or certified organic. Jersey, Guernsey, and Normande milk is preferable to that from Holstein and Friesians.

2. Skim milk and other low-fat and pasteurized milks are processed foods. They can make you fatter and sicker. Avoid them.

3. For those who don't tolerate milk and have spent at least six months without consuming it, start with a half teaspoon daily of homemade yogurt from raw, pastured goat's milk. Titrate up as tolerated.

4. For children who tolerate milk, raw milk (from a certified source) modulates epigenetics and offers both short- and long-term health benefits, including reduced allergies and infections from increased microbial diversity, enhanced enzyme activity, and intact proteins.

5. Low-heat boiling preserves milk's benefits better than high heat. Avoid milk processed by ultrapasteurization (UHT).

6. The fats found in pastured cream can help you lose weight rather than gain it. Full-fat milk also has better nutrition and flavor. Look for the creamline on top—the yellower, the better. Unprocessed whole milk is rich with essential fatty acids, CLAs, vitamin D, beneficial cholesterol, and other nourishing fats. Grass-fed butter is your friend.

7. Fermented dairy products have impressive associations with good health and even extreme longevity: yogurt, kefir, and cheeses are the best tolerated, most bacterially biodiverse ways to consume milk.

## CHAPTER 12
# Knowing the Chicken Before the Egg

I began keeping chickens because I wanted eggs that came from healthy, well-treated animals. The fabulous eggs they produced would have sufficed, but somewhere along the way, I became mesmerized by the chickens themselves, from their almost musical communication to the way they trick one another out of getting the best scraps, to the way they reliably know exactly one hour before sundown to go to their roosts and sleep. Studies done on chicken intelligence show that they are equal to preschool-age children in empathy, self-control, and even numeracy.[1] Sure, some are as dopey as you might imagine— no different from humans!—but others walk over to me and cluck until I pick them up and pet them. I always say someone forgot to tell them that they're chickens and not dogs!

Chickens eat just about anything—scraps from meals, foraged greens and seeds, plenty of bugs and worms. But they always prefer fresh foliage over scraps. And when I say fresh, I mean still *alive*, as in still attached to the living plant. If I drop plants clipped seconds earlier from my garden, they forsake those clippings for the live stuff every time. They instinctively know that living food is higher in nutrition, phytochemicals, and other elements of secret chicken ambrosia.

They transform these scraps and dirt candy into luscious eggs with bright golden yolks. Talk about the Rumpelstiltskin Effect! My eight chickens give me as many as 55 eggs a week, depending on the season. They also act as built-in composters for my garden. Their nitrogen-rich droppings, mixed with the carbon-rich wood chips we layer over their run, become microbial- and nutrient-dense perfectly balanced fertilizer for my garden. This, of course, draws lots of worms and bugs and microbes to the soil, which allows for more (and better) fruits and veggies to grow, and then becomes more forage and scraps for them. It's a perfect cycle.

You don't have to keep chickens to recognize that honoring a chicken's natural habits and habitat makes for healthier animals, and, in turn, healthier humans.

Egg yolks from pastured chickens are filled with fabulous nutrition: essential fats like omega-3s and omega-6s, as well as CLA, healthy saturated fats, cholesterol (yes, cholesterol!), plus vitamins and minerals. They are the most concentrated source of choline, which plays a wide range of roles in neurological health and is particularly crucial for brain and memory development in pregnancy, nursing, and toddlerhood. Eggs from pastured hens contain significantly more naturally derived omega-3s than eggs from factory hens.[2,3] Adequate levels of omegas (in the ideal ratio with omega-6s, 4:1) improve symptoms from asthma, ADHD, seizures, depression, and cognition.[4,5] I mention this proper ratio because in purely grain-fed, indoor animals (which we'll talk more about in a bit), the ratio may be 14:1 or much more.

Hens that spend time in the sun lay eggs with yolks three to six times higher in vitamin D than eggs from confined hens.[6] Yes, you can actually obtain your daily vitamin D by consuming pastured eggs rather than supplements! This crucial vitamin, best known for its role in building strong bone, is also a gene transcription factor that boosts immunity, improves mood, reduces blood pressure, and lowers risk of cancer as well as autoimmune, neurological, and psychiatric disorders.[7] Deficiency may play a role in autism.[8,9] But vitamin D in eggs comes only from hens free to graze fresh greens and bask in the sun. Healthy chickens, healthy eggs, healthy people.

Pastured eggs have higher levels of $B_{12}$, folate, and vitamin E. Eggs also are a uniquely abundant source of two carotenes, lutein and zeaxanthin, antioxidant vitamins essential for macular protection, the part of the retina responsible for central vision. They also have a protective effect against colon cancer, with an enhanced benefit in younger people.[10] The deeper the yellow-orange color of the yolks, the more antioxidant power they have.

Eggs and their yolks—like real milk, cream, and butter—went

through a period of being demonized (*Too much cholesterol! Too much saturated fat!*). But scientists, doctors, and consumers are finally recognizing their value as a perfect food.

## THE REAL DIRT ON CHOLESTEROL

What is cholesterol—aside from that sinister compound associated with heart disease and premature death? Cholesterol is a steroid manufactured in the liver and used to build healthy cell membranes. It's so critical for infant brain development that mother's milk concentrates both cholesterol and unique enzymes that aid in its absorption from the intestinal tract. Children need cholesterol in their diets to fuel their rapid brain growth. Though the brain is only 3 percent of the body's mass, 20 percent of cholesterol makes its way there to play a pivotal role in insulating, protecting, and nourishing the neurons there.[11] It is critical for formation of synapses—the connections between your neurons that allow you to move, think, learn, and form memories.[12] In fact, in 2013, the FDA began to require consumer warnings that certain cholesterol-lowering medications could cause memory decline and other cognitive issues. It should also come as no surprise that cholesterol deficiency has been linked to the development of autism, Parkinson's disease, Alzheimer's, and ALS.[13,14] Children with autism have lower cholesterol levels than their neurotypical peers. People suffering from psychiatric disorders—from depression to violent behavior to suicide-completers—tend to have lower cholesterol levels.[15,16]

Cholesterol is also the body's repair substance. When arteries sustain damage, cholesterol steps in to patch things up and prevent aneurysms. It's the raw material from which our bodies make vitamin D, cortisol that helps us manage stress, as well as estrogen, progesterone, and testosterone that help regulate puberty and sexual function. In addition, cholesterol transports sulfur groups that are essential for building glutathione, the "garbage truck" of the cell that binds and carts out toxins and free radicals. These powerful antioxidant properties help to protect the body from cancer. Cholesterol helps the body—and brain—function well.

Paradoxically, low—and not high—cholesterol is associated with earlier death.[17,18,19,20,21] In fact, high cholesterol is associated with longevity, including lower incidence of infection and cancer.[22] After all of cholesterol's negative press, it may sound crazy that people with higher cholesterol levels live longer, but it's been corroborated repeatedly.[23,24] This may partly have to do with cholesterol's potent immunomodulating function.[25,26] In 200 children aged newborn to 20 years, those with allergic disorders (including asthma) had lower total and LDL cholesterol than the others.[27] And in a large study of more than 68,000 deaths, it was low cholesterol that predicted an increased risk of dying from gastrointestinal and respiratory illness.[28]

Eating eggs doesn't even confer the cardiac risk we've assumed for many years. Researchers who took a close look at the egg-eating habits and heart health of 118,000 people found that nondiabetic people who ate five to six eggs per week had a *lower* risk of heart disease than those who ate one or less egg per week.[29] Imagine that!

Cholesterol essentially became a "problem" when doctors developed the ability to measure it. They demonized it, restricted it, and medicated people to reduce levels. Cholesterol was "bad," so naturally eggs were "bad." Though eggs are a complex food rich with countless beneficial compounds, soon eggs were equated with cholesterol in the same way that milk became "calcium," carrots "vitamin A," and oranges "vitamin C." **We must learn and relearn: whole foods are far more than the sum of their parts.**

LDL in particular has been demonized as "bad cholesterol," despite the fact that LDL's role is to deliver life-sustaining cholesterol to our cells. The real problem is actually when triglycerides increase—in part a result of consuming excess sugar and processed carbohydrates—which leads to smaller, denser LDL that are prone to oxidization and glycation. *Oxidized and glycated LDL* is the real danger,[30,31] which may be better addressed by reducing sugar and processed carbohydrate consumption rather than restricting unprocessed, nutrient-dense sources of cholesterol.[32,33,34]

We really don't know what the upper limit of "normal" cholesterol is for each individual. Current recommendations—which dictate that one in four Americans requires statins—are likely inaccurate. And we must keep in mind that members of the medical panel that made those recommendations were criticized by the *New York Times* for conflicts of interest. Interestingly, the majority of panel members received money from one or more pharmaceutical companies that produce cholesterol-lowering medications.[35,36]

To sum up, eggs are a delicious way to consume unprocessed cholesterol, which is associated with a long and healthy life. The industrial way agribusiness raises and feeds hens makes its eggs and us sick, but eggs themselves are not inherently unhealthy. Ultimately, cholesterol, along with other nutrients in pastured eggs, benefits our body, immune system, and especially our brains.

## WHY HEALTHY CHICKENS MATTER

Usually outsiders aren't permitted to enter CAFOs, but I once was able to tour a facility abroad. As I entered the dim, warehouselike, multi-level building, all I could see were chickens from floor to ceiling: kept in wire cages piled high, packed six hens to a cage, with just enough space between them for eggs and waste to drop. They had pale, droopy combs, a sign of nutrient deficiency. These chickens had intact beaks, unlike many U.S. chickens who are de-beaked because they peck one another to death under the stressful, crowded conditions. The strong smell of ammonia made the chickens cough, even with enormous ten-foot-by-ten-foot fans circulating the air (without which the birds would quickly die from their own fumes). Artificial light shone to mimic longer days, since chickens naturally lay more eggs in summer than winter. I later learned that these conditions were actually far superior to those in the United States.

Chickens induced to lay ever more eggs develop "layer fatigue." Because it's physiologically impossible for them to absorb enough calcium to produce so many eggshells, calcium leaches from their bones. Their bones eventually break, and they can become paralyzed and die. Unlike free-range chickens who can live 10 years or more, very few caged layers survive past 12 months of age, when they're simply thrown out.

Even smaller-scale so-called free-range or cage-free facilities can cram hundreds of chickens into one large space. In order to get free-range certification, producers must only include coops with a small door that opens onto a five-foot-by-five-foot fenced-in outdoor pen. Most chickens, however, are too uncertain of what lies on the other side and never venture through. Small producers tell me that their chickens, too, end up in the garbage after their most productive laying is over. "No one these days would buy them," they say.

The producers are referring to a time when older hens traditionally became stew birds. Their less tender meat required longer cooking, but their flavor was considered vastly superior to typical broilers. Moreover, their feet and necks are still exceptional for soup and their fat is excellent for cooking.

I don't recommend eating CAFO birds or their eggs. Commercial chicken feed is comprised largely of GMO corn (carbohydrate) and GMO soy (protein), which increases the egg's omega-6 fat content to unhealthy ratios—leading to a more reactive immune system in us. Other elements in soy-fed chickens' eggs include detectable soy isoflavones, which lead to higher estrogen content and possible greater reactivity for soy-sensitive kids. Genetically modified, high-pesticide soy or corn in feed also potentially exposes us to whatever genetic and epigenetic material the chicken consumed. We are what we eat eats.

Other ingredients in chicken feed are chicken feathers, which are also used as fertilizer for crops, even though feathers—like hair—hold remnants of toxic exposures. A 2012 study tested U.S. and Chinese feather meal and found antibiotic residues in both, as well as acetaminophen (from Tylenol, for poultry fevers); diphenhydramine (from Benadryl, used for poultry anxiety); and norgestimate (a sex hormone). All these also become part of the soil that grows our veggies.[37]

Commercial layers are susceptible to disease due to their cramped, stressful living conditions and thus receive regular doses of antibiotics, which happen to also promote faster growth and more productive laying. More than 25 million pounds of antibiotics are administered to chickens for such "nontherapeutic" purposes a year. Here again, this chronic, preemptive use of antibiotics has led to the rise of resistant superbugs—meaning most antibiotics are becoming useless against these bacteria. In eggs tested for deadly food-borne pathogens, all pathogens detected were resistant to one or more drugs. Over less than 20 years, the number of antibiotic-resistant salmonella has gone from 1 percent to *more than 30 percent,* leading to recalls after eggs sickened thousands.

## EGGS: NOT JUST AMAZING ON THE INSIDE

When a hen lays an egg, her body secretes a naturally antimicrobial protective coating called "bloom," which prevents bacteria from traveling through that porous shell. It also helps prevent moisture and carbon dioxide loss that would lead to an overall degradation in the quality of the egg. When the bloom is intact, eggs stay good for much longer than washed eggs. Unwashed eggs don't require refrigeration because of the bloom. And shells have their own value, hard enough to protect the embryo inside, but porous enough to allow in whatever the growing chick needs. Many traditional cultures grind the mineral-rich shells into food for themselves or their animals. (I recycle crushed eggshells in my garden or in my hens' scraps as a calcium source.)

American producers wash their eggs in an attempt to get rid of disease-causing bacteria. In Europe, however, E.U. egg marketing laws state that Class A eggs—those found on supermarket shelves—must not be washed or cleaned in any way. This mandate is in place to encourage good practices on farms; it is in the farmers' best interest to produce the cleanest eggs possible, as no one will buy unwashed eggs that are dirty. Regulators also understand that washing eggs damages the bloom, which they know would *increase* the risk of contamination. Even contaminants in water used to wash the eggs, for instance, could seep through the porous shell. E.U. law stipulates that eggs "should in general not be refrigerated before sale to the final consumer." The regulations explain that "Cold eggs left out at room temperature may become covered in condensation, facilitating the growth of bacteria on the shell and probably their ingression into the egg."

In the United States, however, the USDA requires that all eggs be rinsed with warm water, washed in detergent followed by chemical sanitizer, then dried. As washing removes the bloom, egg producers in the United States compensate by spraying eggs with a layer of mineral oil so that eggs could sit in cold storage for up to a year.

## What You Can Do

You can buy eggs from farmers you know—whether at their farms or the farmer's market. As more and more people raise backyard chickens, perhaps you can obtain eggs from a neighbor . . . or even keep chickens yourself. I recommend honoring chickens' natural laying cycle. They lay most of their eggs in the spring and summer, and fewer in the winter. I serve eggs in warmer months more than in colder ones.

## A GOOD EGG/HEALTHY CHICKEN

Words like "free-range" or "cage-free" unfortunately don't guarantee that chickens were allowed to forage bugs and plants in the sunshine and fresh air. Neither does organic certification, though it does mean that the chickens aren't being administered chronic hormones or antibiotics and that the feed is GMO free.

- Buy from a farmer's market, a farm, or a CSA. Purchase great eggs from someone who keeps chickens in your neighborhood. In all of these cases, find out how growers raise their chickens. Visit at least once, if possible, at a time prearranged with the grower.
- Words like "pastured chicken" as well as USDA organic labeling are ideal.
- Make sure chickens have free access to fresh air and sunshine, bugs in the dirt, and fresh pasture to forage.
- Keep in mind that chickens are omnivores and like to eat bugs, worms, small rodents, and even meat or fish scraps (though obviously not chicken parts). "Vegetarian feed" may not offer

chickens everything they need nutritionally unless the animals are allowed outside to scratch and forage. Vegetarian feed is superior to refuse from industrial meat facilities however.

- Look for labels that say **"Certified Humane," "Animal Welfare Approved," and "No Antibiotics,"** which ensure humane treatment—no beak or toe clipping.
- A helpful resource is http://www.cornucopia.org/organic-egg -scorecard/.

# TAKE HOME

1. Feed your children plenty of pastured eggs for a great source of vitamin D, cholesterol, choline, essential fats, and phytonutrients.
2. Good-quality eggs—especially yolks, yolks, yolks—are worth their weight in gold. Forgo the egg white omelettes and take advantage of the Rumpelstiltskin Effect!
3. The quality of the egg depends on whether it came from a "happy hen" who lives as she is meant to—frequently outdoors, foraging on healthy pasture, supplemented with good-quality (organic) feed.
4. Eat them lightly hard-boiled, roasted, poached, and sunny-side up as well as in omelettes, quiches, and frittatas. Serve them over soups, burgers, veggies, or rice. Enjoy occasional custards and puddings, too! NOTE: Keeping the yolk intact and cooking lightly optimally preserves the egg's nutrients and delicate fats and cholesterol.
5. Request stew hens from egg farmers you trust so that older laying hens aren't thrown out—and discover how exceptionally flavorful, tender, and delicious they are when braised or stewed in coq au vin or chicken ragout.

## CHAPTER 13
# Fish: From the Water

As eating meat went out of vogue in the 1980s due to fears of cholesterol, saturated fat, and heart attacks, fish became the new healthy "meat." At first, this move seemed smart. The essential fatty acids found in fish, including omega-3 fatty acids critical for brain health and function, benefit every system in the body. They can alleviate mental illnesses, including depression, bipolar disorder, and aggression,[1,2,3] and childhood neurological conditions such as ADHD.[4,5] They may reduce risk for sudden unexpected death in epilepsy (SUDEP).[6,7] Symptoms of inflammatory disorders improve with omega-3 consumption, including asthma,[8] rheumatoid arthritis,[9] systemic lupus erythematosis, cardiac disease, and diabetes complications. Essential fatty acids (EFAs) like omega-3s and -6s can't be synthesized by the body, only derived from diet.

But there's one big caveat with eating fish. As with other food sources, it's only as good as its aquatic terrain and the way it's farmed or caught. Manure, fertilizers, and pesticides from large factory farms wash from streams and rivers into the ocean. Industrial waste and emissions, garbage, and even medications find their way into our water. This damages the ocean—poisoning underwater ecosystems and fish populations—and pollutes our water, our food, and us.

We don't eat fish with any thought to the population size, seasonality or the life cycle of a fish. Certain fish are best caught in the winter, others in the summer, some young, and some older. Wild salmon have a life cycle, which involves traveling from river to sea to meet and feed in northern waters for one to seven years before returning to spawn in their river of origin. Yet the demand for fish never abates or changes, and overfishing affects the balance of the ocean ecosystem by depleting resources that sea life needs to stay healthy. **The ocean is not a source of unlimited abundance.**

Effective ocean stewardship may put healthy, sustainable seafood on the table for the long term. In the meantime, here's what you need to know about eating fish.

## MERCURY IN FISH

Many doctors recommend avoiding tuna if you're pregnant or nursing. As per the Environmental Defense Fund, I recommend avoiding tuna of any kind, at any time. No canned tuna. No tuna salad. No spicy tuna maki or ceviche or tuna steaks. Mercury bioaccumulates, meaning it works its way up the food chain. Fish that eat other fish inherit their meal's mercury content. So tuna (and swordfish and shark), which occupy the top of the oceanic food chain, accumulates the most mercury. When you eat tuna, you absorb and retain that mercury.

But tuna isn't the only problem. **A 2009 U.S. Geological Survey study detected mercury contamination in** *every fish* **sampled in nearly three hundred streams across the country.** More than 25 percent contained mercury at levels exceeding the EPA's recommendation for people who consume average amounts of fish, and more than 66 percent exceeded the EPA's level of concern for fish-eating mammals.

Fish is not inherently high in mercury, nor is our water. The mercury is there because of unregulated industrial dumping and emissions from coal-burning power plants. At last measure, 67 percent of the total mercury in the atmosphere comes from the United States.[10]

Why does it matter if we're exposed to mercury? Because our bodies convert inorganic mercury to the more highly toxic methylmercury. Even trace levels of the toxic metal can impede brain development and cause myriad health problems. In a study of people who ate a significant amount of fish and showed symptoms consistent with mercury poisoning—fatigue, headaches, decreased memory, and joint pain—all had blood mercury levels well above the EPA's safety threshold of 5 micrograms per liter. Like lead, mercury harms in very small doses. According to the CDC, 16 percent of American women of childbearing age have blood mercury levels high enough to increase the chance of harm to their fetuses. Such exposure has been linked to adverse effects in language development, cognitive function, and general intelligence,[11] as well as lower scores for attention, eye-hand coordination, and other fine motor responses.[12]

Mercury also harms older children. Researchers observed a delay in transmission of auditory brain signals in 14-year-old subjects associated with mercury exposure from eating fish in their diets.[13] I've heard pediatricians say that a patient's mercury level is in the "normal range." But the only laboratory delineation is between environmental (i.e., incidental) and occupational exposure. **There is no normal range for mercury or any toxic metals, because no level is known to be "safe."**

Interestingly, the health benefits of eating fish can be impressive enough to mask the effect of high mercury exposure, and the debate continues as to whether omega-3 benefits outweigh harm from mercury.[14] Yet the problems associated with mercury and other toxins are also quite clear, and large-scale studies don't detect "canaries in the coal mine" very well. If five thousand children are exposed to mercury, the ones with Coke and Twinkie genes and wide-open drains may detoxify it promptly. But others—often those already suffering with toxicity or chronic illnesses—accumulate mercury. While some kids show illness immediately, others may be asymptomatic until sometime down the road when their total toxic load—including mercury—reaches critical levels. There's good news, though: While most patients who confess to regularly eating high-mercury fish like tuna have measurable blood mercury levels, those levels often drop after avoiding fish after just one month. Reducing exposure is the first step to detoxifying heavy metals.

Children who eat fish regularly—no matter the kind—should be tested for blood mercury levels. Though blood levels don't reflect your child's cumulative mercury exposure over time—blood merely serves as the vehicle that delivers mercury to either be excreted or stored in liver and brain—a positive blood test indicates exposure in the diet right now. Any level of mercury has potential to cause issues. If your child has a detectable mercury level, eliminate *all* fish for one month, then retest.

Any woman thinking about getting pregnant, as well as her partner, should have her mercury levels checked *before pregnancy.*[15] She should take a good-quality, sustainably harvested fish oil supplement daily—third-party tested for metals—if she is avoiding fish. In some couples I've counseled who are experiencing prolonged infertility or multiple miscarriages, reducing mercury levels has helped them conceive and carry a baby to term.

Mercury is not just limited to large deep-sea fish like tuna or swordfish. That said, cod, salmon, haddock, herring, and sardines are considered "low-mercury fish." Shrimp also have lower levels.

## SALMON: NO LONGER THE MIRACLE FISH

After decades of overfishing, commercial Atlantic salmon is no longer wild. Whether it's called Canadian, Irish, Scotch, or Norwegian, "Atlantic salmon" is always farmed and, unfortunately, rarely in a sustainable, responsible way.

Normally, wild salmon have beautiful, pink flesh from the shrimp they eat. But farmed salmon are "feed-intensive"—requiring at least *three pounds* of feed for every pound of flesh they produce—so it's prohibitively expensive to feed them their natural diet. Instead, producers opt for cheaper grains like corn (often GMO), meat offal from slaughterhouses, and other "refuse" to provide calories. As a result, caged salmon's flesh is an unappetizing gray, so they're also fed dyes to give their flesh an appealing pink color. Because salmon are overcrowded and eat feed never intended for fish, they're vulnerable to a plethora of infestations, so they're bathed in antibiotics and pesticides.

Farmed fish consistently have higher levels of toxins than wild fish: polychlorinated biphenyls (PCBs)—neurotoxic, hormone-disrupting chemicals banned in the United States since 1977—carcinogenic dioxins toxaphene and dieldrin, which result from chlorine paper bleaching and incineration of PVC plastic, and mercury. This is because wild fish are also ground into feed for farmed fish, which concentrates the contamination present in wild fish. Uneaten feed and fish waste litter the ocean floor beneath these farms, generating populations of microbes that consume oxygen vital to shellfish and other bottom-dwelling sea creatures. You ingest these drugs and chemicals two ways: when you eat farmed fish, and again because they contaminate other fish through build-up in sea-floor sediment.

In this way, industrial farm fishing raises environmental concerns similar to those of feedlot livestock. Meanwhile, the FDA is in the process of approving genetically engineered salmon to be raised off Panama and sold, unlabeled, to unsuspecting consumers.

**In order to replenish healthy fish, we must both reduce our consumption and simultaneously push world governments to protect and rebuild fish populations and water ecosystems.**

## A GUIDE TO EATING FISH

*Fish to Definitely Avoid (particularly for children, teens, men and women planning to conceive, or women who are pregnant/nursing):*

- **Tuna steaks or canned tuna:** Tuna's levels of mercury and PCBs are so high that the Environmental Defense Fund (EDF) recommends not eating this fish at all.
- **Farmed salmon and tilapia:** Most farmed salmon (everything labeled "Atlantic salmon" is farmed) are fed fishmeal, given antibiotics, and have levels of PCBs high enough to rate a health advisory from the EDF. Their squalid conditions also threaten wild salmon trying to swim to their ancestral spawning waters. Tilapia are dosed with hormones, antibiotics, and pesticides, and they are fed corn, soy, and even animal feces.[16]
- **Chilean sea bass:** An endangered species, Chilean sea bass (aka Patagonian toothfish) has been fished to near depletion in its native Antarctic waters. Trawlers and longlines used to catch

them have damaged the ocean floor and hooked albatross and other seabirds. The EDF has issued a consumption advisory for Chilean sea bass due to high mercury levels.

- **Largemouth bass:** Once a wild freshwater fish of choice in the United States, it's been overfished and now measures dangerously high in mercury.
- **Grouper:** High mercury levels in these giant fish have caused the EDF to issue a consumption advisory. Groupers can live to be 40 years old but only reproduce over a short amount of time, making them vulnerable to overfishing.
- **Orange roughy:** Like grouper, this fish lives long but reproduces slowly, making it vulnerable to overfishing. Seafood Watch points out, "Orange roughy lives 100 years or more—so the fillet in your freezer might be from a fish older than your grandmother!" This also means it has high levels of mercury, which has led to health advisories. Children—and women thinking about getting pregnant or who are pregnant—should avoid.
- **Atlantic cod:** A general name for white-fleshed fish, cod became the "it" fish for fast-food and frozen dinners. However, huge corporate fishing operations with giant factory ships overwhelmed smaller fishing fleets, obliterating cod populations everywhere. Even after severe restrictions on cod fishing for more than 15 years, recovery has been limited. The average 20-pound cod of a couple generations ago has been replaced by 3-pound "scrod," or pan-size cod. Pacific cod is in healthier shape, but that won't last if the world demand for cod directs its focus there. Limit cod intake.
- **Imported shrimp:** About 90 percent of shrimp comes from countries with poorly regulated seafood industries. Imported farmed shrimp comes loaded with contaminants: antibiotics; residues from chemicals used to clean pens; filth like mouse hair, rat hair, and insects; and *E. coli*. Less than 2 percent of all imported seafood (shrimp, crab, catfish, etc.) gets inspected before sale—another reason to buy domestic seafood from sustainable sources.

- **Imported catfish:** Nearly 90 percent of imported catfish comes from Vietnam, where there's widespread use of antibiotics and pesticides that are banned in the United States. The two varieties of Vietnamese catfish sold in the United States aren't technically considered catfish by the federal government and therefore aren't held to the same inspection rules as other imported catfish.
- **Eel:** This fish, which frequently winds up in sushi dishes, is highly contaminated with PCBs and mercury. The fisheries are also suffering from pollution and overharvesting. Consider squid instead.
- **Atlantic halibut and other whitefish:** Flounder, sole, and halibut caught off the Atlantic coast are often heavily contaminated and have been overfished since the 1800s. According to Food & Water Watch, populations of these fish are as low as 1 percent of what's considered sustainable.
- **Shark:** When fewer sharks are around, their prey—cownose rays and jellyfish—increases and subsequently depletes scallops and other fish. As predatory fish, shark are extremely high in mercury.

## Other Fish with High Toxic Load

**Oysters (Gulf of Mexico)**
**Marlin**
**Pike**
**Walleye**
**White croaker**
**Swordfish**

## Better Choices for Occasional Consumption

- **Anchovies and herring:** These small oily fish are nutrient-dense, high in omega-3 fatty acids and calcium, and are less contaminated because they eat fewer fish. There are enough of these fish for humans to eat them, if we are careful and support sustainable fishing practices. My kids love eating sardines as a snack on crackers. Once parents get over their *own* yuck factor, they often discover their kids love these tangy fish. They're high in umami and add rich flavor to salads, sandwiches, and even veggies.

• **Wild-caught Pacific salmon:** Less toxic than farmed salmon. However, it would be impossible to meet the world's demand for salmon with just wild-caught Alaskan salmon. Eat sparingly.

*Also*

**Organically farmed Arctic char**
**Pollack**

**When buying any farmed fish,** ask your fish supplier its buying policy to ensure it sources fish only from farms with high environmental and welfare standards. **Best choices are fish farmed to organic standards or in closed systems,** which reduce negative environmental impacts associated with open-net pen or pond systems.

## HOW MUCH FISH DO YOU NEED?

The world's current wild catch comes to about 170 billion pounds a year, which is about the weight of the entire population of China.[17] This is six times more fish than we ate 50 years ago. **The medical profession, however, currently recommends that each person eat two servings of fish per week, one oily fish and one whitefish, which would mean that we would actually need to harvest 60 billion pounds *more* fish than we are catching now. It's just not possible.** This is why I recommend significantly limiting fish intake until better, more sustainable methods are in place. Meanwhile, eat alternate sources of omega-3 fatty acids from pastured land animal products, augmented by fish oil or algae. Here are my recommendations:

1. **Eat low-mercury fish only once a week or less.** Children, teens, and pregnant women should avoid mercury-containing fish, but if

total avoidance is impossible, eat it once a month at most. Choose either very small fish or those grown in minimally polluted areas like the Arctic, Antarctic, or Alaskan waters. Check websites that evaluate fish health and sustainability like Monterey Aquarium or Seafood Watch for current recommendations.

2. **Find sustainably sourced fish oil.** As much as I prefer that we derive all our nutrients directly from the food, cod liver or fish oil is a traditional food that provides our bodies with omega-3 fatty acids with less contamination. Fish oil provides EPA and DHA (docosahexaenoic acid), which are necessary for cognitive development, healthy vision, and more.

   The best companies source sustainably caught fish and employ third-party testing by batch for heavy metals such as mercury as well as PCBs, antibiotics, and other toxins. Remember that some amount of bioavailable omega-3 fatty acids such as DHA and EPA can also be derived from eggs, meat, and dairy products *if raised entirely on pasture.*

# TAKE HOME

1. Eat fish infrequently—not more than once a week.
2. Ideal fish are anchovies, sardines, and Spanish mackerel, occasionally salmon. Avoid tuna, swordfish, sea bass, tilefish, and other large or bottom-feeding fish.
3. Look for sustainable fisheries on websites like Seafood Watch and Monterey Aquarium.
4. Source omega-3 fatty acids from a combination of sustainably harvested fish oil that's third-party tested for purity, or pastured eggs and butter. Omega-3s from vegetable sources—including walnuts, flax, and purslane—are less bioavailable for us, though still beneficial.
5. Many fish contain mercury, which can contribute to health issues. If you serve fish once a week or more, ask your doctor to test your child's blood mercury level. A level over three implies current exposure—try stopping fish for one month and retesting.

## CHAPTER 14
# Water: What We Drink

*In the wildness is the preservation of the world.*
—HENRY DAVID THOREAU

When I visited the Valley of Longevity in Ecuador, I had a transformative experience through the very simple act of quenching my thirst. We were winding through perilously narrow mountain roads in a rickety bus when we noticed small, sparkling waterfalls apparently sprung straight from the rocks. We begged the driver to stop. The water was frigid, crystal clear, and sweet. Everyone filled their water bottles and even drank straight from the source. Every danger I'd heard about "wild" water ran through my mind. In my head, I could hear my husband saying, "Were you *trying* to get parasites?!" But this water was the freshest, most cleansing water I'd ever drunk in my entire life. Everyone felt more vibrant. We all changed after drinking that exquisite wild water.

Drinking sweet water from the source used to be something all children—all people—had the opportunity to enjoy. Mountain water—fresh, untreated, untouched—tastes so delicious because of a natural underground filtration system through which water travels so slowly it can take thousands of years. It sheds toxins, soaks up minerals, and ultimately emerges from mountains as icy springs. Indeed, our bodies have evolved to depend upon water as a source of diverse trace minerals (hence the term "mineral water!").

In recent decades, however, drinking wild water has become taboo, even "dangerous." As a child growing up in the suburbs, I'd been taught it could make you sick, or even kill you. People said rivers were polluted with fertilizers and toxins from dumping, and streams teem with giardia and other parasites.

## POLLUTION: WHAT'S IN OUR WATERWAYS?

- **Medications and personal care products:** In 1991, researchers at the U.S. Geological Survey discovered "intersex fish" in the Potomac River in the eastern United States. They found male smallmouth and largemouth bass with immature eggs (males of these species don't typically have eggs). In a subsequent 1999 study, researchers tested 139 streams around the country and found that *80 percent of samples* contained residues of drugs like hormones (the culprit behind the sex-changing fish), plus painkillers, blood pressure medicines, or antibiotics.[1]

  Animals and humans excrete medications into water through sewage and farm runoff into watersheds. Sewage treatment plants aren't able to remove most pharmaceuticals from wastewater, and no government safety limits exist for levels of those pharmaceuticals in drinking water.

- **Fertilizers, pesticides, and herbicides:** Rain or snow melt carries pesticides from agricultural fields, golf courses, parks, and residential properties through storm drains and into reservoirs, endangering wildlife and stressing water treatment facilities. Fertilizer's nitrates and phosphates wash into rivers and lakes and feed surface algae, which subsequently bloom, blocking sunlight and oxygen from reaching deep marine life. Most marine life either leaves or dies, resulting in massive "dead zones."

- **Heavy metals and other compounds:** Lead, arsenic, mercury, sulfur, petroleum, asbestos, and oils leach into water from improper disposal of household and industrial waste or agriculture. Lead, found in groundwater and well water from years of use as a pesticide, inhibits metabolic processes in the body and brain. It's also in the tap water of older buildings and homes owing to lead pipes and joint seals. No level of IQ-lowering lead is considered safe for children.[2] Arsenic, used excessively during the last hundred-plus years as a farm pesticide and growth agent in chickens, has seeped into groundwater. Now, we drink it. Chronic low-dose and even trace exposure have been implicated in neurocognitive problems, respiratory problems, cardiovascular disease, diabetes, and cancers of the skin, bladder, and lung.[3,4,5]

Industry, farms, and health-care facilities are primary sources of water pollution. Many industrial facilities still dispose of waste into rivers, lakes, and oceans. Others overwhelm sewage treatment facilities and contaminate our watershed. These exposures directly and cumulatively affect our health. A research arm of WHO has declared glyphosate, the major ingredient of Monsanto's Roundup, as a "probable cause of cancer." Also, studies show that children with higher urinary levels of the pesticide dichlorophenol—a chlorine compound in pesticides that kills bacteria (including in our microbiomes)—have increased risk of food allergies.[6]

- 100 percent of U.S. streams have detectable levels of at least one pesticide;
- 50 percent of shallow wells have detectable levels of pesticides;
- 25 percent of private wells contain at least one contaminant at levels of potential health concern;
- 90 percent of the 139 municipal water systems sampled by EPA in 2003 to 2004 contained detectable levels of atrazine; 50 percent had levels exceeding EPA standards.

## Fracking Fracks Up Your Water

Hydraulic fracturing, or "fracking," is the process of drilling and injecting fluid into the ground at a high pressure to fracture shale rocks and release natural gas. A growing energy source in the United States, fracking has become of tremendous concern to health professionals, farmers, and hydrologists because it uses unconscionable amounts of water resources (approximately 40,000 gallons per fracturing) and irrevocably contaminates clean water. "Fracking fluid" is a mixture of up to six hundred chemicals, including known carcinogens, endocrine disruptors, and toxins such as lead, mercury, uranium, methanol, formaldehyde, ethylene glycol, and hydrochloric acid, all of which seep into our water supply. The oil and gas industry isn't required to disclose the exact chemicals used in the fracking process, but they are sourced from industrial waste.[7] In Pennsylvania, the state actually **placed a gag order on physicians to prevent them from sharing the contents of fracking fluid,** deeming it "proprietary," even to sick patients affected by toxic chemicals.[8] A physician challenged this law in federal court, but lost.[9] There are currently five hundred fracking wells in the United States, and there have been more than one thousand documented cases of water contamination next to areas of gas drilling as well as cases of respiratory, neurological, and other damage due to ingesting and bathing in contaminated water. Many farmers oppose fracking because it contaminates the soil, air, and water around the wells—especially because wells will inevitably leak—which hurts the health of their families, livestock, and plants. Fracking also causes earthquakes.[10] But some are using oil and fracking wastewater to water crops—especially in places like drought-plagued California.[11] When will industry stop using farmland as a dumping ground for their toxic waste?

The good news is that some communities and even states are banning fracking. After tenacious lobbying by hundreds of thousands in New York State (including testimony from yours truly), the governor banned fracking in the entire state in 2014.

Tune in to what's happening with fracking in your area—including infrastructure like pipelines—and raise your voice to protect kids' health.

## THE REAL DIRT ON BOTTLED WATER: WORSE THAN TAP WATER?

Capitalizing on public concern about water quality, industry is marketing bottled water as pure and safe. But don't be fooled. The claims are not what they seem to be.

Oversight of bottled water is lacking. As a packaged food product, bottled water is regulated by the FDA, whose rules are more lax than the limits imposed by the EPA for tap water.[12] Yet about 70 percent of bottled water never crosses state lines for sale, which exempts it even from FDA oversight. Many states claim that they regulate bottled water—though most have few or no resources dedicated to policing—but about one out of five states don't. And FDA regulations don't apply to bottled water used in beverages like "sparkling water," "seltzer water," "soda water," "tonic water," or "club soda." These beverages, considered "soft drinks," are exempt even from bottled-water standards, other than vague sanitation rules without specific contamination limits.

Studies done on bottled-water quality reflect this lack of regulation. The National Resource Defense Council analyzed more than a thousand bottles from 103 brands of water. **Nearly one in four of the bottled waters violated state contamination limits for bottled water in at least one sample,** most commonly for arsenic or certain cancer-causing, man-made ("synthetic") organic compounds. About one fifth of the water contained synthetic organic contaminants—such as industrial or plastic chemicals (e.g., toluene, xylene, phthalate, adipate, or styrene).

On the other hand, municipal water systems in the developed world are well regulated. In the United States, for instance, municipal water falls under the purview of the more stringent Environmental Protection Agency and undergoes regular inspections for bacteria and toxic chemicals. **Check out the Environmental Working Group's national drinking water database to see how your community's water scores.**

## Plus

1. **All that plastic can make you sick.** Especially at very high or very low temperatures, plastic bottles leach toxic breakdown products into their contents. Flexible and durable, BPA is used in clear, hard plastics (especially polycarbonate) as well as in a plethora of daily items like dental sealants, hospital blood bags, cash register receipts, and the lining of tin cans. Compounds like BPA and

DEHP have been shown to have estrogenic activity. Estrogen plays a key role in everything from bone growth to ovulation to heart function. Too much or too little, particularly in utero or during early childhood, alters brain and organ development in unpredictable ways. Elevated estrogen levels increase a woman's risk of breast cancer and can alter onset of puberty. Estrogenic chemicals found in many common products have been linked to a litany of other problems in humans and animals. Naturally occurring estrogens bind with proteins in the blood, limiting the amount that reaches estrogen receptors. But research shows that BPA bypasses the body's natural barrier system and penetrates cells of laboratory mice. Scientists have tied BPA to ailments including asthma, cancer, infertility, low sperm count, genital deformity, heart disease, liver problems, and ADHD. Even BPA-free plastics share many of the same—or worse—estrogenic activity.[13] And these plastics have epigenetic effects. In this case, you ingest the plastics and instead of poisoning you, they reprogram your DNA and cause disease in your children and grandchildren, hurting them instead. The less plastic in your life, the better!

2. **Bottled water is a terrible value.** People spend as much as ten thousand times more per gallon on bottled water than tap water. If a 20-ounce bottled water costs a dollar, it works out to five cents an ounce for what is no better (if not worse) than tap water. Gasoline is only two cents an ounce, assuming a cost of $2.50 a gallon. The water business already has become more lucrative than the oil business!

3. **Bottled water means more garbage.** Bottled water produces up to *1.5 million tons of plastic waste per year*. More than 80 percent of bottles are simply thrown away instead of recycled. Plastic waste now comprises vast eddies of plastic trash that spin endlessly in the world's major oceans,[14] killing and contaminating birds and fish that mistake plastic garbage for food. In 1960, only 5 percent of seabirds had plastic in their stomachs, whereas now 90 percent do. Plastic's slow decay rate means the majority of all plastics ever produced isn't going anywhere soon.

4. **Bottled water means less attention to public systems.** Ever notice how water fountains are less available than 20 years ago? This is in great part due to the advent of bottled water. **We should maintain high-quality water fountains that allow everyone access to fresh, clean water all the time.**

5. **The corporatization of water.** Water is the "Blue Gold" of the twenty-first century. Thanks to increasing urbanization and population, shifting climates and industrial pollution, fresh water is becoming humanity's most valued resource. The bottled-water industry commoditizes access to safe and affordable water. Multinational corporations are pushing communities to sell groundwater and distribution rights wherever possible. Peter Braeback, Nestlé's chairman, actually said, "The one opinion, which I think is extreme, is represented by the nongovernmental organizations, who bang on about declaring water a public right. That means as a human being you should have a right to water. That's an extreme solution." Nestlé is currently bottling water in drought-stricken California and selling it at a hundred times the price.

## Other Thirst-Quenchers to Avoid

*Sports drinks:* Many children involved in athletics are offered sports drinks for "rehydration." These drinks often contain artificial dyes, flavorings, and HFCS, which are the opposite of beneficial to children's health. So far, no scientific evidence demonstrates that sports drinks improve hydration.[15] Yet sales of sports and energy drinks in schools are increasing. With full-calorie sodas phased out from many schools, beverage manufacturers heavily promote sports drinks as a "healthier" alternative.

*Soda:* Made from unfiltered water mixed with myriad chemicals and HFCS or aspartame, soda contributes to kids being sick, hyper, violent, and fat.[16,17,18]

*Juice from cans and bottles:* Pasteurized and bottled juices offer few benefits. Even "no sugar added" juices, have added fruit sugar.

## What Should I Drink?

There's no shortage of delicious options to quench your thirst—and most cost less money than the ongoing purchase of bottled concoctions. Here are my top picks:

- **Filtered tap water:** This is the ideal drink for children (and the rest of us). It should make up the majority of what we imbibe. Sometimes I hear from families that their kids don't like the taste of water. It's no wonder. Some tap or bottled water tastes like chlorine or chemicals or just dead, as though it's been sitting around for days even though it's right from the tap. Filtered water, on the other hand, can have a fresh, clean taste. I recommend filtering tap water to remove heavy metals or pharmaceuticals that regular municipal filtration doesn't catch. Plus, it's a way to mitigate effects of fluoride, which we'll talk about in a bit.
- **Tap water:** Though I prefer filtered tap, straight tap is still better than bottled water. It can be worthwhile to privately test your water if you are concerned about exposures or to simply know what's in your water.
- **Coconut water:** Rich in minerals and electrolytes, coconut water is so similar to our plasma that it's actually been used as an IV plasma replacement. When fresh and unpasteurized, it offers natural electrolytes and hydration.
- **SodaStream:** For those who want something fizzy—or to wean from soda—buy a SodaStream (the Penguin model offers glass bottles instead of plastic). You can mix the "soda" with some juice or stevia leaf as you wean your family off sweet drinks.
- **Cocoa:** Yes, the comforting winter treat! Fair-trade, sustainable cocoa (or better yet, cacao) mixed with water, milk, or a milk alternative, and a dash of natural sweetener like honey or maple syrup is delicious and nourishing.
- **Tea:** My favorite. It's delicious and packed with phytonutrients, and the unending variety keeps things interesting. My kids each have a Klean Kanteen thermos (a nonplastic reusable water

bottle) that gets filled with their tea of choice each day, so they can take a healthy drink to school.

## Teas I Have Known and Loved

Tea is the ultimate superfood, truly perched at the intersection between food and medicine. Many aromatic teas (peppermint, ginger, chamomile) have the effect of regulating our autonomic nervous systems. Teas like tulsi, lemon balm, linden, and chamomile help soothe and relax. Many of those teas also support digestion (chamomile, ginger, peppermint, marshmallow), detoxification (dandelion, nettles), and improve focus (skullcap, green tea). They also nourish by providing electrolytes, vitamins, minerals, and phytonutrients.

Instead of juice, soda, or highly sweetened bottled drinks, set fresh herbs or tea bags in a pitcher to sit in the sun for several hours (or simply add hot water), add raw honey or maple syrup (or no sweetener), and refrigerate. Take it along to school or work in a reusable bottle. Or join your child for a warm cup of tea after school or before bed to process the day. My kids have access to our hot water carafe and 20 to 30 types of tea.

## TIP

### Reuse, reuse, reuse

For drinking on the go, invest in a reusable canteen or water bladder. Stainless steel and cushioned glass options are best. Klean Kanteen, Lifefactory, and others offer lid options (even bottle or sippy cup adapters!). Ensure the bottle isn't lined with BPA or another plastic. Water bladders are lightweight, and excellent for hiking and camping. Opt for a rubber version. Wash carefully and then dry it by propping it open, or simply store it in the freezer between uses. Don't drink from plastic.

## FILTRATION 101

### The Ideal Filter Removes

Arsenic, fluoride, chlorine, bacteria/viruses/parasites, heavy metals, nitrates, radon, VOCs, sediment, medications, and copper.

### And Retains

Trace minerals, which provide flavor and necessary nutrients.

### Types of Filters

**Carbon and sediment filters** like Brita and Pur are inexpensive, "entry-level" options that eliminate spores, fungi, parasites, and bacteria, but not heavy metals or fluoride. They require frequent replacement.

**Ceramic water filters** often combine (1) charcoal to remove toxins and organisms and (2) an active alumina filter to remove fluoride. They filter thousands of gallons, yield mineral-rich water, and last longer than carbon filters. Cost, higher initially, is lower per gallon. Easy to install and gravity-fed, these filters take up the space of a coffeemaker.

**Reverse osmosis filters** force water through a membrane under pressure, removing everything but $H_2O$. Reverse osmosis removes impurities *and* important minerals. These $A_2RO$ systems require that you add a remineralizer to balance the water for consumption. Each gallon of water creates three to five gallons of wastewater, not an option if water is scarce. Very expensive, slow, and large, they require a storage tank and a professional plumber to install.

**Water distillers** use heat to create steam, which condenses to purify the water. They effectively kill bacteria and remove impurities, but also demineralize water, like reverse osmosis. Drinking distilled water can create a mineral imbalance in the body.

**UV systems** use high-frequency light to irradiate bacteria. They're expensive and require a power source.

**Water ionizers** filter then ionize to make water alkaline. The idea is that the water will, in turn, make the body more alkaline (versus acidic) to reduce risk of disease. They're expensive, the water requires remineralization, and more peer-reviewed research is needed to support the claims.

## WHAT'S THE BIG DEAL ABOUT FLUORIDE?

We all need it, right? After all, it's added to our water, our toothpaste, even our dental treatments. It turns out that most developed countries—including 97 percent of Europe—don't fluoridate water. Mass fluoridation has raised concerns among scientists, doctors, and governments across the world.

Fluoride's initial claim to fame was as an industrial pollutant, a by-product of increased aluminum use in everything from electrical wiring to food wrappers, beverage cans, and cookware, to automobiles and airplanes.

Normally, fluorine resides safely in the Earth's crust, naturally bound with aluminum, copper, and iron. But once it transforms into its ionic state, it wreaks all kinds of havoc in both the environment and our bodies. As the most reactive of all elements, fluorine disrupts hydrogen bonds in our DNA and acts as a free radical, attacking molecules, damaging enzymes, and compromising or disabling certain biological reactions. "Because of this, the aluminum industry disabled many with fluorine gas emissions from their factories," reports the U.S. Department of Agriculture. "Airborne fluorides have caused more world-wide damage to domestic animals than any other air pollutant."

A post-WWII campaign to fluoridate drinking water was less public health innovation than public relations tactic sponsored by industrial producers of fluoride—including the government's nuclear weapons program.[19] A tenuous link was made between dental hygiene and water fluoridation to "prove" that fluoride compounds were innocuous, thereby heading off lawsuits by sick factory workers and others poisoned by industrial fluorine gas pollution.[20] It worked, and created markets to stimulate fluoride production to boot.

Everything we add to the public water supply directly improves its safety or quality—except fluoride. Fluoride is classified as a drug and added to water as "medical treatment." The dose of this particular drug cannot be controlled, however, because different people consume different amounts of water. **No other drug in the world is administered—especially to children—without a specific dose.** Yet there is no ongoing official monitoring to evaluate levels of exposure or side effects that could be related to fluoridation. A 2007 review in the *British Medical Journal* states, "There have been no randomized trials of water fluoridation"—currently the standard for all drugs.[21] The FDA itself classifies fluoride as an "unapproved drug."[22,23] Somehow, we've all just accepted that it's good for us. Meanwhile, 90 percent of fluoride added to public water supplies is not pharmaceutical grade but silicofluorides, an arsenic-contaminated industrial waste product from the phosphate fertilizer industry. Drink up!

We're also exposed to fluoride through beverages we drink, like soda or juice; mechanically deboned meat; crops and animals watered or fed with fluoridated water; and pesticide residues. Bottle-fed babies consuming formula made with fluoridated water may get three hundred times the fluoride of breast-fed babies.[24]

This matters because fluoride can have harmful effects on both body and brain. Excess fluoride exposure causes dental fluorosis, resulting in white streaks, brown stains, pits, or broken enamel. As of 2010, *41 percent of kids ages 12 to 15 had some form of dental fluorosis*, according to the CDC.[25] Fluoride suppresses thyroid function—at one time it was a drug used in Europe to reduce thyroid activity. It accumulates in the body—especially in children who have immature kidneys—up to 80 percent in the bones and pineal gland.[26]

Fluoride also increases oxidative stress, which can interfere with cell signaling from growth factors, hormones, and neurotransmitters. As a result, fluoride causes developmental neurotoxicity, which can persist over generations.[27] When researchers evaluated the results of 27 different studies, 26 showed that high-fluoride drinking water was associated with an average IQ of seven points lower in children.[28] **These findings were at water fluoride levels under the EPA's**

**allowable level of 4 mg/liter**. Subsequently, fluoride was classified as a neurotoxicant in a 2014 *Lancet Neurology* article.[29]

But is fluoridation effective? Not to the degree we've been led to believe. According to the WHO, industrialized countries that rejected water fluoridation experienced a decline in dental decay similar to fluoridated countries. In nearly 40,000 U.S. children, the National Institute for Dental Research found little difference in tooth decay among children in fluoridated versus non-fluoridated communities.[30] Several studies concur.[31,32] A 2009 NIH-funded study tracking six-hundred-plus children found no significant link between fluoride intake and tooth decay, concluding that "achieving a caries-free status may have relatively little to do with fluoride intake, while fluorosis is clearly more dependent on fluoride intake."[33] A 2015 review questioned the quality of pro-fluoride studies, noting "little contemporary evidence that has evaluated the effectiveness of water fluoridation for the prevention of caries."[34]

The bottom line: **Any cavity prevention attributed to fluoride can be achieved with topical fluoride**[35] or better yet, excellent nutrition. Ingestion is not necessary to prevent cavities and may be cumulatively harmful. Get that water filter and vote to ban fluoride in water!

## ALL WATER IS CONNECTED

Taking steps to protect water is as important in building healthier terrain as drinking clean water. Filtering and keeping plastic bottles out of our oceans are no longer issues when we keep our water supply clean. Here are some simple practices:

- Conserve water by turning off the tap when running water is not necessary. Even where water isn't scarce, used water flows to treatment facilities that run on unsustainable energy and require chemicals.
- Imagine that whatever you throw down the sink or toilet is headed right for a river or ocean. Find alternative disposal

methods for paints, oils, and medications, such as "pharmaceutical take-back locations" or your local police station. Educate local pharmacies, hospitals, nursing homes, and community members to stop disposing of drugs down the drain.

- Use environmentally friendly household cleaning agents and toiletries. Don't use on your skin or in your home what you wouldn't eat. I like coconut oil with baking soda for cleaning teeth; and vinegar, baking soda, and lemon juice for cleaning the home. Dr. Bronner's or Seventh Generation are other good options.
- DON'T use pesticides, herbicides, and fertilizers on your lawn, and don't use them in your home. A recent study found the use of indoor pesticides—pest control, flea foggers, flea and tick collars, and roach and ant sprays—were associated with a 47 percent increased risk for childhood leukemia and a 43 percent increased risk for childhood lymphomas. Outdoor pesticides used as weed killers were associated with a 26 percent increased risk for brain tumors.[36] Diatomaceous earth or boric acid can help with roaches and ants. Learn to appreciate diverse grasses in your lawn!
- Native plants and trees in your garden preserve soil nutrients and other compounds from washing into nearby water sources. Plant them. The more, the better.
- Don't throw litter in or near rivers, lakes, or oceans. Pick up litter you do see.
- Minimize (or eliminate) your use of plastic.
- Keep water public. Prevent privatization of universal resources like fresh water.
- Stand up and protect your waterways. Support meaningful action toward sustainable cleaning of our waterways and putting an end to damaging drilling practices. Taxpayer money should be going toward actions that benefit the citizens. We all have a responsibility to leave our children a planet with water as clean as (or cleaner than) the water we began with.

# TAKE HOME

1. Ideally, water offers a source of rich minerals, which comprise its flavor.
2. Filtered tap water is the most accessible way to drink clean water in cities.
3. Avoid bottled water: It's more expensive than gasoline but lower in quality than most tap water, which is cheaper and has far better regulation. Plus plastic bottles pollute our inner and outer terrains.
4. Your water filter should have the capacity to remove heavy metals like lead, arsenic, and aluminum, as well as compounds like fluoride.
5. Fluoride is a neurotoxin and should not be ingested. If your city adds it to the water, let it know you'd like your tax dollars to go elsewhere, for the sake of your child's brain. For those who desire fluoride for dental health, topical use (in toothpaste) protects teeth equally to fluoridated water, and with less risk.

## CHAPTER 15
# Simple Pleasures:
# Healthy Sweets, Fats, and Umami

F ood offers not just energy and nutrition, but also pleasure. Combining pleasing tastes—sweet, fat, and umami—from nutrient-dense sources, with other nutrient-dense, living foods is a way to combine "business and pleasure."

Tastes send various messages to the brain. Just as bitter foods alert us to the possibility of poison and activate the body's defenses, sweetness indicates that food contains sugar and carbohydrates, which provide quick energy and calories; saltiness and umami tell us necessary minerals will maintain our proper electrolyte and mineral balance; and the mouthfeel of fat tells the body that a bundle of energy and dense nutrition is coming. Processed foods attempt to trick the body with synthetic forms of these real foods without offering their amazing benefits.

## HEALTHY SWEETS

How many times have we as parents allowed our kids some junky treat, then felt guilty and promised ourselves we'd do better? There are alternatives to the junk. While refined sugar and artificial sweeteners offer no benefits, nature provides unprocessed plant-based sugars for our enjoyment and good health.

You've probably heard all sweets are damaging to your health. Not so. Naturally occurring sweeteners benefit the body in unexpected ways. While refined sugar, corn syrup, and agave nectar contain essentially no antioxidant activity, raw honey, evaporated cane sugar, date sugar, dark muscavado, maple syrup, and blackstrap molasses have high levels of phenols and antioxidants—in spades.[1] Ultimately, some healthy sweeteners boost your antioxidant intake to a level greater than eating a serving of blueberries. Moderation is key; a little goes a long way. And always read the label, as industry is always looking for a way to spin products to you and your children. Be suspicious of "natural sugars" or "healthy sweetener" claims on processed foods because much industrial processing robs plants of their benefits. Avoid low-nutrient sweeteners: refined sugars, "raw sugar," and even agave nectar, as they are nearly devoid of antioxidant and nutritional benefits. The quality of your sugar is critical—so find small-scale or local producers who care about their products.

### Maple Syrup

Maple syrup, rich in minerals, vitamins, amino acids, and phyto-chemicals, is produced by boiling sap collected from the sugar maple tree (and some other maple species). As recently as 2014, previously unidentified beneficial phytonutrients were found in maple syrup.[2,3] Biological studies of maple syrup extracts suggest that its unique combination of compounds reduces inflammation. And believe it or not, its antioxidant value is higher than a serving of strawberries or oranges.[4] Animal studies suggest that pure maple syrup protects the liver, helps to prevent cancers like breast and colon, benefits the mi-crobiome, and has the ability to reduce plasma glucose levels.[5,6,7,8] The phytonutrients in maple syrup and even maple bark extract counteract any negative effect from its sugars, and are being investigated as a way to prevent and even treat type 2 diabetes.[9]

I particularly like using organic maple syrup as a substitute for sugar when baking, to sweeten otherwise unsweetened breakfast por-ridge, or to drizzle over yogurt and kefir. Don't be fooled by Aunt Jemima and other HFCS-containing imitators. Get the real deal only—the darker (grade B or darker) it is, the more nutrient-rich—for delicious flavor and health benefits.

## Blackstrap Molasses

This dark, thick sweetener remains after the sugar is extracted from raw sugarcane. Sugarcane—must be bad, right? Not so fast! Sugarcane is a plant rich in nutrients and phytochemicals. More on that below. Suffice it to say that blackstrap molasses has more antioxidant properties than any other sweetener—five times more than a serving of raspberries and blueberries.[10] Also, minerals abundant in molasses—including magnesium, calcium, and potassium—play critical roles in healthy carbohydrate metabolism, among other metabolic processes. For instance, magnesium deficiency has been correlated with insulin resistance,[11] calcium supplementation has been shown to increase insulin sensitivity,[12] and low potassium levels have been associated with increased risk of developing diabetes, particularly in young African-Americans.[13] Blackstrap molasses is an exceptionally dense source of other nutrients, too. As a side benefit, it works like a charm to keep the bowels regular, even in some of the toughest cases of constipation. Add some molasses daily to your oatmeal or smoothies, mix it into sauces or marinades (I like it on chicken or steak, or in stir fries), or just dissolve it in hot water and add to drinks.

## Date Sugar

Date sugar is simply dried dates—which are about 50 to 70 percent sugar—ground into coarse powder. Because the sugar is compromised of the whole fruit, it has the nutrient profile of dates—considerable amounts of fiber, minerals, vitamins, and antioxidants.[14] Date sugar doesn't readily dissolve in liquids but can be substituted measure for measure for brown or granulated sugar in baking.

## Evaporated Cane Sugar

As we've discussed, unprocessed sugarcane is a plant that, like all plants, has tremendously beneficial antioxidant compounds. Some powerfully inhibit brain lipid peroxidation—one of the major avenues by which sugars damage the brain.[15] One study showed that ingesting evaporated cane sugar can improve metabolic function and reduce glycemic response, while another study showed that *fermented sugar-cane juice kills human leukemia cells.*[16] While vast amounts of sugar do no one any favors, a bit of evaporated cane juice may help to maintain our health. Use it to replace white sugar for an occasional treat.

## Honey

Raw honey has exceptionally high concentrations of enzymes (over five thousand that we know of) and provides an outstanding source of energy. It contains amylase, which helps digest food, and traces of bee pollen, which is rich in amino acids, minerals, and vitamins. Honey benefits the immune system, liver, and brain. It's been studied as an effective treatment for infections, allergy, coughs, asthma, wounds, and neuroinflammation—even diabetes.[17] Raw honey reduces the chronic sneezing and runny nose associated with allergies. Honeys from specific trigger plants (for example, birch trees) can *relieve* allergy to those particular plants—acting almost like a natural allergy shot.[18] Honey has proved *as effective as over-the-counter medications* in reducing sick children's coughs and helping them sleep through the night.[19] Honey stirred into coffee is more effective than treatment with steroids or over-the-counter cough medication for persistent postinfectious cough. It's even being tested in an aerosol form for chronic asthma with promising results.[20] Honey also facilitates wound healing, from mild to severe.[21] Honey has powerful antimicrobial properties.

Honey is even being explored as an antidiabetic agent.[22] The phytochemicals in honey improve glycemic control and reduce oxidative damage.[23] Honey flavonoids protect struggling pancreatic cells that can't make insulin.[24] Animal studies reveal that a dose of honey and metformin lowers glucose more than metformin alone, also protecting organs that are vulnerable to complications in diabetes, like the eyes, brain, and testes.[25] Low-dose honey also decreases complications in type 2 diabetes.[26]

Honey also promotes detoxification, protecting liver and kidneys from effects of numerous toxins, including cadmium,[27] Tylenol,[28] and melamine.[29,30] Honey acts to turn off microglial activation—the cell danger response—which has powerful implications in neurological conditions. **Honey does this because it's more than just "sugar," but a complex mix of living compounds that interact with the body in unique and powerful ways.**

**A note on buying honey:** Most honey found in the supermarket is "commercial" honey, meaning it's likely been pasteurized for easier filtering, a cleaner look, and to kill any yeast that might cause fermentation. Yet even fermentation boosts honey's natural benefits. Heating honey, on the other hand, damages its delicate volatile compounds and destroys many enzymes responsible for activating vitamins and minerals in the body.

Most suppliers warm honey only slightly to avoid this damage. Raw honey looks cloudier than supermarket honey bear versions, and contains elements including particles and flecks of bee pollen, honeycomb bits, and propolis. Propolis is a resinous substance that bees collect from trees and flowers that reinforces the hive but also prohibits harmful bacterial or fungal overgrowth—and confers those benefits on us. Over months, raw honey may granulate and crystallize to a thick consistency but can be gently rewarmed to reliquefy.

No strict legal requirements exist for labeling honey "raw," but you should seek out raw honey from a local apiary. Without knowing your source or testing pollen, it's impossible to know whether honey comes from a legitimate source. Chinese companies have been dumping tons of their honey into the U.S. market after ultrafiltering it at high pressure through extremely small filters to remove pollen. Chinese honey—often contaminated with outlawed antibiotics like chloramphenicol—can't be traced without its pollen.[31] Imported honey can also be mixed with unhealthy, cheaper sweeteners like high-fructose corn syrup.[32]

Raw honey varies considerably, ranging from glass-clear to dark mahogany and from watery to chunky to crystallized solid. Darker honey is higher in antioxidants and has more intense flavor. Differences in flavor stem from the flowers on which the bees forage for nectar. Engage your kids in taste-testing many varieties. Seek out apiaries that commit to humane treatment of bees and pesticide-free forage (or keep bees yourself!).

Warning: Do not feed honey to babies younger than 12 months of age, as it can cause botulism.

## Chocolate

Cacao is a plant with potent health benefits. Its chief phyto-chemicals are the alkaloids theobromine (translated: drink of the gods) and theophylline (literally: love of the gods). Not surprising given how passionate many feel about this plant! Less stimulating than coffee or tea, cacao is also nourishing and filling and its bioflavonoids induce mild euphoria, relaxed focus, and ease of function. It lowers blood pressure, protects the heart, improves lipid profile, enhances cognition and memory, and protects you from inflammation and cancer.[33] Theophylline ultimately became a pharmaceutical for treating asthma by relaxing and opening airways. A square of good-quality, fair-trade dark chocolate is an excellent treat. I adore powdered cacao in raw milk, almond or coconut milk, or water, with a bit of maple syrup or muscavado (don't totally mask the bitterness with sweet!), and one or more of the following: cinnamon, ginger, vanilla, cayenne, or orange extract. Heat, froth in the blender, and drink.

## HEALTHY FATS: EVERYTHING WE'VE THOUGHT ABOUT FATS IS WRONG

Fats make food delicious. In addition to the unique flavors of fat—from butter to olive oil to bacon fat to sesame oil—they evenly disperse other flavors like lemon, salt, pepper, and spices. Fats retain moisture in foods and prevent them from drying out when baking or roasting. And fat is nutrient-dense and nourishing.

We've thought of fat as something to avoid, but children's bodies and brains need a constant supply. Their nervous systems are composed of more than 60 percent fats. The brain is built from lipids—or fats—and deficient or disordered lipids lead to disordered brains. Lack of fatty acids plays a significant role in depression, bipolar disorder, schizophrenia, violent behavior, ADHD, autism, and seizures.[34]

It's a myth (or a gross oversimplification) that eating fat makes us fat. Aside from it being purposely masked in processed foods, eating nourishing fats is more likely to prolong satiety and reduce our food intake.

Synthetic trans fats have gotten a bad rap, for good reason. But conjugated linoleic acids (CLAs)—the natural ruminant trans fat found in grass-fed butter and milk fat, along with fat-soluble vitamins A and D—have potent anticancer properties. They also reduce obesity risk,[35] protect from atherosclerosis,[36] reduce inflammatory markers in autoimmune disease,[37] and help heal the damaged gut in celiac disease.[38]

Saturated fats, too, offer health benefits—despite their infamous reputation. Once upon a time, we were told that the best fats were polyunsaturated; monounsaturated fats were just okay; and saturated fats were evil. We imagined that for all time, "healthy" people only ate olive oil. Now we know that natives of tropical islands who ate more than 50 percent of their fats from coconut oil were lean, healthy, and long-lived. Yet when some islanders switched over to more "healthful" polyunsaturated fats, their dense LDL cholesterol shot up and beneficial HDL dropped.

Further, coconut oil fights viruses, raises HDL, and helps prevent neurological illness. Saturated fats like the lauric acid found in coconut oil have been shown to improve, not worsen, lipid profiles like triglycerides.[39] Coconut oil also reduces abdominal fat when compared to soybean oil.[40] The so-called good oils, like processed corn, safflower, and sunflower oil, actually lower beneficial HDL, increase inflammation, and predispose us to cancer. Lard and bone marrow, rich in monosaturated fat, lower LDL and maintain HDL.

## THE ORIGIN OF THE MYTH THAT SATURATED FAT IS EVIL

People have always eaten fat from their animals. They saved lard from pigs and tallow from cows and ate every bit of fat from their chickens, geese, or ducks. Fat was valuable.

The demonization of saturated fat originated with the food industry.[41] In 1911, Crisco was created from a combination of naturally saturated fats—tallow, lard, and coconut oil—and was heavily marketed to compete with lard and butter from farms. By the 1940s, however, Crisco switched to hydrogenated cottonseed oil, corn oil, and peanut oil to reduce costs. Hydrogen was added to liquid oil (hydrogenization) to turn it into solid fat, mimicking the texture that butter, lard, and coconut oil gave to processed foods. Blamed in the 1950s as having triggered the new epidemic of coronary heart disease, Crisco claimed that saturated fats—rather than the chemically altered hydrogenated (trans) fat it preferred to use—were the problem. Its aggressive public relations campaign stuck. From then on, saturated fats were seen as "bad" and polyunsaturated fats (corn and later soybean) as "healthy," leading to the rise and reign of partially hydrogenated cottonseed, soybean, and safflower oils. To achieve the desired texture in processed foods, more of these replacement fats were required and more damaging fats were passed on to consumers. Ultimately, synthetic trans fats harmed human health in the extreme.

Eating animal fats has been particularly demonized. Olive oil is the "it" fat at the moment; many people use nothing else. But it is expensive, requires shipping great distances for many, and isn't good for higher-heat cooking. Moreover, it only offers certain lipids and our cells require diverse fats—from mono and polyunsaturated to saturated.

When I was young, my mother would only serve chicken soup after cooling it, so she could skim and dispose of all the fat from the top. She told childhood stories of waiting by the stove to eat that fat, called schmaltz, on bread, which she called a "heart attack sandwich." Now we know that the schmaltz—undoubtedly from pastured chicken in those days—was not just delicious but filled with beneficial fats. Next time you roast a pastured chicken or make a grass-fed hamburger, use the drippings to sauté greens. Let me know if any greens are left!

## WHAT FATS SHOULD WE EAT?

It's pretty simple, actually.

- Animal fats are healthy if the animals were raised outdoors eating pasture under healthy, humane conditions.
- Plant-derived fats are healthy if they were grown organically and cold pressed without solvents.

Healthy plant fats are rich in phytonutrient content. Animal fats are healthy when the animals have eaten rich amounts of phytonutrients *and* have had contact with sun, fresh air, fresh water, and rich soil. Beneficial fats are processed as little as possible. There is no specific prescription of how much fat one should or shouldn't eat; it is individual. Most traditional cultures eat an average of 30 to 50 percent of calories from fat.

### Avoid Oxidized Fats

Hydrogenated, partially hydrogenated, and refined oils are all oxidized fats. Oxidized fats can't be used for energy or structural needs, and often contain harmful toxic compounds. They also contribute to the formation of free radicals, which cause damage to healthy fats in your body. Any fat that's overheated—for example, the oil in your skillet that's started to smoke—is oxidized and can contain other harmful compounds. Saturated fats—coconut oil, butter, lard, schmaltz, or tallow—have higher smoking points and therefore are less likely to oxidize. The good news is that it's safe and healthy to consume easily oxidized fats in their original packaging—as plants and seeds—rather than extracting them, which renders them vulnerable to oxidation. If you're buying oil, opt for cold-pressed over solvent-extracted oils, and cook at lower heat.

Here's a list of fats to seek out at the market.

## Animal Sources

- **Butter and ghee**: When derived from animals that consume high-quality pasture from high-quality soil, butter becomes a "superfood." Its fatty acids boost immunity, inhibit growth of pathogenic fungi, and disable viruses and other pathogenic organisms. Its high quantities of CLA protect us from obesity and cancer. Fat-soluble vitamins A, D, E, and $K_2$ are essential for building healthy brain, bones, and body. Even with all the calcium in the world, without sufficient $K_2$ (found only in milk from grass-fed cows) bones can't calcify efficiently.

  Ghee is clarified butter that has been simmered until most of the water has evaporated. It's stable at room temperature for years. (Some ghee has lasted for a hundred years!) Because milk solids are also removed, ghee can be tolerated by some dairy-allergic people. Ghee has been used medicinally by Ayurvedic practitioners for thousands of years to reduce inflammation, aid digestion, and help transport medicinal herbs. Organic grass-fed ghee is easy to find in stores but it's also easy to make at home.

- **Tallow** is fat from beef or lamb. It rarely develops free radicals or becomes rancid. Palmitoleic acid as well as stearic acid show promise as a treatment for type 2 diabetes by stabilizing blood glucose and insulin levels and reducing inflammation in fat tissue.[42] Stearic acid also reduces dangerous visceral fat tissue.[43] Additionally, grass-fed ruminants produce fat with substantially higher omega-3 fatty acids and beta-carotene than conventional counterparts. Rendered tallow can keep in your fridge for months. A little goes a long way—use a spoonful to sauté vegetables. Some specialty shops carry this, or simply use drippings from roasts.

- **Lard** is rendered pig fat, similar to tallow but with more saturated fat and higher propensity to become rancid if not handled properly. It, too, contains palmitic acid (with noted antimicrobial properties). It's great for high-heat cooking and exceptional for baking.

- **Schmaltz** is rendered chicken, duck, goose, or turkey fat and—when these animals are raised on pasture—is excellent for cooking. Think the chicken soup remedy. We always roast veggies and sometimes even sprouted quinoa or another grain along with our roasting chicken to absorb the healthy juices. The fat slows the insulin spike associated with carbohydrate consumption and stabilizes blood sugar—plus it's delicious. Schmaltz serves as a delicious spread on crackers or sourdough bread.

## Plant Sources

- **Coconut oil** offers tremendous antimicrobial activity thanks to lauric and capric acids. It has been used effectively against measles, herpes, influenza, strep, staph infections, clostridia, listeria, and even HIV and hepatitis C when dosed medicinally. In the digestive system, palmitic acid boosts key antibodies and has been studied as an oral vaccine adjuvant, intended to stimulate the immune response to a desired antigen.[44] Coconut oil's medium-chain (as opposed to very long, long, medium, and short) fatty acids nourish energy-producing mitochondria most efficiently, which can improve seizures and many neurological conditions.[45] It also aids weight loss and even can benefit diabetics by normalizing blood glucose levels after a meal.[46]

  Coconut oil is solid at room temperature, but liquefies as it warms. The best-quality coconut oil is unrefined (that is, "virgin"), made by shredding and cold-pressing coconut while it's fresh, fermenting it while the oil and milk separate, then gently heating it to remove moisture. A second kind is expeller-pressed, which is usually deodorized for those who dislike the taste and smell of coconut. Removing the aromatic compounds, however, impacts the oil's health benefits.
- **Olive oil** is rich in antioxidants, which helps prevent it from turning rancid. The oil requires very little processing and retains its vitamins and minerals, phytonutrients, antioxidants, and healthy fats. Olive oil also contains oleic acid, which regulates

clotting in the body, balances cholesterol levels, and reduces inflammation contributing to allergies, asthma, autoimmune disease, and cancer. And it is delicious. Unfiltered olive oil is intensely flavorful and nutrient-dense.

Avoid olive oils labeled "100%" or "pure," since those terms carry little meaning. Go for the extra-virgin instead. Less reputable distributors blend their olive oil with other oils and it's difficult to taste the difference.[47] According to an investigation of 186 olive oils, many of us are spending big bucks for an adulterated product 69 percent of the time, even from trusted and popular stores.[48] Imported olive oil is most likely to be pure when bottled and sold directly from the grower on family farms, rather than bought from a middleman or distributor who buys in bulk and combines oils from many growers to sell to corporate bottlers and distributors. If you are curious about your olive oil, UC–Davis Olive Oil Center accepts samples for testing. It is best unheated or used for sautéing at low heat.

- **Sesame oil**, made from sesame seeds, is exceptionally nutrient-dense. When the seeds are pressed into oil, their antioxidants work synergistically with others, like vitamin E, to enhance our health. A source of zinc and magnesium, sesame oil benefits skin, hair, and bone. When swished in the mouth, it reduces bacteria that cause cavities.[49] Sesame oil prevents hyperlipidemia, hypertension, obesity, and diabetes, and it protects the brain by reducing neuroinflammation.[50] It also helps prevent cancer.[51]

## A Heads-Up on Certain Vegetable Oils

Corn, soybean, canola, and cottonseed oils are nearly always genetically modified and are only recommended if certified organic due to excessive pesticide residue. Cottonseed is not even regulated as a food and therefore doesn't meet minimum safety regulations for consumption, yet it is still permitted as an ingredient. Even organic, these oils are best avoided.

They're also high in omega-6 fats. While omega-6s are essential for health in ratio to our omega-3s (the ideal ratio is 4:1), we can become susceptible to inflammation when we consume too many omega-6 fatty acids. Too much soy and corn make their way into our diets through processed foods and restaurant fare, high omega-6 fatty acids contribute to allergies, asthma, autoimmune, and neurological conditions, and even increase our cancer risk.[52,53] High omega-6 fatty acids have even been linked to violent behavior.[54]

Most unrefined vegetable oils tend to oxidize when cooked, yet refined oils have chemical residues with fewer redeeming nutrients. Even safflower and sunflower oils are often refined, so it's best to enjoy the seeds themselves rather than the oils. Minimally processed palm kernel and palm fruit oil—packed with beta-carotene and other antioxidants—are not unhealthy per se, but have problems in their harvesting. Their popularity has led Indonesia and Malaysia to clear-cut 18 million acres of biodiverse tropical forests, threatening extinction to orangutans. Unless the palm oil is explicitly labeled as certified fair trade, it is best avoided.

## Healthy Sources of Omega-6 Fatty Acids

Omega-6 fatty acids aren't always "bad." Yes, when they're out of balance with omega-3s, they can promote disease states from cancer to autoimmune disease. But you and your children need them to stay healthy. The key is to derive them from healthy sources that maintain a balance (around 4:1).

- **Sunflower seeds:** Omega-6 fatty acids in a nutritious package—and a great snack!
- **Flax seeds and hemp seeds:** These seeds, or their oils, are wonderful sources of omega-6 and -3 fatty acids. Use them unheated only—in salad dressings, drizzled over veggies, or mixed into granola. (Hemp seeds naturally offer a 4:1 ratio of omega-6 and -3. I love sprinkling these on salads or veggies.)

- **Grapeseed oil:** This neutral-flavored oil is rich in vitamin E. It's best used cold or over low heat to avoid oxidation. Make sure to buy it organic because grapes are often heavily sprayed with pesticides.
- **Evening primrose oil:** This oil can have a beneficial effect on hormonal balance as well as skin and seizure disorders.[55,56]

## UMAMI

Umami translates from Japanese as "yummy deliciousness," and it is usually found in foods that have been cooked, fermented, aged, or even have a bit of mold (think aged cheese or steak). Otherwise known as the "fifth taste" (besides sweet, sour, salty, and bitter), umami offers a deep, savory, satisfying flavor that enhances enjoyment of food. From babies to adults, umami stimulates the orbitofrontal cortex, our reward pathway—which means eating it satisfies us. Both umami and sweet likely signaled to our ancestors that foods were rich in nutrition and energy. The elements of umami benefit us with intense enjoyment of our food. We have a taste receptor for umami, which detects certain amino acids including glutamic acid, i.e., glutamate (not to be confused with monosodium glutamate—the synthetic version that food manufacturers add to foods).

At low levels, glutamate acts as a neurotransmitter essential for normal brain function, including learning and memory. But a rush of concentrated glutamate overstimulates the brain and can trigger neuroexcitatory events like migraines, seizures, tics, and even anxiety and focus or behavioral issues in vulnerable kids. Even those who are sensitive to tiny amounts of synthetic MSG, however, usually can tolerate moderate amounts of foods with natural umami.

Babies start their love affair with umami beginning with amniotic fluid in the womb. Their exposure continues with their mother's glutamate-rich milk—ten times more than in cow's milk. Umami flavor in breast milk elicits a relaxation response in babies, likely due also to the amino acid theanine. Theanine—another component of umami also found in tea and chocolate—has calming properties that can help even the most sensory and agitated of children.

TIP ─────────────────────────────────────────

Umami foods require less salt—because glutamate enhances flavors in food—and yet dramatically decrease our perception of bitter. They therefore make ideal "companions" for harder sells like dark greens, especially for picky eaters and "supertasters." It's why kids obsess over ketchup or soy sauce! Season dishes with condiments like umeboshi vinegar or organic tamari, and use flavorful, mineral-rich foods like bone broths, mushrooms, seaweed, and nuts to quietly transform foods from bland or bitter to compelling.

Other umami foods include fermented fish or soy, cured meats or cheese, soups from meat or bones, vegetables or fungi, umeboshi vinegar (the pickling brine from making umeboshi plums), and products from ripe tomatoes. Here's a more complete list of foods that you can add to your family's repertoire:

## Umami from the Sea

- **Seaweed:** Kelp, kombu, dulse (red algae), and nori seaweed are rich in minerals, but can be a source of heavy metals or radiation due to their incredible binding properties, so enjoy in moderation.
- **Fresh fish:** Anchovies, sardines, scallops, squid, mackerel, shrimp, roe, and anchovy paste.
- **Smoked or fermented fish**: Gravlax and bonito.
- **Fermented fish sauce:** Also known as nam-pla, nuoc mam tom cha, yu-lu, and ishir. Worcestershire sauce also has natural umami.

## Umami from the Land

- **Mushrooms:** Varieties like shiitakes, morels, maitakes, turkey tails, and reishi can flavor vegetarian broths richly with a meaty umami—and powerful health benefits.

### Tonics

Mushrooms exemplify how foods can be tonics, reverberating through our entire systems to create balance and harmony in the body, and, ultimately, build resilience. Many (though not all) tonics come from roots, berries, and mushrooms and have compelling, earthy flavors that work in hot, soothing soups and beverages: mushrooms, astragalus, licorice, hawthorn berries, cacao, and green tea, too. These foods and beverages whisper to the deepest levels of our beings and act as our epigenetic allies, protecting us from harm, minute to minute, day by day.

Mushrooms, as one example, are seemingly miraculous tonics. I'm not referring so much to white mushrooms here as to medicinal (and edible!) mushrooms like morels, maitake, shiitake, turkey tail, reishi, and others. They transform our internal terrain and create a physiological shift from bad to good and good to better. They are safe and gentle for children who are wrung out, fatigued, and inflamed. No pharmaceutical I'm aware of has the diverse range of action of mushrooms in reducing inflammatory and autoimmune disorders while simultaneously enhancing immune function against "bad players" like HIV, hepatitis C, herpes, and others. (Kind of like steroids and antimicrobials wrapped in one, and without the side effects of either.) The turkey tail mushroom suppresses inflammatory response, enhances the microbiome, and appears to be a powerful adjunct to cancer therapy.[57] Reishi promotes cellular resilience, longevity, and self-repair.[58] Elders in East Asia have lived well past a hundred years of age because they consume tonics made from red reishi mushrooms—which boost glutathione, protect mitochondria, and facilitate detoxification.[59] Shiitake and maitake dramatically enhance immune function.[60] Mushrooms even are good sources of vitamin D![61] They also offer nervous system benefits: neuroprotection, more restful sleep, less irritability, and a sense of well-being.[62,63] All this in a day's fare! If you don't like to eat mushrooms, simmer a handful in water for 6 to 10 hours, then use as a stock for a healing soup that's filled with umami.

- **Tomatoes:** Glutamate and adenylate increase tenfold as tomatoes ripen. Ketchup and tomato sauce have concentrated umami flavor.
- **Vegetables:** Celery, cabbage, potatoes, peas, spinach, and asparagus.
- **Nuts:** Walnuts, almonds, and sunflower seeds.
- **Corn:** The only grain that has significant umami in its unfermented state. Eat only organically grown to avoid pesticide residue.
- **Fermented roots, fruits, and vegetables:** Pickled ginger, cabbage (sauerkraut), cucumbers (pickles), capers, olives.
- **Fermented soybeans:** Soy sauce, organic nama shoyu, or wheat-free tamari. Soy sauce traditionally undergoes multiple fermentations over nearly three years (which is why you want one that's aged, with no need for cheats like sugar, alcohol, or preservatives). Miso, tempeh (fermented soy bean cakes), and fermented tofu like Chinese furu are also options. Tempeh and furu are called "Chinese cheese."
- **Green tea:** Gyokuro and sencha are rich in umami as well as relaxing theanine. Matcha is a popular powdered green tea that's whipped in warm water and served in a large drinking bowl.
- **Rice vinegar:** Delicious sprinkled over veggies or used in a salad dressing.

## Umami from Animals

High-protein foods like eggs, milk, and meat (especially organ meat) have great potential for umami and can be enhanced through cooking, ripening, drying, curing, salting, smoking, and fermenting. Chicken, duck, turkey, game, and veal are highest in umami; beef and lamb the least. Other foods high in umami include mayonnaise (homemade from real eggs and olive oil, not sugar and soybean oil), aged cheese, blue cheese, Parmigiano-Reggiano (Parmesan), bacon, sausage, ham, pastrami, and corned beef (nitrate-free). Liver is high in umami because it has high amounts of that powerful antioxidant and detoxifier, glutathione. Keep in mind that organ meats, exceptionally dense in nutrients and umami, can also concentrate toxins—especially liver, which filters the blood—so it's worth finding a pastured, organic source.

### Soups

Soups are an inexpensive source of unlimited umami and dense nutrition. To harness the greatest flavor, cook meat and poultry with vegetable bits or fish with seaweed. Soup transforms refuse into a meal—bones, skins, feet, fish heads, and the tops and ends and skins of vegetables that would normally be thrown out. Keep in mind that the most nutritious parts of our food are often parts we toss. Get over the "yuck" factor and make nutrient-dense concoctions with peelings and trimmings. One recipe for dashi—the grandmother of umami—simply calls for simmering water left from boiling potatoes with smoked shrimp head powder. It can be as simple or complex as you want. Be creative!

## ABOUT SALT . . .

Salt has needlessly gotten a terrible rap over the years, mostly because industry has quietly loaded chemical sodium chloride into the most apparently innocent of processed foods. But our appetite for salt is driven by our body's needs, not the foods we eat. A specific range of sodium, among other electrolytes, is needed to maintain adequate blood flow to the body's organs; our brains determine when more or less salt is necessary. When our adrenal glands pump higher amounts of stress hormones, they activate our salt cravings. These cravings also reflect the body's demand for increased electrolytes like sulfur as well as macro- and trace minerals—from salts of magnesium and calcium to zinc, copper, selenium, iodine, molybdenum, boron, and others—that many children need in spades due to excessive depletion of these minerals from soil and water. These minerals help build bones and teeth and act as cofactors in countless critical metabolic reactions throughout the body.

As such, high-quality salt is an essential part of every child's diet. Unless otherwise noted, the sodium in table salt or added to processed food is industrial NaCl, the salt equivalent of processed food. Sea salt, however, is a superfood of sorts. It adds upward of 75 trace nutrients and electrolytes beyond simply sodium to your reserves. A child with excessive salt cravings may require medical evaluation for certain disorders, but otherwise children should use sea salt to taste.

NOTE: Iodine is a nutrient critical for thyroid and brain health. Chemical table salt is fortified with some iodine—often not enough—but sea salt and salt in processed foods are not. In any case, I recommend getting your child's spot urine level tested, and administering an iodine supplement if indicated.

# TAKE HOME

1. Animal fat can be your friend—specifically when it's pastured and unprocessed. Be brave—render fat from chicken or duck skin (and enjoy the crispy bits of skin as a snack), save lard from frying bacon or tallow drippings from your roast—and keep it in a jar to spoon out when you want to fry or sauté. No need to feel guilty—enjoy deep nourishment and fantastic flavor. A little goes a long way.

2. Pastured butter and ghee are filled with dense nutrition. Some dairy-reactive children may tolerate small amounts of ghee.

3. Unheated and unprocessed vegetable fats like sesame and coconut oil are delicious and healthy. To ensure you're getting the quality you paid for, buy domestic olive oil from single producers or olive oil co-ops; buy foreign only from family farms that bottle their own product.

4. Minimally processed sweeteners—maple syrup, raw honey, date sugar, and blackstrap molasses—have impressive nutritional and antioxidant benefits, including the potential to stabilize blood sugar and counteract diabetes. Cacao and dark, minimally processed chocolate act as tonics in drinks and desserts. Enjoy them in moderation.

5. Umami bases and condiments, prepared traditionally, enhance the appeal of food, from broths to tomato sauce to fish sauce to tamari to Parmesan cheese. They reduce the perceived bitterness of greens. As condiments, these can lure even the pickiest of eaters to sample what they otherwise wouldn't.

6. Sea salt and other good-quality salts contains electrolytes, sulfur, essential macrominerals like magnesium and calcium, and countless trace minerals necessary for proper metabolic function in the body. Sprinkle these salts to taste. Examples of other sources of dense minerals are bone broths, seaweed, and blackstrap molasses.

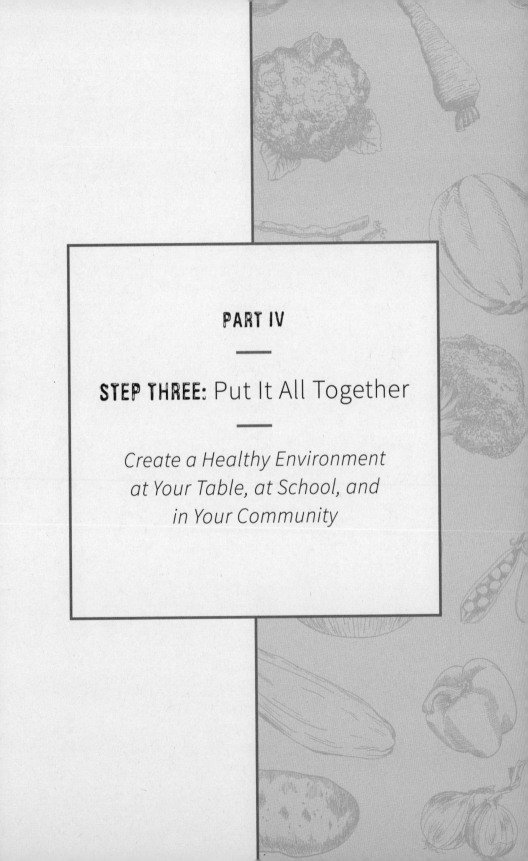

# PART IV

—

## STEP THREE: Put It All Together

—

*Create a Healthy Environment
at Your Table, at School, and
in Your Community*

*Better than any argument is to rise at dawn*
*and pick dew-wet red berries in a cup.*

—WENDELL BERRY

My summers and holidays as a child began with my friends and me taking off on our bikes to meet up with other neighborhood kids. We popped home for lunch and then headed out again until parents yelled that it was dinnertime. Then it was out again until dusk. We spent our days outdoors, rolling down grassy hills, exploring creeks, playing hide-and-go-seek, and sucking the nectar from honeysuckles. We made mud pies in the summer and snowmen in the winter. At the end of the day, we came home muddy and grass-stained, or cold and pink-cheeked. We were truly "free-range kids."

Most children today don't live this way. They are often disconnected from the natural world. They spend days sitting indoors in classrooms with 20 minutes for running around on blacktops (or artificial turf)—if they're lucky. If one kid misbehaves, a teacher may rescind recess for all, which means no outdoor time all day. At home, they then toil over hours of homework, to be rewarded with an hour or two of screen time before bed. Many children no longer interact freely and intimately with nature also because of their parents' fears: of dirt, UV radiation from the sun, germs, potential injury, and stranger danger.

Yet numerous studies show that exposure to nature and soil enhances mood, cognition, and quality of life. Digging in dirt isn't only fun, it makes your children smarter and happier. Children who spend three hours outdoors daily are much more likely to have perfect vision than kids who spend the same amount of time indoors.[1] The vitamin D that they absorb through their skin from the sun promotes immunity in critical ways that oral vitamins cannot fully imitate. Studies show that children who spend recess time in a green environment,

271

rather than on cement or blacktop, subsequently perform better on tests in the classroom.[2]

We have an opportunity to reconnect to a source of living nourishment grounded deeply in nature and reclaim our children's vibrant health and happiness. Now that you know the *why* behind my recommendations, it's time for the most important part: the *how*. As a working mom of three, I understand the wide divide between good intentions and best practices. But as you incorporate new foods and habits into your routine, they become second nature—and fun! The foundation for healthy children comes down to two simple concepts: healing from the inside out (buying and cooking good food) and healing from the outside in (being in nature). Or what you might call "treating your kids like dirt"!

## CHAPTER 16
# Healing from the Inside Out:
# Cooking Better Food

We spent the last six chapters talking about the best foods to feed your children, but ultimately, it is simple: Kids need to be deeply and fully nourished. When they eat fresh, whole, living foods (whether plants or animals) grown in fertile soil with mineral-rich water, they can support their physiology and development, and put some in reserve for when challenges come along. These foods can include the following:

## YOUR SHOPPING LIST

### Fats

| | |
|---|---|
| Butter** | Olive oil* |
| Coconut oil* | Schmaltz** |
| Flax oil* | Sesame oil* |
| Ghee** | Sunflower seed oil* |
| Grapeseed oil* | Tallow** |
| Hemp oil* | Tree nut oils like walnut, |
| Lard** | macadamia, hazelnut* |

*Unrefined, cold pressed, and organic*
**From pastured animals*

### Seasonings

| | |
|---|---|
| Annatto | Cayenne |
| Apple cider vinegar | Cilantro |
| Black or green cumin | Gemasio |
| Black pepper | Herbamare |

Kelp

Oregano

Organic wheat-free tamari or
nama shoyu (soy sauce)

Paprika

Rosemary

Sage

Sea salt

Thyme

Turmeric

Umeboshi plum vinegar

## Make a Spice Station

Set up your spices in a visible place in your kitchen. Get your children involved in making meals by asking them to pick out seasonings that look interesting to them. Even if they're just asking for "the red one" or "the green stuff," it's a great way to pique their curiosity about new flavors. Turmeric contains curcumin, one of the most powerful antioxidants and anti-inflammatories known.[1] Black cumin seed has been shown to effectively treat everything from asthma to seizures to cancer.[2,3,4] The Koran even refers to it as "the cure for everything except death." Cayenne helps with pain syndromes.[5] Rosemary has such powerful aromatic phytochemicals that simply inhaling its aroma boosts memory.[6] Spice up your food!

## *Teas*

Alfalfa

Chamomile

Ginger

Green

Hibiscus

Lemon balm

Licorice

Linden

Oatstraw

Passionflower

Peppermint

Red clover

Rooibos

Rosehip

Skullcap

Tulsi

## Whole foods

| | |
|---|---|
| Fruits and vegetables from the entire color spectrum (organic or biodynamic when possible) | Seeds, nuts, grains, and beans (sprouted) |
| | Raw honey, maple syrup, date sugar |
| Pastured, organic meats | A small selection of minimally processed foods to use for snacks, packed lunches, etc. |
| Pastured, organic eggs | |
| Pastured, organic dairy | |

### The Superfood Myth

People always ask me which "superfoods" I recommend, expecting me to name exotic foods like goji berries, acai juice, or yacon. My take? *All* foods raised in a responsible, nutrient-dense way possess characteristics associated with superfood. To qualify as a superfood, your body has to really love it and want to change for the better as a result. Dandelion is a perfect example. Nutrient-dense and bitter, it's good for the gut and the microbiome; the gallbladder, the liver, and detoxification; and blood sugar stabilization. It helps flush the kidneys and reduce the pain response. It's a powerful antioxidant and it helps fight cancer.[7] You can eat all of the parts: flower, leaves, and root. And dandelions grow everywhere, so you can gather them . . . for free!

There's no need to travel to the corners of the world to find "magic food." Your superfoods may be growing wild in your backyard, hiding under a rotting log in the forest, stocked at your farmer's market or CSA, munching on lush grasses in not-so-distant pastures or laid that day by foraging hens in your own backyard! Fresh, whole foods have superpowers when grown in the way nature intended, exposed to the elements—sunshine, high-mineral water, rich soil, bugs, worms, and the whole crew of miracle workers above- and belowground. I point patients to specific foods to emphasize particular healing benefits, but it's best to enjoy a wide array of nutrient-dense foods for the diverse "superpowers" they offer.

Here's a snapshot of the healing journey and the foods that aid it:

1. **Empty the basin:** Remove allergens and food toxins as possible, as well as factory-farmed food and industrial chemicals. Drink clean water.
2. **Heal the gut:** Introduce therapeutic remedies such as bone broths infused with astragalus; aloe gel; bitters; teas such as chamomile, licorice, or fennel; soups; sauerkraut; and kefir.
3. **Balance the immune system:** Enhance vitality with maitake, reishi, and other mushrooms; ginger, teas such as red clover and alfalfa, and spices such as turmeric and black cumin seed. Homemade goat milk yogurts (if dairy is applicable) are helpful, too.
4. **Detoxify:** Help the body cleanse its systems with foods such as organic dandelion root tea or young dandelion greens, cabbage, stinging nettles (handle with care or you will be stung!), artichokes, raspberries and other berries, beets, and the whole color spectrum of fruits and vegetables.
5. **Nourish the cells** with nutritive teas, soaked and sprouted nuts and seeds, sprouted grains, cacao or chocolate, some pastured meat, tallow/lard/schmaltz/duck fat, coconut oil, squash, and sweet potato.
6. **Regulate neurological function** with remedies that calm, such as passionflower and lemon balm tea, that promote focus like green tea, and that enhance brain plasticity like brassicas (kale, Brussels sprouts, broccoli sprouts, cabbage). Offer diverse healthy fats.

## GROCERY SHOPPING

I recommend you limit your grocery store shopping to those foods that you can't get from a farm or farmer's market (more on this in a bit), such as dried goods and other pantry staples. Here's what to keep in mind when you go:

- **Don't bring your kids:** Grocery stores are no places for children. Supermarkets—and the food companies represented there—strategically set traps to capture your child's attention. From packaging (cartoon characters and celebrities) to product placement (the shelves at a child's eye level are prime real estate) to checkout line displays of candy while you stand there with nowhere to go. If you can—and I realize it's not always up to you—leave the kids at home.
- **Read labels:** Trying to corral your kid at the store makes it very difficult to focus on what's written on a food label. It takes the utmost concentration, even for the most experienced parent. Remember, labels are difficult to read on purpose.
- **Look out for these red flags:**
  1. MSG: hydrolyzed anything (yeast, vegetable protein, soy protein, etc.), autolyzed anything, anything "caseinate," natural flavors (sometimes)
  2. Aspartame or other artificial sweeteners: NutraSweet, saccharine, Splenda
  3. Food dyes: anything FD&C, yellow or red number anything, any color
  4. Preservatives: science lab words. Things you don't see on the list of ingredients in cookbooks or can barely pronounce.
  5. High-fructose corn syrup: corn syrup, corn sugar
  6. Partially hydrogenated fat: cottonseed oil, soy oil, corn oil, canola oil, "vegetable" oil

## Meal Planning

With reasonable advance planning, you can employ these principles without turning your life upside down.

- **Start seasonal:** What delicious ingredients are available right now in the season and place where you live? I wouldn't choose to eat fresh tomatoes in the cold Northeast during December; I'd choose a dish that features meats or root vegetables with dark, leafy kale. On the other hand, in summer, my family rejoices in the abundance of organic heirloom tomato varieties available at the farmer's market (or from our own garden!) that we fit into as many recipes as possible for the short months of tomato season. Arrange meals around what is freshly picked, whether from the garden, store, farmer's market, or CSA. Consider Google your friend for coming up with recipe ideas. When we first joined a CSA 12 years ago, kale and Napa cabbage rotted in my crisper because I had no idea how to prepare them. Now, I hop online for inspiration. Adjust your cooking style to the seasons, too. Think about hearty soups and Crock-Pot meals in the winter and salads or grilled veggies in the summer.

- **Love your leftovers:** Make the most of dinner prep by making slightly more food than you normally would and stretching those leftovers over the course of the week. If we've had roast chicken on Sunday, I'll make leftover chicken thighs into a potpie, and the carcass into slow-cooked soup with veggies and spices. I might skim some of the fat off the top and use it to flavor veggies. Throwing a meal in the Crock-Pot before leaving in the morning means dinner can be ready by the time you're home from a busy day. A little leftover broth might become the cooking liquid for a pot of grains. Those grains can then become the base for taco night along with some black beans, spices, salsa, and chopped veggies. Freezing surplus also stretches leftovers.

- **Think about ingredients:** Because I cook from scratch, I consider the foundations of a meal as I shop. Produce, including dried fruit, whole grains, meat/fish, eggs/dairy, oils, nuts/seeds/beans, spices, fats. With these components— and my easy recipes—meal options are limitless.

- **Limit processed foods:** Our processed food supply is restricted mainly to crackers made with seeds, occasional gluten-free or sourdough breads, and rare treats like organic tortilla chips, plantain chips, or small-batch sorbet or ice cream.

## FARMER'S MARKETS AND CSAs

I call farmer's markets my "natural Prozac" because I always leave happier than I arrived. I connect with growers and food-makers, take in the fragrant fresh vegetables and herbs, vivid fruits, mushrooms, eggs, and meats, as well as the carefully crafted cheeses, decadent jams, and other goods. Freshly picked produce smells and tastes fantastic as opposed to what you buy in stores, which has been bred to look handsome, uniform, and last for weeks.

*Do* take your children to farmer's markets instead of supermarkets. Explore together. Say hello to the farmers and ask questions about their work as well as their growing practices. Take samples of foods. See what your kids like. Give them a "farmer's market allowance" and let them make decisions about what to buy for the week. Create parameters: One thing they've had before and liked, one thing they've never had before that they are interested in trying, and, of course, a treat.

NOTE: Most farmer's markets have specific requirements about how far the food can travel and what can be sold. Beware of imitations, i.e., "farm stands" that get their produce from the same suppliers as the grocery stores but sell it along the road or at a fruit stand.

Community Support Agriculture (CSA) is a model where individuals support a local farm for the whole growing season in exchange for boxes of the farm's weekly harvest. It's a subscription for superfresh food. CSAs can offer fruits and vegetables, eggs, meat, even dazzling flowers. To find a CSA program near you, go to http://www.localharvest.org/csa/ and type in your zip code.

## OTHER SOURCES FOR GOOD FOOD

### Foraging

> *A weed is a plant whose virtues have not yet been discovered.*
> —RALPH WALDO EMERSON

In unsprayed areas, such as (hopefully) your own lawn—or untamed areas—look for dandelion leaves, flowers, and roots. We forage in our yard for rose hips, plantain leaves, wood sorrel, or lamb's-quarter. Learn what's around you and get the phytonutrient boost of wild food on nature's tab. **Always positively identify what you are eating.** Books such as *The Forager's Harvest* (Samuel Thayer) and *Edible Wild Plants* (John Kallas) are good guides.

### Grow Your Own!

Start a plot in your backyard or in a community garden, using Seed Savers' heirloom seeds for a punch of flavor and nutrition, or cuttings from friends or local nurseries. Start by "building" soil by adding compost (which can be bought or made from your own food waste and yard scraps). Plant seeds or seedlings and see what happens. Check out Chapter 16 for much more information on this, as growing your own food is one of the best ways to reap the health benefits from spending time outdoors.

If you don't have outdoor space to plant, grow herbs and greens on your windowsill, balcony, or roof. We have grown tomatoes, basil, mint, and a small avocado tree along with a worm compost bin in our New York City apartment. It can be a little messy, but it's worth it when you see your kids' excitement as they watch the seeds sprout, the leaves unfold from the stalks, and eventually pick their very own harvest.

## FEEDING YOUR FAMILY WHEN
## NOT EVERYONE EATS EVERYTHING

### *Dealing with Food Sensitivities*

To address my family's sensitivities, I've cooked meals that are gluten/corn/soy/dairy/citrus-free. It sounds extreme, but it is really not that difficult. We've never had a shortage of foods that everyone can eat and enjoy. Most guests in our home gush over our food without ever knowing that they are eating "free-from" food. We have plenty to choose from: meat or fish, beans, veggies in all forms, most fruits, rice, potatoes, quinoa, and other nongluten grains.

While the learning curve can be steep when cooking for food-allergic or food-sensitive kids, shopping and cooking become second nature after the initial transition.

Anyone can cook; no training is necessary. Making meals for a family requires only basic ingredients, basic equipment, some simple tried-and-true recipes, and—every once in a while—flights of imagination. Cooking at home started as a necessity for my husband and me; as doctors in training with kids and little income, we didn't have money to eat out or buy prepared foods. Once we detected our son's soy allergy and discovered that nearly every restaurant used partially hydrogenated soybean oil in its food—which could trigger a weeklong episode of breathing difficulties and missed work—cooking was the only option.

With a couple of good knives, a cast-iron skillet, and a few stainless-steel pots, you can prepare delicious recipes. Gadgets are fun but completely optional.

### Fun Gadgets: Getting the Best Bang for Your Buck

**Slow cooker:** For bone broths and one-pot meals that cook all day while you're working or otherwise occupied.

**High-speed blender:** Expensive, but worth it for all of the ways it makes homemade food tasty and easy. They can last for more than a decade. Make smoothies, homemade frozen yogurt, soups, and nut butters, and grind wheatberries to make fresh flour. Think Vitamix or Blendtec.

**Dehydrator:** Preserve your harvest of fruit and veggies at the height of the season, or make inexpensive homemade kale chips or healthy fruit roll-ups from actual fruit!

**SodaStream:** To make your own fun fizzy beverages at home.

**Food processor:** A major time-saver for quick slicing and dicing of veggies or fruit.

## MORE REASONS COOKING IS GOOD FOR YOUR FAMILY

### It Is Healthier . . . Physically

In a study comparing those who cooked dinner to those who ate out, researchers found that young people who eat home-cooked food eat more healthfully. They consumed significantly more fiber, fewer carbohydrates and calories, and less salt and sugar.

### It Is Healthier . . . Emotionally

University of Michigan researchers found that *the amount of time kids spend eating meals together at home is the single biggest predictor of academic achievement and fewer behavioral problems*—more important than time spent in school, studying, attending religious services, or playing sports.[8] Wow. More frequent family meals increased the odds of a child's positive social skills and engagement in school and decreased the likelihood of problematic social behaviors.[9]

### It Saves Money

For the same amount of money (or less) that you spend on take-out, you'll get better-quality food when you cook at home. Unless you seek out restaurants that share a philosophy of quality, organic food fresh from the farm—and thankfully there are more of these than there used to be—you are likely eating monocrops, factory-farmed meat, and partially hydrogenated oil, all for a higher price than if you'd purchased far better ingredients yourself.

## Tips for Starting a Family Meal Practice

- **Start slowly.** If your family is not used to eating together, start by planning one or two family meals in a week. Sit down together for a family meal, homemade or otherwise. A weekly favorite take-out meal may first bring everyone together, unplugged. Gradually increase until you have at least one family meal every day. If this is impossible because you or your partner work late or your kids are enrolled in sports or other activities, then try for breakfast, or even a special weekend snack. If that's impossible, it may be time to reprioritize activities.
- **Sit with your children.** Your physical presence matters. Be together at the table where you can make eye contact with your child. Ask your child what is happening in his life and encourage him to share by recounting things—serious or silly—that happened during his day.
- **Unplug.** No phones, TV, iPads, Nooks, Kindles, and whatever else I'm forgetting. Not for kids, not for parents. This is not easy. There are days I find this very difficult, especially if something important is going on with a patient or I'm exhausted and want to check out after a long day. But your brain needs a break as much as your kids need you to be present. No books or newspapers either, unless you are using those as a way to be together.
- **Keep it positive.** Make mealtime a refuge from the demands of the day for both you and your kids. Try to avoid criticizing table manners or nagging at the table. Share positive things that have happened, or interesting things

you are considering. Maybe talk about plans for something fun for the family to do together. Tell jokes. Paradoxically, sometimes the most difficult or secretive kids open up when they have a low-pressure venue to share with the family and are not put on the spot.

- **Include activities** to keep kids emotionally engaged if needed. This can range from the corny—playing telephone, spelling bees, mental math—to more edgy choices if you have tweens or teens. Some kids love to be read to. I used to read *Harry Potter* at the table (each character with a different voice and accent), which made everyone look forward to hearing me sound ridiculous!

- **Ignore family protests.** Tell your kids this: "I love you and it is important to me that we spend some time together each day enjoying food." Stay neutral, don't get angry, and be present. Remember, you are the rock for your kids, who are going through all the tumult of their days.

- **Ask everyone to help prepare the meal.** Assigning (or better yet, accepting volunteers for) various tasks means that everyone plays a role. Cooking will be quicker, and children like to eat what they helped plan and prepare. With advance notice, some teens really enjoy preparing a special meal—they like to be trusted and enjoy the good feedback, and you don't have to cook. Win-win! Don't forget to clean up as a team as well.

- **Create special family meals or rituals for certain nights or once a month.** Make homemade pizza together. Taco night. Salad bar night with an ice cream bar for dessert. Do a taste-test night: make three different salad dressings or smoothies and find out which one people like most. See if they can guess ingredients. Let one child plan an entire surprise meal once a month and help shop for the secret ingredients. Be his or her *sous-chef*.

> • **Invite other friends or family over for some meals.** Most kids (though not all) enjoy festive meals. Invite guests to make the experience more compelling. No screen time still applies!

## INTRODUCING NEW FOODS

I know that getting your children to eat beneficial foods isn't as simple as preparing them and setting them on the table. I first introduced kale to my very picky three-year-old son, knowing he liked spinach and broccoli, but that kale could be tougher and more bitter. When he said he didn't want it, I casually told him he would have to eat just two bites, and if he didn't want to eat more, he needn't. He took a cautious bite and looked at me. "I like it this much," he said, holding his fingers about one inch apart. "Okay," I said neutrally, turning my focus back to my plate. Next thing I knew, he had eaten all the kale on his plate. He became a kale proponent, making up games like, "Which do you like better: juicy kale or kale soup with vegetables?" It isn't always this easy, but keep in mind that most kids eventually come around. Here are a few rules for helping your child enjoy different foods:

**Rule One: Start early.** Though it's never too late to change, new studies show that our early food preferences, particularly for fruits and vegetables (or conversely, sugary snacks and drinks), begin in the first year of life. And they can be long-lasting. Infants who preferred healthy foods were found to still enjoy them at six years old.[10]

**Rule Two: Let your child surprise you**. Don't preemptively yuck your kid's yum. Parents often tell me, "It's never going to happen" about foods I recommend . . . before their kid ever tries them. Consider: At least 50 percent of parents in my practice are sure their children won't take it. Guess what? Ninety-nine percent of kids prescribed fish oil take fish oil successfully. I have patients who beg for their bitter tonic!

**Rule Three: Have a positive attitude.** Overcome whatever trepidation, anxiety, or dislike you have for certain food. Many parents confess to me that they themselves don't like vegetables. Join your child on this adventure and get excited to try some delicious new foods.

**Rule Four: Teach your child about being adventurous and brave.** For a child who doesn't want to try something, frame it as an adventure into new, exciting frontiers. If he or she is worried about the experience, talk about how being brave means doing something even though it's difficult. Tell them you're proud of them when they try new things.

**Rule Five: "Not everything has to be your favorite."** Sometimes good enough is fine. We've given kids the impression that every morsel of food must be absolutely delicious to them. But that's not always going to be the case.

CHILD: Ugh, I don't want X.
ME: I'm sorry to hear that. Did you like last night's dinner?
CHILD: Yes.
ME: What about the night before?
CHILD: Yes, make-your-own-tacos are my favorite!
ME: Great! Well, I'm sorry that X is not your favorite. But not everything has to be your favorite. Eat what you can, and hopefully tomorrow will be yummier for you.

**Rule Six: Be a badass.** Feeding children is primal—it embodies deep meaning for us as caretakers. Being positive is important, but you also have to stand your ground. This is difficult for a lot of parents, but it pays off in the long run.

**Rule Seven: Offer foods again and again (and again).** Studies have shown that it can take as many as 20 to 30 tries to get a child to accept a new taste. Not to mention tastes change—one month's yes is another month's no. Often parents say to me: "I stopped sending vegetables or fruit to school with my child because they just came home untouched." My response? "If you don't send it, they *can't* eat vegetables or fruit." Don't stop offering!

**Rule Eight: "Hunger is the best sauce."** Ma from Laura Ingalls Wilder's *Little House on the Prairie* said it best. There's nothing like hunger to make a kid warm to a new food. I put out veggies—raw or cooked—while I prepare dinner. As the smells of food waft through the house, hungry kids pop by the kitchen to grab whatever's handy. That platter of broccoli sautéed with garlic may well disappear by dinnertime. I used to be annoyed that my kids ate all the vegetables before dinner . . . until I realized "MY KIDS JUST ATE ALL THE VEGETABLES!" As a solution, I made more vegetables. Win-win.

**Rule Nine: Don't make food a battle.** When offering new dishes, begin by including a food you know your picky child will eat. You can't force-feed your child and you don't want this to become a control issue. It doesn't mean that they get breakfast cereal or PB and J every night for dinner, though—if they choose not to eat a given meal, they can wait for the next meal.

**Rule Ten: Don't take your children's eating personally**. Maybe you made a delicious dinner after a long day's work and they only ate the rice. Maybe they only picked at your smiley face omelet with zucchini for eyes and a red pepper smile. It's not a personal rejection of your love or your value as a parent. It sucks to put out that kind of effort and get a "meh" in return, but avoid giving up, feeling hurt, or spitting accusatory comments like "You *never* eat healthy food" or "You can eat fast food every night for all I care."

**Rule Eleven: Make one meal for the family.** I am a working parent who makes a fresh gluten-free, dairy-free, soy-free dinner for her food-allergic family every night. I am not, however, a short-order cook. I make one nutritious and delicious (I'm told) meal for everyone, and frankly, I'm done for. Yet parents tell me about the different meals (yes, entire meals!) they prepare for each kid in the house and then another for themselves! The best way to get kids involved in new foods—and to preserve your sanity—is to make dinner for everyone . . . *once.*

**Rule Twelve: Phase in new foods.** Sometimes an enthusiastic parent will leave my office and do a complete makeover of the family kitchen within 24 hours. Then they come back having given up, despondent that no one was on board with the switch. These changes are important and positive. But food is a doorway to a deeper place for many people—comfort, pleasure, attachment, wanting to be loved, to look good, and even confidence in the ability to provide. So telling your partner that you've thrown away everything in the kitchen, or telling your kids that they can't eat any of the foods they love anymore may invite more pushback than necessary. Start by talking about it. Then replace foods incrementally. Replace fast-food French fries with homemade ones, or eventually mix it up with sweet potato fries. Rotate old favorites with new dishes. Replace pasta with whole grains like sprouted rice or quinoa, cereal with slow-cooked oatmeal, instant ramen with chicken soup plus slippery mung-bean noodles. Slow and steady wins the race.

## TROUBLESHOOTING: SCHOOL LUNCHES, HEALTHY SNACKS, AND NAVIGATING "JUNK TRAPS"

### Keeping Snacks Healthy

We used to eat regular crackers. Then we transitioned to rice crackers, then to really funky, tasty crackers made mostly out of seeds. Sometimes it clicks immediately, and sometimes it's a process—unless your child is ill and needs a more dramatic change right now, you have some leeway. Tackling snacks can be difficult, especially if your kids crave the processed stuff. You can start out small, replacing Doritos with organic tortilla chips, then maybe plantain chips. Packaged cookies may lead to homemade cookies or maple-coated nuts. Here are some suggestions for navigating snack time:

- **Buy lots of fresh fruits and vegetables that kids like:** Berries, melon, carrots, celery, apples, cucumbers, grape tomatoes, pears, snap peas, mangoes, kiwi, grapes, even kohlrabi and turnips are kid-friendly foods. Make sure they are all ready for eating (for example, cube melons, slice carrots). Silly things like using a crinkle-cutter can make a difference for a picky eater. I know a little girl who was compelled to eat all sorts of vegetables because they looked "fancy." If your kids like pickles, a quick and dirty way to get veggies into them is to cram slices of raw turnips, beets, carrots, and other root veggies into your pickle jar with just the leftover juice. Let it sit for a week and then you have a jar of delicious pickled veggies for snacks and condiments.

- **Just add dips:** Cultured cream cheese, hummus, bean dip, nut or seed butter, homemade jam can all elevate a fruit, vegetable, or cracker. My kids sometimes like just a spoonful of almond, hazelnut, or sunflower butter.
- **Make snacks available any time of day:** Keep healthy snack foods in a specific place in the fridge or pantry so your kids can help themselves whenever they're hungry.
- **Other snacks to have on hand:** hard-boiled eggs, cheese cubes, yogurt (buy plain and add fruit, honey, nuts, cinnamon, etc.), nuts, seeds, granola, dried fruit, chickpeas.

## Other Ways to Make Snacks More Fun

- Drizzle fruit with a little raw honey.
- Serve frozen yogurt with a big bowl of berries, nuts, granola, dark chocolate chips, and shredded coconut.
- Make-your-own smoothie bar with different frozen and fresh fruits and veggies, along with some cocoa, cinnamon, nutmeg, lemon and orange rind, coconut water, almond milk, kefir, etc.

## When Junk Happens

Sometimes I hear this from families: *Johnny refuses everything except red Popsicles.* Question: "Does Johnny earn money, go to the store, and buy red Popsicles? If the answer is no, remember you can control the "junk" that's entering your house. (Though admittedly this requires both parents to be on the same page.) That said, sometimes junk happens. When my daughter was seven, she attended a friend's birthday party. At pickup, the mom commented (smugly) that my daughter had gorged herself on candy to the point of near vomiting. My response? "That's fine. Now she'll know how it feels when she eats too much candy." Indeed, my daughter volunteered afterward that she had eaten too much candy and felt sick.

You and your kids will always be presented with situations where there's a lot of unhealthy food being dangled in front of you. Here's how I cope:

- **Bring your own treats:** When we'll be in places with a high likelihood of junk, I always bring a bag with some "acceptable" treats, i.e., additive-free items—seaweed snacks, plantain or potato chips, all kinds of dark chocolate treats (chocolate-coated nuts, ginger, raisins, etc.), maple candy, honey straws, dye- and corn syrup–free lollipops, fruit leather made from real fruit, homemade almond macaroons, or ginger chews.
- **Offer swaps:** Halloween, birthdays, celebrations at school—it seems that we use any excuse to flood children with candy. I've heard of well-heeled schools that have regular "lollipop" or "ice cream days" to make school seem more "fun" (rather than including more time outdoors, more hands-on activities, less homework). To help sweeten the deal for kids forking over their booty to you, offer something in exchange. Forgo homework for a day, instead, bake something homemade together, go somewhere special together.
- **Another tactic,** especially on Halloween, is to let your child pick some candies from the mix. With the remainder:
  Trade some for additive-free options you can live with.
  Trade for money: each candy for a penny, nickel, dime, or quarter.
  Leave them as an offering for the "candy fairy" in exchange for a small surprise trinket and sparkles under their pillow.
  Build something out of candy. I've seen kids design really creative edifices to admire instead of eat.
  Perform experiments with candy: What happens if you soak it in water? Vinegar? How long does it take the dye to diffuse?

## SCHOOL LUNCH

School lunch has become the front line of the battle for healthy food. And it makes sense when you consider why and how schools started feeding kids to begin with.

Children used to walk home from school to eat a "hot lunch," and then return. But modern public schools—modeled after factories—began exploring "feeding programs" after social scientists, nutrition experts, government researchers, welfare groups, parent/teacher organizers, and ladies' charity leagues wanted to end nutritional in-adequacies among school-age children. Parents were informed of the connection between diet and academic achievement, hot school lunches were organized and served, and legislation ensued. As school lunches caught on, so did corporate food-service outsourcing, and, ultimately, the debate over "good school lunch." And while nutritionists, parents, school boards, and corporations debate, most kids are provided with awful lunches (as in, pizza counts as a vegetable).

Corporations—who lobby to supply food to millions of children—serve lunches of processed food for profit. Yet this issue doesn't always blip on parents' radars. I know parents who are incredibly particular about what their children eat, what they wear, who they play with, and what they read, but when I ask what they eat at school they just say, "school lunch."

But health, behavior, or learning issues that result from eating processed, chemical-laden junk during the day follows your child home. Consider this: Surrendering school lunch to junk is like losing five full meals a week (sometimes ten if school breakfast is included) to corporations with little interest in your children's well-being.

Let's also talk about *when* children are eating and how much time they have to do so. As schools have grown but cafeteria space hasn't, lunch begins as early as *9:30 in the morning*. Teens may have been at school since 7 a.m., but since teachers forbid students from eating in classes later, kids are forced to push through on cortisol to survive the day.

Lunchtime was once an hour long. Now, lunchtime can be only 30 minutes, so children—even younger ones—have to put away their books, get to a cafeteria, obtain food, eat, clean up, and return to class all in 30 minutes! My children often came home with their lunch half-eaten because they "didn't have time to eat." Figure in a few stolen moments of socializing and some kids come home starving with a full lunchbox.

A study conducted by the Johns Hopkins School of Public Health found that these factors meant children ate healthier foods:

1. Quieter cafeterias (outside is great for this) or an alternative quiet lunchroom for those who prefer it

2. Food cut into pieces (apple slices, carrot sticks, etc.)
3. Longer lunch periods, especially with recess tacked on the end
4. Teachers or adults eating lunch in the same cafeteria

## PACK YOUR OWN

Preparing parts of lunch for kids the night before saves time and means your family will eat healthier meals.

Rotate new foods until you have a sense of what your children enjoy. Again, it's okay that not everything you serve will be a favorite, and it may take several tries before foods come home eaten. But don't give up. The goal is not to pressure kids to eat foods they don't want, but to get them excited about the food so they'll try it. If you stop sending vegetables because they come home uneaten, you're ensuring your child won't eat veggies. Instead, get creative.

### Brainstorm

**Salad**: Veggies and chicken/meat strips, taco ingredients, nuts and seeds, cheese, sliced hard-boiled eggs, salmon candy

**Rice bowl**: Sprouted rice, quinoa, or other grain with beans, seeds, or nuts, poached egg, fish or meat, and assorted veggies with a tasty dressing

**Frittata or quiche**

**Chili**: Veggie or meat (some grated sweet potato builds great texture and flavor)

**Veggie sushi**: Nori stuffed with brown rice or quinoa, avocado, and other veggies

**Snacks**: Cut veggies with dip (hummus, cultured cream cheese, bean dips), fruit, plantain chips, kale chips, seaweed (best from Atlantic sources)

**Treats**: Dark chocolate, maple candy, honey and cinnamon–coated nuts, almond macaroons, chocolate-covered coconut, chocolate mousse, pumpkin custard

**Leftovers from dinner**: Best and easiest lunch ever!

## Other Supplies

Use a metal tiffin lunchbox to avoid plastics and reduce waste

Wax paper bags instead of plastic

Klean Kanteen water bottles or thermoses for tea or soup

Notes with inspirational or quirky quotes, cartoons, and wacky sketches go a long way!

## MEALS AT A GLANCE: YOUR CHEAT SHEET FOR HEALTHY EATING

**Breakfast:**

- **Eggs**. Any form! Poached, scrambled with veggies, hard-boiled (great for storing in the fridge and grabbing for on-the-go).
- **Oatmeal**. Steel-cut is best, thickly cut is next best—best soaked with a bit of yogurt then slow-cooked overnight in a Crock-Pot. Bob's Red Mill makes gluten-free oats, which most but not all GF kids tolerate.
- **Sourdough or GF French toast**. You can make this in advance and freeze, then stick it in a toaster during morning rush time.
- **Sourdough pancakes or waffles** (gluten-free options are available). Prepare the batter in advance and store in the fridge for up to one week. Serve with cut-up veggies.

\*****Don't get stuck on "breakfast"**: Breakfast doesn't have to include traditional breakfast foods. I know kids who eat steak or soup for breakfast. For example, a traditional breakfast in Colombia is bone broth and hot chocolate!

**Lunch:**

- **Dinner leftovers** (my favorite!)
- **Cheese and veggies**
- **Sprouted hummus or bean dip with veggies and seed crackers**
- **Soup or chili in a thermos**
- **Salad with cheese, egg, meat, or beans** (send dressing on the side if your child doesn't like soggy lettuce)

- **Melted cheese on sourdough toast**

*Make sure to rotate through some fun add-ins:

- **chocolate-covered nuts, seeds, or fruit**
- **seaweed snacks**
- **plantain chips**
- **homemade cookies or muffins**
- **square of dark chocolate, plain or with mint**
- **crystallized ginger** (it's spicy but some kids love it)
- **maple candy**

**Dinner:**

- **Chili**
- **Make-your-own-tacos** (or taco salad)
- **Burritos** with high-quality sprouted tortillas plus cheese, sour cream, beans or meat, mushrooms, onions, lettuce, tomatoes, salsa. Some kids love pickled jalapeños.
- **Hearty soups,** for instance, bone broth chicken soup with chunks of chicken, a bit of ginger, and tons of cut-up veggies, or a thick lentil or split pea with salad on the side and sourdough bread for dipping. Puree soups for kids who are prone to pick out the veggies, and remember that adding a touch of cream (even coconut cream can work) to carrot or squash soup can make the difference between turned-up noses and full bellies.
- **Meat sauce and sautéed veggies served over sprouted quinoa**
- **Frittata with sautéed veggies, with or without cheese**
- **Marinated chicken breast with sweet potato fries and garlic sautéed broccoli**
- **Greens such as kale, collards, Swiss chard, bok choy in olive oil or schmaltz with garlic and salt or with a splash of umeboshi vinegar**
- **Carrots, zucchini, leeks sautéed in olive oil or butter**

*Mix it up. Breakfast for dinner is always fun

*At every meal: Always include at least one vegetable (or two) along with a fruit. Cut them up for your child. Remember: Studies show that bite-sizing produce increases the likelihood of kids eating them.

**Snacks:**
- **Sprouted nuts or seeds,** including those baked with a bit of maple syrup or honey, or spices
- **Roasted kale chips**
- **Cut-up fruits and veggies with drizzles or dips**
- **Smoothies made with fruits and veggies**
- **Plantain chips, or fried green or sweet plantains**

**Drinks:**
- **Water**
- **Homemade tea** (iced or warm) with or without a touch of sweetener or milk
- **Homemade lemonade sweetened with maple syrup**
- **Hot cacao drink with almond (or other) milk and a spoonful of blackstrap molasses**

## Sample Menu

Day One
- Breakfast: sourdough French toast with cinnamon, maple syrup, a fruit and veggie, tea
- Snack: carrot sticks with dip and nuts
- Lunch: squash-and-lentil stew with quinoa, cut veggies and fruits, plantain chips, some dark chocolate–covered almonds
- Dinner: chicken with olives, honey, and garlic; black cumin quinoa; salad

Day Two
- Breakfast: Crock-Pot oatmeal with fresh berries, sliced veggies
- Lunch: baked potato covered with cheese and sautéed veggies, cut veggies and fruits, a coconut macaroon, kale chips
- Dinner: make-your-own taco salad with guacamole, beans, cheese, salsa, and spices

Day Three
- Breakfast: eggs with sautéed onions and veggies, salsa on the side

- Lunch: rice and beans mixed with sautéed veggies, organic tortilla chips and salsa, cut-up fruits and veggies, a square of dark chocolate
- Dinner: roast chicken with veggies left in timed oven, squash pie, cabbage salad

Day Four
- Breakfast: boneless sardines or mackerel in olive oil with a splash of umeboshi vinegar, seed crackers, cut veggies and fruits
- Lunch: slices of leftover grass-fed roast with quinoa and greens, cut veggies and fruits, dried mango, sprouted sunflower and pumpkin seeds mixed with dark chocolate chips
- Dinner: chicken potpie with veggies, sautéed kale on side

Day Five
- Breakfast: smoothie of fruits mixed with yogurt or with a scoop of almond butter plus water, cut veggies
- Lunch: chopped salad with bite-sized veggies and sliced hard-boiled eggs, roasted salty nuts and seeds to sprinkle over top, blue potato chips, chocolate-covered ginger or fruits
- Dinner: bone broth or mushroom-based soup with hearty veggies, yucca, and millet

Day Six
- Breakfast: fried egg, red cabbage sauerkraut, cut veggies
- Lunch: hummus with carrots and other veggies, seed crackers, roasted and salted seaweed, cut fruits, pumpkin custard
- Dinner: ground beef chili (with carrots, celery, peppers, and grated sweet potato), quinoa, Brussels sprouts

Day Seven
- Breakfast: sourdough or sprouted toast with almond butter and raw honey, fruits and veggies
- Lunch: rice or quinoa bowl with tons of veggies and fixings (including sliced chicken or beef, nuts, spices), bliss balls
- Dinner: veggie frittata, salad, sweet potato fries

## CHAPTER 17
# Healing from the Outside In

*Those who contemplate the beauty of the earth find reserves*
*of strength that will endure as long as life lasts. There is something*
*infinitely healing in the repeated refrains of nature—the assurance*
*that dawn comes after night, and spring after winter.*
—RACHEL CARSON, *SILENT SPRING*

There's a reason most people feel happier when they're walking near trees and plants, or sitting on a beach. It's no accident that people escape to the countryside or seaside for restorative time or vacations. Simply being outside in nature offers tremendous physical, mental, and emotional benefits. This chapter is dedicated to partnering with the most powerful healing force of all: nature.

## RESTORATIVE ENVIRONMENTS ARE HEALING

*Restorative environments* are natural places that allow the renewal of personal adaptive resources to meet the demands of everyday life.
    Consider:

- Exposure to nature scenes, more so than urban environments, improves stress levels and mood, and enhances positive emotions, improves cognition, and sharpens focus.[1] Just looking at nature can improve attention.[2]
- Children playing in natural school playgrounds (on grass versus concrete or rubber surfaces) showed fewer attention and concentration problems, and improved cognitive and physical functioning than children playing in less natural school playgrounds.[3]

- Children perform better on tests when exposed to green spaces,[4] and schools with more green space have higher test scores.[5]
- Several studies show that natural settings might have restorative effects that include increased performance on tasks requiring attention and cognitive processing. Time in green space also improved working memory and reduced inattentiveness, even for kids with ADD.[6,7,8]
- One study showed that spending time in the forest can reduce repetitive negative thoughts and rumination, risk factors for depression.[9] And note, for teachers and parents, nature even makes us more cooperative.[10]

## FOREST BATHING

The concept of shinrin-yoku, or forest bathing, has become an integral aspect of preventive medicine in Japan over the last 30 years. There, doctors recommend deriving healing from spending time walking, meditating, and doing activities in the forest as part of a preventive care plan.[11] The practice has been well studied, with measurable improvements in health that include:[12,13,14]

- **Stress:** reduced "fight or flight" activation of the sympathetic nervous system, lowered adrenal stress hormones, lowered blood pressure
- **Immunity:** increased natural killer cells and anticancer proteins, decreased inflammatory markers
- **Sleep:** better sleep and better energy
- **Cognition:** improved focus (even in children with ADHD)
- **Mood:** happier and increased sense of well-being
- **Resilience:** faster recovery from illness or surgery

The forest can offer tremendous balance to children and help them to focus and function, optimally to be happier and healthier, and to be more resilient. Nothing man-made, pharmaceutical, or otherwise, comes even close to offering this array of benefits . . . for free!

**Take Away:** *Parks, schoolyards, green spaces, and most important, wilderness are not simply optional places for leisure and sport; they facilitate physical, mental, and social health in profound and fundamental ways that cannot be imitated or replaced.*

> *Take a walk or a hike in nature each day.*
> *Help your kids plan and build a fort, pitch a tent, or construct a teepee outside.*
> *Build a temporary labyrinth with sand outside, and walk it with your child.*
> *Do homework sitting on a rock, under a tree, or in a fort, tent, or tree house.*
> *Go for a scooter or bike ride in a park before or after dinner.*
> *Give your kids a patch of land to grow whatever they want to grow: a food garden, a butterfly garden, or a rare plant garden.*
> *Speak up for wilderness and green space in your community.*

## Soil Microbes Make Us Happy, Healthy, and Smart

Our relationship with bacteria-rich soil can improve our mood. When cancer patients were treated with a microbe found in soil, they reported improved quality of life and happier mood.[15] A subsequent study showed it improved survival in those with melanoma.[16] This soil bacteria, *Mycobacterium vaccae*, boosted serotonin levels in mice as effectively as antidepressant drugs did.[17] The mice learned more quickly and were more alert and better focused as well.[18] Encourage your kids to make mud pies—or better yet, make them together. Doctor's orders!

## EARTHING, AKA GET YOURSELF IN THE DIRT

Throughout history, humans mostly walked barefoot or wore footwear made of animal skins and slept on the ground or on skins. The ground's abundant free electrons were able to enter our bodies, and every part of the body could equilibrate with the electrical potential of Earth. This stabilized the electrical environment of all organs, tissues, and cells. *Earthing* (or grounding) refers to the benefits—including better sleep and reduced pain—we derive from being connected to these conductive systems that transfer Earth's electrons from the ground into our body.

Earthing helps to set our biological clocks by regulating our body rhythms, which impact sleep quality and cortisol secretion.[19] Earth's electrons can also reduce pain and balance our sympathetic (fight or flight) and parasympathetic (calming) nervous systems.[20]

In short, running barefoot outside, lying in the grass watching clouds or reading, or sitting on a rock are actually fantastic for your health and well-being.

## LET THE SUN SHINE

Slathering kids in sunscreen has become a part of everyone's summer routine. Science tells us, however, that we may not be doing them a favor. As with our fear of dirt, germs, and outdoors, we've developed a fear of sunshine. Yet a 2014 study at the Karolinska Institute that followed 30,000 women over 20 years found that the women who assiduously avoided sun exposure were significantly more likely to die than those who didn't.[21] That's right. More sun exposure meant they were *less* likely to die.

Most of us know of the benefits of vitamin D, a steroid hormone that modulates more than three thousand genes and proteins, including absorption and transport of calcium, phosphorus, and magnesium for bone mineralization and growth; cell growth and healing; and critically, immune function. It supports sleep and mood by promoting serotonin and melatonin production. Vitamin D decreases inflammation and may modulate autoimmune diseases. One randomized study of more than one thousand women showed a 77 percent reduced risk of cancer throughout four years in those being supplemented with vitamin D and calcium over those only getting calcium.[22]

University students who had sun exposure were happier than those who avoided sun.[23] Yet scientists felt that benefit could not be fully attributed to vitamin D levels. Cells throughout the body, including the skin and eyes, are sensitive to blue light from the sun, which in turn regulates hormones, appetite, stress, sleep cycle, and other important elements of hypothalamic function. It stimulates melatonin release, which helps us fall asleep, acts as a powerful antioxidant, increases gut motility (which can help reflux), and even mitigates depression. The hypothalamus and the pituitary gland influence the adrenal glands, which control cortisol production. These important effects on brain activity, which increase alertness, improve cognition, and boost mood and vitality, are independent of vitamin D production. We've quantified just some of what the sun offers. Getting outside in the sun benefits us on many levels.

What about the dreaded UV rays? Ultraviolet light in excessively high doses can cause DNA damage and increase risk of certain skin cancers, which is why it's critical to avoid sunburns. But some daily sun is not necessarily bad: Workers who spent more time in the sun had lower risk of melanoma than those who were outside intermittently.[24] Chronic sun exposure may offer protection from melanoma,[25] as well as psoriasis and multiple sclerosis. And phytochemicals in botanicals, applied topically and taken orally, help protect us from the damaging elements of UV rays—just as they do in plants themselves—while allowing us to benefit: from sesame and coconut oils,[26] pycnogenol (pine extract),[27] red clover sprouts or tea,[28] green or black tea,[29] and others.

Protect children from sunburns by staying covered or in the shade during the strongest hours of sun—that's a great time to explore forests or play in forts. When necessary, use a sunshirt with UV protection or apply natural sunscreen. Check out the Environmental Working Group's ratings for the safest sunscreen options. Balance a healthy respect for the power of the sun, with partaking of its benefits.

## The Real Dirt on Artificial Turf: Why Use Toxic Turf When Grass Is Great?

Many parents and educators argue that children spend considerable time outdoors participating in sports. While exercise and time outdoors both have considerable positive impacts on children's health, many children spend their outdoor time on synthetic turf—another example of industry finding a lucrative way to dispose of toxic waste.

1. **Tire scraps are toxic and may make kids sick.** Most synthetic turf fields use crumb rubber from recycled tires as "infill" or cushioning material. Crumb rubber contains myriad toxic chemicals, such as the carcinogen called carbon black. Every synthetic turf field contains forty thousand ground-up rubber tires; this expands the surface area that can release toxic chemicals inhaled or absorbed in skin, especially open wounds. Human exposure routes include inhalation, skin, and accidental ingestion, all of which occur during normal play.

   Synthetic turf fields can contain high levels of lead in its green pigment. As aging fields deteriorate, the plastic material becomes powder, releasing lead in more absorbable form. Lead, a potent neurotoxin, alters the developing brain even in tiny amounts.[30] Further, more and more cases of leukemia and lymphoma are being reported in students who have played on synthetic turf fields.[31]

2. **Temperatures on synthetic turf fields can rise to unsafe levels.** The surface temperature of synthetic turf fields on sunny days can reach 160 degrees or higher. High-powered water cannons with lots of water are required to cool surface temperatures to safe levels. On hot days, this must be done repeatedly to reduce risk of serious heat-related illness in athletes. Further, turf contributes to climate change. Synthetic turf fields, like tar roofs, contribute to the "heat island" effect. Finally, these fields, made from petroleum by-products, do not convert carbon dioxide into oxygen and store carbon in their biomass as their grass-field counterparts do.

3. **Synthetic turf requires the use of disinfecting chemicals.** A synthetic athletic field must be disinfected regularly to remove body fluid as well as bacteria that otherwise would be removed by rainfall and the natural processes of soil. The

disinfecting chemicals are registered pesticides that present their own health risks.

4. **Synthetic turf blocks the benefits of earthing**. The electron transfer of earthing discussed above cannot penetrate the tire crumb that makes up turf. Kids who play on turf are not benefiting from this regulating effect of being outdoors.

**Take away**: *Dispose of these materials and put down wood mulch or ground cover. Do not play on synthetic turf fields that contain ground-up rubber tire infill. If there is no other option, shower immediately after leaving the field and change clothing, including socks and shoes, where tiny rubber crumbs can hide.*

## YOUR NATURE PRESCRIPTION

*Live in each season as it passes; breathe the air, drink the drink, taste the fruit, and resign yourself to the influence of the earth.*
—HENRY DAVID THOREAU, *WALDEN*

## LEVEL 1

- **Grow herbs in planters or outdoors**
- **Join a community garden**
- **Spend 15 minutes outside: climb a tree, roll down hills, lie in the grass**
- **Use essential oils and smudges in the home**
- **Shop at the farmer's market**

### Start Small

Get a pot and soil, and grow herbs from seed indoors, or bury a ginger-root and watch it sprout. Your kids will love watching the plants grow;

it creates relationship with nature through the act of caring for and harvesting the plants.

## Building Community Through Collective Gardens

If you feel overwhelmed by growing food alone, start by seeking out a community that has a collective approach. Contribute time to caring for a garden with others in exchange for some of the harvest. This can be an opportunity to grow food, learn, find your tribe, and build community, and not shoulder the entire burden alone.

Together, you can write a letter about your project and ask people to donate surplus seeds, plants, tools, soil, and money. There are free plants all over the place wherever you live. Train your eye to see them. Some garden nurseries get new stock every week and will allow a regular pickup of donations throughout the growing season. Most seed companies only send out donations once a year, in fall or winter. Organize an annual seed swap and include giveaway tables of donated seed packets from organic seed companies. Check out the organization Foods Not Lawns.

### Nature's Aromas

Scent is a powerful way to connect with nature. Volatile aromatic compounds from plants enter directly into our primitive nervous system—bypassing any neurological processing—which links us to memories and past experiences. The *aroma* of rosemary has been shown to enhance memory and focus.[32] We even have scent receptors covering our skin that promote wound healing when we come into contact with certain plant-based volatile compounds.[33] Our healing relationship with plants is complex.

**Houseplants or cut flowers, grasses, or boughs of evergreens:** There's a reason we send flowers and plants to people when they are sick, experience a loss, or celebrate. Plants smell wonderful and make us feel good. Keep plants—houseplants, branches of ever-greens, wildflowers—in frequented rooms in your home in all seasons.

**Smudging:** Traditional cultures burned bundles of sage, sweetgrass, cedar, and other aromatics as medicine for lungs, nervous system, and skin.[34] They used smudging to bring plants and nature into their homes and to "clear the air." Research shows that beyond simply inviting good feelings, it literally disinfects the air—lowering levels of diverse organisms in the air by 94 percent within an hour and lasting for up to a month afterward.[35] Smudge sticks are easy to buy from local herbalists or online, or better yet, to make with your children. Light them, blow them out so they smolder, and allow the scent to permeate your home. (Don't forget to put them out safely afterward.)

**Essential oils:** These can bolster our immune systems, brain function, emotion, sleep, and more. They have excellent anti-microbial properties as well, especially in combination.[36] Sample different options and see which ones make you feel great. Then add a few drops to the bath, an ultrasonic humidifier or diffuser, or to some coconut oil to massage into your body, and enjoy. Someone once gave me a cotton ball with a few drops of pep-permint essential oil in an empty baby food jar for my severe nausea when pregnant—it really helped! I've also used two to three drops of peppermint oil in a cup of ice water, then doused a compress to apply to the forehead of kids with a headache or fever. Three to four eucalyptus drops in the shower or bath are wonderful to clear congestion. I love a couple of drops of lav-ender on a pillow for relaxation, and Thieves Blend (cinnamon, clove, lemon, tea tree) to help fight infection. In fact, my sixth-grade son's science fair experiment compared bacterial growth after applying Thieves Blend, soap or hand sanitizer from his hands on a petri dish. Thieves (an antimicrobial) won by a land-slide. That's my go-to "hand sanitizer."

### Inspire Kids about Food and Nature Through Reading

*James and the Giant Peach* by Roald Dahl
*Fantastic Mr. Fox* by Roald Dahl
*Bread and Jam for Frances* by Russell Hoban
*Farmer Boy* by Laura Ingalls Wilder
*Little House on the Prairie* by Laura Ingalls Wilder
*The Lorax* by Dr. Seuss
*A Seed Is Sleepy* by Dianna Aston and Sylvia Long

### LEVEL 2

- **Plant your own garden, berry bushes, or a small orchard**
- **Start a compost heap**
- **Visit a farm**
- **Read a book about permaculture gardening**
- **Order heirloom seeds**
- **Spend time walking and exploring forests**
- **Go camping**

*One of the most important resources that a garden makes
available for use, is the gardener's own body. A garden gives
the body the dignity of working in its own support.
It is a way of rejoining the human race.*
—WENDELL BERRY

### Gardening 101

Gardening is one of the best ways to reap the benefits of being in nature. You're exposed to elements that nourish your body and your children's—growing things helps interest kids in digging in the dirt—plus you get the freshest food. It can be as easy or involved as you desire. Some people imagine that the only way to cultivate a garden means tremendous effort and expense: tilling, planting rows of tomatoes and peppers and strawberries, seedlings, watering and fertilizing and weeding regularly, then harvesting. That's just one way to do it.

A much more realistic—and beneficial—alternative is to practice *permaculture,* an approach to growing that imitates natural systems and takes advantage of nature's incredible ability to sustain itself. Rather than trying to control nature, we piggyback on nature's boundless energy and foster a relationship. In this model, we are merely facilitators, becoming part of a web of soil, sun, rain, and diverse plants, microbes, insects, and critters. This relatively self-sustaining system is also called a "food forest," which will produce many perennials as well as some annuals. It means there are two clients: the people who live there and the land itself.

*Companion planting* means planting certain crops next to others to discourage pests and weeds, and to encourage healthy soil.

## Plant-feeding Hedges or Trees

Feeding hedges (called "fedges") provide fruits with few duties on your part. We planted a hedge of raspberries, serviceberries, gooseberries, blueberries, and elderberries with little subsequent effort beyond pruning and harvesting. Fedges planted in a curved pattern can protect crops from critters, deflecting them from snacking on the plants inside the circle.

Feeding trees can provide fruit or nuts, pollen for bees, seasonal shade, privacy, windbreak, and—critically—leaves that eventually turn into mulch to build soil. In dry areas, orchardists plant trees in small depressions in soil, connected by a net pattern of shallow trenches, to collect rain and soil runoff. Dwarf trees are available in most varieties and are easier to maintain for those of us who prefer to remain earthbound.

## Composting 101

Compost plays many roles: it recycles waste, preserves soil nutrients, creates fertile humus, boosts microbial life, and offers opportunity for exercise because occasionally we must turn it, and eventually, spread it. Wait until you have three feet's worth of material to compost so the microbes are able to raise it to the minimum necessary heat to break it down: It should include layers of 50 percent green (grass clippings, fresh plant trimmings, kitchen waste, and—yes, I know it is technically brown but it falls into the green category for our purposes—manure), and 50 percent brown (dried leaves, hay, straw, wood shavings). Some people will add a little fishmeal or blood meal for extra nitrogen if they are worried that they don't have enough "green." The heap (which most prefer to keep in a container of sorts to avoid attracting rodents) should be moist like a wrung-out sponge. Some people who are more fanatical will add small amounts of soil from wilder areas to inoculate the compost heap with more microbial biodiversity. I even visited one small-scale permaculture farmer who used composting toilets and a year later had rich compost from "humanure" for their family's crops (though personally I recommend applying humanure to nonedible plants, as it can concentrate our bodies' waste toxins). In the end, the beauty of compost is that you have transformed waste into something fantastically valuable . . . for free!

## Building Soil, AKA the Real "Black Gold"

You don't have to grow your own food to care about building soil fertility. After all, in the same way our entire skin is considered one organ, so is Earth's skin one organ. All soil is connected. Soil is an amazing entity—a fertile, alive place filled with possibility. One teaspoon of pasture soil might contain a billion bacteria, a million fungi, and ten thousand amoebae. Soil is where the dead are brought back to life. Decomposing organic debris and minerals weathered from stones feed vibrant living plants and organisms, which process dead particles in the soil and recast them as living matter. Fertility of the soil comes from the richness of this cycle and not from a bag of synthetic fertilizer.

The life in soil builds upon itself. Soil that is rich with nutrients and microbes means more plants, and more kinds of plants. The diverse plants attract diverse insects, which provide food to more species of birds and other creatures that feed upon them. Microbes are attracted to the living and dead matter that results. Diversity begets diversity. And diversity is abundance for all, including those at the top of the food chain.

Nature builds soil from two directions: the top down, and the bottom up. From the top, leaves fall from above to become part of the earth. We can mulch over that organic matter, to build mature soil filled with organic matter, microbes, and critters, ready to nurture healthy plants. From the bottom up, plant roots build soil by pulling nutrients from deep in the earth and siphoning them to the surface for other plants to use. When we harvest plants, we remove some of those nutrients from the soil, which ideally we return through compost, mulch, or natural fertilizer.

### Don't Waste Time Raking Leaves

Yep, you heard me. Fallen leaves are free food and microbiome for your soil, food and habitat for the critters—salamanders, chipmunks, earthworms, snakes, others—necessary for healthy soil. Certain butterfly species pass the winter as pupae within those leaves, and birds feed on bugs and worms there in spring. Dead leaves suppress weeds, break down into compost that enriches soil, and keep roots safe and warm throughout winter. If you must clear the leaves, don't use loud, polluting leaf blowers and don't send the leaves to the landfill in plastic bags—instead rake the leaves (don't forget to jump in them) and compost them for use around trees, shrubs, and other plants. Feed your soil!

### LEVEL 3

- **Keep chickens (or other livestock)**
- **Work to start an edible schoolyard or an outdoor classroom**
- **Plant a green roof or vertical garden**
- **Take a class on foraging and preparing wild plants with your child**

- **Send your soil to be tested and feed it accordingly**
- **Learn about biodynamic growing**
- **Build a tree house or outdoor fort**

## Chickens 101

Keeping chickens for eggs is quite simple, and it is far easier than caring for many other pets. To have a steady supply of delicious eggs—and yes, they do taste better than store-bought—you need only a few things to get started:

- Investigate local laws and ordinances. New York City, for example, allows unlimited chickens (within limits of health, hygiene, and animal protection), but no roosters (whose crowing can be a nuisance).
- Build or procure a henhouse, with space calculated to the number of chickens you intend to keep, protected from the elements (hot sun, cold winds, rain, and snow). It can be as simple or decked out as you desire.
- Obtain organic, non-GMO feed and nontoxic bedding, like pine shavings or straw.
- Obtain chicks or chickens.

## Keeping a Family Goat or Sheep

Keeping cows, sheep, or goats is not just for farmers. Dwarf or small-breed Jersey cows require little more than half an acre of land (and can be rotated between neighbors). They provide maximum two to three gallons of milk a day, which can be shared. Goats graze in just about any kind of rocky or hilly terrain, and they are solar-powered lawn mowers, offering free fertilizer and milk to boot. They are hardy, adapt well to heat and cold, require little space, and are inexpensive to keep. A goat averages three quarts of milk a day for ten months a year. Sheep offer similar benefits, plus wool.

## Nature Education and Edible Schoolyards

Nature is the ultimate teacher for us all and provides a superior classroom to anything money can buy. Every school should offer a food- and nature-based curriculum to equip children with the knowledge that every human who walks this planet should have—how to be custodians of land and wildlife: building soil, identifying trees and plants, planting, growing and harvesting sustainably, and preparing food. Such an education complements and can integrate science, math, literature, and art.

Now that we know the health and cognitive benefits of being in nature, imagine children who sit for hours at desks staring at smart-boards instead moving around outside, learning by doing, in contact with trees, plants, sunshine, and fresh air. How would nature awaken their focus, creativity, curiosity, and passion? How could it improve their executive function, stress levels, and mood?

Many projects like this are already in practice. Since 2005, chef Alice Waters's Edible Schoolyard Project has been teaching children about foods they can grow, pick, and prepare themselves. Using the garden as a classroom, children create healthy, filling meals from soil to seed to plant to plate. The program has been so successful that it's branched out to more than 3,500 locations worldwide. Wellness in the Schools also offers similar opportunities in New York City. Investigate to see if there are similar programs in your area, or start one. Your children will thank you!

## Taking Action

We cannot raise another generation of consumers. The word "consume" means to destroy (as in a consuming fire) or to waste. Our children instead must become a movement of creators who know how to work with, rather than against, the elements of the natural world. We can create a very different future for ourselves, our communities, and the Earth by the way we buy, grow and eat and by how we educate our children.

# TAKE HOME

1. Eat dirt! Eat food that grew in rich organic, biodynamic soil. Eat freshly picked veggies that aren't power-washed. Prepare and cook foods with peels on if they are edible.
2. Grow food in dirt! Spend time feeding soil with compost and mulch. Don't use chemical fertilizers or pesticides—allow plant diversity in your lawn. Use leaves and bits of cut grass and compost to build healthy soil ecosystems that create rich soil and abundant plant and wildlife. Use ground cover that gives back nutrients to the dirt and doesn't need mowing.
3. Bathe in dirt! Spend as much time as possible outside. Kick your kids outside (without their sunscreens). Encourage them to play in the dirt. Join them if you are so moved! Make mud pies, and don't be afraid to take a bite or two. Spend hours a day in forests and parks, on mountains, and play sports on fields instead of turf.
4. Protect dirt! Let your community and legislators know that you value the quality of air and water and that you want to preserve our soil, trees, and nature. This doesn't make you an environmentalist per se, just a smart human being. Legislators and leaders experience political and financial pressure all the time from industry; they must hear the voices of their community often. And as the Dalai Lama says: "If you think you are too small to make a difference, try sleeping with a mosquito." Let's keep our principals, doctors, communities, legislators and leaders awake!

*We need the tonic of wildness. . . . At the same time that*
*we are earnest to explore and learn all things, we require that*
*all things be mysterious and unexplorable, that land and sea be*
*indefinitely wild, unsurveyed and unfathomed by us because*
*unfathomable. We can never have enough of nature.*

—HENRY DAVID THOREAU

# RECIPES

These are some favorite recipes that are used in regular rotation in my household. And take note: It was my kids who voted on which dishes to include! Nothing here is complicated. I'm not a chef. I'm a fan of easy and fast—especially after a long day of work. Yet these recipes pack a ton of delicious flavor. If I'm going to take the time to cook, I want everyone to eat with minimal argument and maximal enjoyment.

Each of these dishes starts with whole, nourishing foods and uses various cooking methods and/or seasoning to transform them into the best version of themselves. They taste like what they are and there's no "hiding" veggies or junking up healthy foods just to make them palatable to kids.

I made an effort to give you general measurements for each dish, but know that I *never* use recipes when I cook (which is why baking is not my forte!). I encourage you to take these recipes merely as suggestions and guidelines; don't get too bogged down by specific amounts. Always feel free to eyeball, taste, replace, adjust, and make it your own.

NOTE: It goes without saying, but all the ingredients called for in these recipes should be the highest quality that you can find—organic, biodynamic, pastured, fresh, and local whenever possible.

## VEGGIE FRITTATA

*Serves 6 to 8*

I love having this dish in my back pocket for when I'm in a hurry to feed everyone, but all I see in the fridge are random ingredients that don't feel like the makings of a meal. Just roughly chop some favorite veggies—any assortment will do—and sauté them while you're beating the eggs, and within 20 minutes you have dinner or lunch. I plan for one to three eggs per person when serving this as a main dish, depending on appetite, but you can easily scale this recipe up or down. It's also delicious cold and is great packed into lunches.

4 tablespoons olive oil or coconut oil or 2 tablespoons schmaltz or lard

2–3 cups assorted vegetables (such as asparagus, cherry tomatoes, onions, leeks, broccoli florets, peas, bell peppers, spinach, or swiss chard), roughly chopped into bite-size pieces

½ teaspoon each salt and pepper

½ teaspoon paprika

12 large eggs

Optional: pastured cheese, grated or in small chunks; pastured, nitrate-free bacon or ham, cut into small pieces

1. Preheat the oven to 350°F.
2. Heat a cast-iron pan or large sauté pan over medium-high heat and add the oil or fat. When it moves easily around the pan, add the vegetables. Sauté until they're just tender, 5 to 8 minutes. Add the salt, pepper, and paprika.
3. While the vegetables are cooking, beat the eggs until frothy in a medium mixing bowl.
4. Reduce the heat to low-medium and pour the eggs over the vegetable mixture, as well as any cheese or bacon you're using. Continue cooking until you can see the eggs at the edges of the pan starting to set. Gently pull back the cooked edges with the spatula so that more liquid runs over the edge. When the egg is mostly set, transfer the pan to the oven and cook for another 10 to 15 minutes, until the top is just golden brown and the eggs have set in the center.

## SWEET AND CRUNCHY BRUSSELS SPROUTS

*Serves 6 to 8*

I've converted a number of greens-averse children to Brussels sprouts lovers with this recipe. It's sweet, salty, just a touch bitter, and generally delicious.

4 tablespoons olive oil or 2 tablespoons lard or schmaltz

10 shallots, peeled and roughly chopped

1–1½ pounds Brussels sprouts, thinly sliced (if you have a slicing option on the food processor it goes very quickly)

2 tablespoons raw honey

½–1 teaspoon sea salt

1. Heat a large cast-iron pan or large sauté pan over medium heat. Add the oil or fat and when it moves easily around the pan, add shallots and sauté until translucent.
2. Toss in half the Brussels sprouts and sauté for 5 minutes or until they wilt a bit. Stir in the honey and salt and mix well.
3. Add the remaining Brussels sprouts, toss with the existing mixture, and sauté for another 5 to 7 minutes. The first of the greens will soak up the honey and fat; the remainder will add a bit of crunch and freshness.

## RED CABBAGE SALAD

*Serves 6 to 8*

People are always asking me for this recipe after eating it at my house, and I'm almost embarrassed to give it to them because it's so simple. But as straightforward as this dish is, it's delicious and somehow manages to taste even better the next day. The cabbage stays crisp as it continues to marinate in the umami-filled umeboshi plum vinegar. This salad is a great way to get purple cabbage and all its fabulous phytonutrients into kids.

½ medium head red cabbage, finely sliced (avoid the wilted prechopped stuff from the store—do it yourself!)

½ cup olive oil

Juice of 1 lemon or 2 teaspoons umeboshi vinegar (if using umeboshi, omit the salt)

1 teaspoon sea salt (but always adjust to taste)

Add the cabbage to a large mixing bowl and top with the olive oil, lemon juice or umeboshi vinegar, and salt (if applicable). Toss well and serve immediately for a fresh, crunchy salad, or marinate for 1 hour on the counter for a more tender, wilted version.

## KALE THREE WAYS

Kale has gotten pretty trendy lately, but it's for good reason: It's a highly nutritious leafy green, filled with phytonutrients that boost brain plasticity for optimal learning and memory. It also has the bitter profile that boosts our bodies' detoxification process. Substitute different varieties of kale or other leafy greens—collards or chicory, for instance—too. Rotating greens allows us to fully benefit from each of their diverse benefits.

### KALE CHIPS
*Serves 4 to 6*

> 1 bunch kale (red, green, lancinato)
> 1 tablespoon olive oil
> Sea salt

1. Preheat the oven to 350°F.
2. Rip the kale leaves into 1- to 2-inch pieces off of the central stem. In a medium-size mixing bowl, toss them with the oil and a pinch of salt (saltiness will concentrate as the kale bakes, so go easy). Arrange the leaves on a baking sheet, making sure they aren't overlapping. Bake until crispy, 10 to 15 minutes.

### RAW KALE SALAD
*Serves 4 to 6*

> 1 bunch lancinato (aka dinosaur or Tuscan) kale leaves removed from stem*
> ½ cup olive oil
> 2 cloves garlic, minced
> ½ teaspoon sea salt
> Optional: dried currants, sprouted sunflower or pumpkin seeds, hemp seeds, Parmesan shavings
> *TIP: **Save stems!** Chop stems finely and throw in the pan first to sauté with that night's veggies; use stems in your next batch of bone broth, or juice them.

Roughly chop the kale leaves into small bite-size pieces. Add the pieces to a medium bowl and coat with oil. Massage—or gently squeeze—the kale for 1 to 3 minutes, or until the oil runs green and the kale is soft. Add the garlic, salt, and any other toppings.

## SAUTÉED KALE
*Serves 4 to 6*

1 bunch purple kale (though any kind of kale will work, or use another leafy green such as collards)

2 tablespoons olive oil or coconut oil or 1 tablespoon lard, schmaltz, or tallow

1 purple onion or large leek, sliced finely

3 cloves garlic, chopped and allowed to sit for 10 minutes *

½ cup bone broth or water (more if needed)

Splash of umeboshi vinegar or juice of 1 lemon

½ teaspoon salt or gomasio

*The superb healing properties of garlic are maintained even after cooking **if the chopped garlic is allowed to sit for 10 minutes first.**

1. Remove the kale leaves from the stems and finely chop both, keeping them separate.
2. Heat a large sauté pan over medium heat and add the oil or fat. When it moves easily around the pan, add kale stems and onions or leeks. Sauté for 2 to 4 minutes. Reduce the heat to low and add the kale leaves and garlic. Cook for another 5 to 8 minutes, depending on whether you like your kale tender or crisp. For "juicier" kale, add a splash of broth or water, increase the heat to medium-high, and cover for 3 to 5 minutes when you add the leaves. Take care not to overcook the kale or it will become bitter and soggy. Sample as you cook!
3. Remove the kale from the pan, and season with the umeboshi vinegar or lemon juice and salt, or a couple of shakes of gomasio.

## HUMMUS

*Makes about 2 cups*

Kids love to dip their foods, and this creamy, satisfying spread tastes best homemade. It comes in handy if your kids are reluctant to eat vegetables—it encourages them to "interact" with their food.

½ cup dried chickpeas, soaked for 12 hours then simmered for
   1 hour (a 15-ounce tetra pack can be substituted in a pinch)
2 tablespoons tahini (sesame paste)
¾ cup olive oil
Juice of 2 lemons or 1 tablespoon umeboshi vinegar (if using the
   umeboshi, you may need less salt)
3 garlic cloves, minced
1 teaspoon sea salt

Combine the ingredients in a food processor or blender and blend until smooth. If desired, add water in ¼-cup increments to achieve looser texture.

### Sprouting Beans, Seeds, and Grains

Allowing grains, beans, and seeds to soak and sprout offers significant nutritional benefits. It makes these foods easier to digest; neutralizes phytic acid, which can block your absorption of key nutrients like calcium, magnesium, iron, copper, and zinc; boosts vitamin C and B complex content; and alkalinizes the body.

## BONE BROTH

*Makes 4 quarts*

Bone broth and stock have always been made from the parts of the animal that could not be used for other purposes, like the chicken carcass from a roast chicken or beef marrow bones, not to mention chicken feet or beef knuckles. Not only do these overlooked bits impart deep, rich flavor to a broth, they also lend amazing health benefits. You can enjoy it as a base for soups and stews, a flavorful cooking liquid for rice and other grains, or a simple mug of something warm.

Think of the broth as a blank canvas for whatever ingredients and flavors you love most—a couple of thumb-size pieces of fresh gingerroot (the peel can stay on if it's organic); a few sticks of dried astragalus root; a handful of medicinal mushrooms such as reishi, maitake, or shiitake; a thumb-size piece of turmeric root or one to two teaspoons of ground turmeric; veggies like squash, celery, onions, and carrots; and other flavoring agents like garlic or fresh herbs such as parsley, thyme, or cilantro. Don't forget that making broth is a perfect opportunity to use vegetable scraps. You can easily scale this recipe up or down—the basic rule of thumb is roughly one pound of bones per gallon of water, but soon you'll be able to just eyeball it.

> 3–4 pounds bones of any type—beef, bison or buffalo, marrow
>   bones, lamb, venison, chicken, duck, goose, turkey, goat, or pork,
>   roasted at 400°F for 50 minutes. Add chicken feet or beef knuckles
>   for more nutrition and flavor. Don't knock it till you try it!
> 1 gallon filtered water
> 3–5 cups assorted vegetables, roots, and fresh or dry herbs
> 10 cloves garlic, peeled

1. In a large stockpot or Crock-Pot, submerge the bones in the filtered water (adding more if necessary). Bring to a low simmer and allow to cook covered for 6 to 12 hours if using chicken bones, 12 to 24 hours (up to 48, if desired) when using larger bones like beef. During the first few hours, skim away any gray foam that rises to the top. This is the time to add mushrooms like maitake or shiitake, as well as astragalus root or ginger.

2. During the last hour of cooking, you can add vegetables—except for garlic and fresh herbs, which you can add toward the end. A good indication that the broth is done is the bones become crumbly—a sign that the minerals are dissolving into the broth.

(Make sure to eat the marrow—in pastured animals the marrow is dense with healthy fats that support immunity.)

3. Strain the broth through a colander or sieve and store in the fridge for up to a week or freeze it into cubes to have handy for future meals. The bits of ginger, reishi, and astragalus have already infused the soup and can be composted.

## BLISS BALLS

*Serves 10 as dessert, or keep in fridge and enjoy over several days*

These make appealing, nutrient-dense treats that boost immunity all year round. A little goes a long way. There are endless variations, including dates, lemon zest, ground nuts, chia or hemp seeds, and so on. Get creative!

16-ounce jar sprouted nut butter, tahini, or sunflower butter
¾ cup blackstrap molasses
¼ cup grade B maple syrup (or ½ cup, depending on desired sweetness)
2 tablespoons reishi powder
2 tablespoons astragalus root powder
2 cups raw cacao powder (or fair-trade powdered cocoa in a pinch)
Unsweetened coconut flakes (optional)

Combine nut butter with maple syrup and mix. Blend in reishi, astragalus, and cacao powder. Use a small melon scoop to form balls, then roll in cocoa and, if desired, coconut. These keep in the fridge for at least a week.

## SQUASH AND LENTIL STEW

*Serves 8 to 10*

This is a great meal—easy and hearty, and the leftovers are delicious to pack up for lunch the next day.

6 tablespoons butter, ghee, coconut oil, or olive oil
1 teaspoon paprika
1 large onion, chopped
2 pounds butternut squash, peeled and cut into ½-inch pieces

1 carrot, chopped

1 celery rib, chopped

4 garlic cloves, minced

1 teaspoon salt plus additional to taste

2 tablespoons minced ginger, peeled

1 teaspoon turmeric

1 teaspoon cumin

¼ teaspoon cayenne (optional)

1½ cups red lentils, soaked and sprouted (see note
on page 318)

8 cups bone broth or water

Juice of 1 large lemon or 2 tablespoons umeboshi
vinegar

Freshly ground pepper, to taste

1. Place a large cast-iron pan or heavy-bottomed pot with a lid over medium-high heat. Add the fat and when it moves easily around the pan, add the paprika. Sauté until the spice is slightly brown and aromatic. Add the onion and sauté until translucent, about 4 minutes, then add the squash, carrot, celery, garlic, and 1 teaspoon of salt. Cook until all the vegetables are tender, about 10 minutes, stirring occasionally. Stir in the ginger, turmeric, cumin, and cayenne (if using) and cook, stirring frequently, for another 2 minutes.

2. Add the lentils and broth or water and simmer, covered, until the lentils are tender, 20 to 30 minutes.

3. Stir in the lemon juice or umeboshi vinegar, season with salt and pepper, and serve alone or with a grain.

## CHICKEN FOUR WAYS

I always like to think about how I can use every part of my food, especially to reap its full nutritional potential. Chicken is a great example: Roast it one night, use the leftover meat for potpies and then use the carcass to make bone broth. Three meals (or more) in one!

## ROAST CHICKEN WITH VEGETABLES

*Serves 6*

> 2 tablespoons chicken fat, duck fat, or 2 tablespoons olive oil
>
> 3 garlic cloves, minced
>
> 1 teaspoon paprika
>
> ½ teaspoon sea salt, plus more to taste
>
> 1 teaspoon freshly ground black pepper
>
> 1 tablespoon blackstrap molasses or honey
>
> One 4-pound chicken
>
> 2–3 cups assorted roasting-friendly vegetables such as yams, potatoes, kabocha squash, carrots, and fennel, cut into 2- to 3-inch cubes

1. Preheat the oven to 300°F.
2. Combine 1 tablespoon of the fat or oil with the garlic, paprika, salt, and pepper, and use the mixture to generously coat the chicken, top and bottom. Drizzle molasses or honey over the top of the chicken. Set aside.
3. Use the remaining tablespoon of fat or oil plus a pinch of salt to coat the vegetables and add them to the bottom of a large Dutch oven. Place the chicken on top, breast-side up, and cover.
4. Roast for 2 to 3 hours, then remove the lid. The chicken will be falling off the bone. Continue cooking until the top of the chicken is golden brown, about 10 minutes.

## CHICKEN POTPIE

*Serves 4 to 6*

This recipe is perfect for any leftover scraps from roasting a chicken. Though, when I do roast a whole chicken, I sometimes add an extra package of legs so I know I'll have enough left over for this delicious dish.

> 5 white or blue potatoes (optional: subtract 2 potatoes and include 1 head cauliflower, 3 turnips, or 3 medium parsnips, roughly chopped)

½ teaspoon sea salt, plus more to taste

5 tablespoons olive oil or 3 tablespoons lard, schmaltz, or tallow, separated

1 large onion, diced

5 stalks celery with leaves, diced

5 carrots, unpeeled and chopped

2–3 cups shredded cooked chicken

6 tablespoons quinoa flour or tapioca starch

2 cups bone broth or stock

1. Preheat the oven to 350°F.
2. Place the potatoes—along with any other vegetables you might be using—in a medium saucepot and cover with cold water. Add a half teaspoon of salt and bring to a boil. Cook until you can easily pierce them with a fork. Drain the potatoes, transfer them to a large mixing bowl, and mash them until smooth. Set aside.
3. Heat a cast-iron pan or Dutch oven over medium heat and add 1 tablespoon of the oil or fat. When it moves easily around the pan, add the onion and cook until translucent, about 4 minutes. Add the celery, carrots, and 1 teaspoon of sea salt and continue cooking for another 5 minutes. Stir in the chicken, remove the pan from the heat, and set aside.
4. In a small saucepan over low heat, warm the additional oil or fat, then whisk in the flour or starch until the sauce thickens. Whisk into the broth or stock and pour over the vegetable and chicken mixture.
5. Spread the mashed vegetable mixture over the top of the chicken and bake for 1 hour or until the top is golden.

## CHICKEN SOUP

*Serves 6 to 8*

One 4-pound chicken (or just legs or thighs, or just the carcass from your roast chicken—no need to get fancy)

2–3 quarts water or bone broth

2 stalks celery, roughly chopped

2 carrots, chopped in half

2 onions, halved

1 yam, roughly chopped

Small bunch of parsley

1 turnip, halved

1 parsnip, halved

1 burdock root, roughly chopped

1 thumb-size piece gingerroot (peel if not organic)

Salt to taste

1 teaspoon ground turmeric

1. Combine the chicken carcass, water or broth, celery, carrots, onions, yam, parsley, other vegetables, and ginger in a large stockpot or Crock-Pot.
2. Bring to a boil, reduce to a simmer, and cook over low heat for 3 hours.
3. Add the salt and turmeric in the last 15 minutes of cooking.

## CHICKEN, OLIVES, AND QUINOA

*Serves 6*

This one-pot dish is the perfect example of how to take simple ingredients to a whole other place with the right spices and seasonings.

1½ cups quinoa or any other sprouted grain, such as einkorn, amaranth, rice, or kasha

4 tablespoons olive oil or 2 tablespoons lard, schmaltz, or tallow

2–3 pounds boneless chicken breast, cut into 1-inch cubes (can be replaced by chickpeas for a vegan version)

3–4 tablespoons raw honey

1 teaspoon cumin

1 teaspoon paprika

1 teaspoon turmeric

Pinch of cayenne (more if you like it a little spicier!)

1 teaspoon salt or to taste

½ cup green olives, pitted and coarsely chopped (best to get the good ones, not canned)

5 cloves garlic, minced (throw in more if you love garlic)

Optional: chopped fresh cilantro, chopped fresh parsley

1. If not pre-rinsed, add the quinoa to a strainer and rinse for at least a minute or 2 to wash away some of the bitter saponins. Transfer it to a medium saucepot and cover with 3 cups of water. Bring to a boil over high heat, reduce heat to low, cover the pot, and simmer until the quinoa is tender and most of the liquid has been absorbed, 15 to 20 minutes. Remove from the heat and set aside.

2. Place a cast-iron pan or large sauté pan over medium heat. Add the oil or fat and heat until it moves easily around the pan. Add the chicken cubes and allow to cook for 1 to 2 minutes without moving them. Stir in the honey, cumin, paprika, turmeric, cayenne, and salt so it evenly coats the chicken. Using a wood or metal spatula, turn the chicken cubes and allow them to brown on all sides, for 7 to 10 minutes.

3. Remove the pan from the heat and stir in the olives and quinoa. Sprinkle with fresh herbs, if using, and serve.

## GRASS-FED ROAST

*Serves 6*

In addition to being nutritionally superior, grass-fed meat cooks differently than its conventional counterpart. Take care not to dry it out, and this recipe will get you juicy, tender meat every time.

1 large roast of beef, veal, goat, or lamb

4 teaspoons raw honey or maple syrup

5 cloves garlic, minced

¼ teaspoon cayenne

1 teaspoon paprika or annatto

1 teaspoon cumin

1 teaspoon turmeric

2 tablespoons lard, schmaltz, tallow, coconut oil, or olive oil

1 yellow onion, chopped

3 carrots, unpeeled and chopped

3 root vegetables of choice (or a combination), such as potatoes, yams, sweet potatoes, or parsnips

3 cups bone broth, stock, or water

Small handful reishi, maitake, shiitake mushrooms (optional)

1 tablespoon apple cider vinegar

1 cup dry organic red wine (optional)

1. If possible, remove the meat from the fridge 1 hour before cooking so it can rest at room temperature.

2. Preheat the oven to 300°F.

3. In a small mixing bowl, combine the honey, garlic, cayenne, paprika, cumin, and turmeric to make a thick paste. Slather it evenly over the meat. Set aside.

4. If you're feeling energetic, brown the meat before making the roast. Set a large Dutch oven over medium-high heat and add the fat. When it moves easily in the pan, add the meat and allow it to develop a crust, 2 to 3 minutes. Repeat so that the roast is browned evenly on all sides. Tongs are helpful for this. Remove the pot from the heat and add all the vegetables, topped by the broth, vinegar, and wine, if using.

5. Alternatively, skip the browning and simply create the rub, coat the meat, and add all the ingredients to the Dutch oven.

6. Cover the pot and transfer to the oven.

7. Cook for 4 hours. Remove roast from the oven and allow it to sit for 10–15 minutes. Slice against the grain and serve.

## HOT COCOA

*Serves 2*

That's right, the treat that so many parents think is on the naughty list. By using good-quality cacao—which is up there on the strengthening and balancing list, with reishi and astragalus as well as cinnamon, which regulates blood sugar—this drink is delicious and nourishing. My kids love sipping it through cinnamon stick "straws"!

2 cups raw milk (or milk alternative such as coconut or nut milk)

4–6 tablespoons powdered cacao or fair trade cocoa

1–2 tablespoons raw honey, maple syrup, or evaporated cane juice

Optional: a dash of cinnamon or nutmeg, a splash of vanilla extract, or even a sprinkle of cayenne

Cinnamon sticks, for serving (optional)

Heat the milk in a small saucepan, taking care not to scald. When it's just under a boil, add all the ingredients and stir. Turn off the heat and whisk well for about a minute, until the cocoa is creamy and thick. This step can also be done in a blender.

## MOLASSES DRINK

Enjoy a delicious drink packed with minerals and antioxidants each day.

1 tablespoon unsulfured blackstrap molasses

¼ cup hot water

¾ cup milk (cow, goat, almond, coconut, rice, etc.)

Optional: ice cubes, a dash of cinnamon, 1 teaspoon cacao powder, honey, or maple syrup to taste

1. Dissolve molasses in hot water, then mix into milk.
2. You can drink it like this, or add cacao or cocoa powder, cinnamon, and honey to taste. Blend with ice for a frothy treat, or drink it warm.

## PUMPKIN CUSTARD

*Serves 4 to 6*

It's my philosophy that dessert should be delicious, and that you shouldn't have to feel guilty that you served or ate them. This is one such magical treat. Pumpkin is a healing food that's grounding and also warming when it's cold outside. You could substitute kabocha or butternut squash, and you could absolutely add this dish to your family's Thanksgiving menu. Yum!

    1½ cups roasted pumpkin (or one 16-ounce can, in a pinch)
    ½ cup milk of choice (cow, goat, coconut, almond, rice)
    ½ cup grade B maple syrup
    3 large eggs plus 1 egg yolk
    1 teaspoon vanilla extract
    1 teaspoon ground ginger
    1 teaspoon ground cinnamon
    ½ teaspoon ground nutmeg
    ⅛ teaspoon ground clove
    ⅛ teaspoon ground cardamom
    ½ teaspoon lemon zest
    Pinch of sea salt
    1 cup heavy cream or coconut milk, whipped (optional)

1. Preheat the oven to 350°F.
2. Whisk together all of the ingredients except the optional cream or milk in a large mixing bowl until completely smooth.
3. Divide the filling evenly among individual ramekins, filling them roughly three quarters of the way. Place the ramekins on a rimmed baking sheet and transfer to the oven. Bake for 25 to 30 minutes. They should jiggle slightly in the center.
4. Allow them to cool to room temperature, then refrigerate for at least 1 hour prior to serving. Serve with homemade whipped cream or coconut milk whipped cream, if desired.

## SQUASH PIE

*Serves 6 to 8*

I've changed a lot of people's minds about squash with this yummy dessert.

    1 small butternut squash, peeled and chopped into 1- to 2-inch cubes
    ½ cup almond milk (or coconut milk or regular milk)
    3 large pastured eggs, beaten

Pinch sea salt

3 tablespoons raw honey or maple syrup

½ cup quinoa flour (or other freshly ground flour or gluten-free flour blend)

3 teaspoons ground cinnamon (or more—we like a lot of cinnamon!)

1. Preheat the oven to 350°F.
2. Add the squash to a medium saucepan and cover completely with water. Bring to a boil over high heat until the squash is tender. Strain and allow the squash to cool slightly.
3. In a large mixing bowl, combine the squash, milk, eggs, salt, and honey. Fold in the flour and 2 teaspoons of the cinnamon.
4. Pour the mixture into a lightly greased 15-inch round cake pan or shallow oven-proof glass casserole. Sprinkle the top with 1 teaspoon of cinnamon, and bake for 45 minutes to an hour, till the top is just browned and the middle is set.

## ELDERBERRY SYRUP

7 cups water

2 cups fresh (or in a pinch, dried) black elderberries

5 cinnamon sticks

½ cup star anise

2 cups raw honey (I get mine from our farmer's market) or evaporated cane juice

1. Pour the water into a large pot and add all the ingredients except the honey.
2. Bring to a boil, then cover and reduce to a simmer for an hour until the liquid has reduced by almost half. Remove from the heat and let cool a bit.
3. Pour through a strainer into a sterile glass mason jar; discard the elderberries.
4. Add 2 cups of honey or sugar and stir well.
5. Cover and seal or keep refrigerated. Enjoy a teaspoon daily to boost immunity.

## DIY Meals and Snacks

Kids love options as well as having a say in what they eat. That's why I really like setting up "bars" for my kids (with all kinds of healthy options) so they can assemble or season their foods exactly the way they want. Here are some ideas:

**Taco bar:** Lay out options, such as organic taco shells or tortilla chips, leftover roast chicken or other meat, sprouted refried beans and rice, chopped lettuce (we mix spinach and romaine lettuce), chopped onions, salsa, pastured cheese, and cultured sour cream. If you prefer to avoid grains, create a lettuce base and put the toppings over it as a "taco salad." We often use plantain chips as a delicious nutrient-dense alternative to taco shells or tortilla chips.

**Seed bar:** Set out a variety of seeds in jars such as sprouted sunflower, sprouted pumpkin, hemp, sesame, and chia and let your kids sprinkle them over salads, oatmeal, or stews, or eat plain.

**Spice station:** Make small containers of healing spices like turmeric, ginger, cumin, cayenne (careful with this one!), paprika, annatto, oregano, rosemary, thyme, cinnamon, cloves, nutmeg, cardamom, and black pepper. Have your kids pick whichever flavors and colors interest them most and let them season their food, whether it's sautéed veggies, plain or puréed chickpeas, or scrambled eggs. You can do the same with chopped fresh herbs like basil, oregano, thyme, and rosemary, too. Enjoy!

# ACKNOWLEDGMENTS

A great many wonderful people in my life deserve thanks for their contributions to this book in ways large and small. First, thank you to my patients and their families. You've allowed me to be an intimate part of your lives and you've committed yourselves to the idea of healing as something larger than just fixing symptoms.

Thank you to a few of my many teachers: Stella Koch, my ninth-grade biology teacher, who likely thought I wasn't even listening, but whose class started me down this path. Dr. Isabelle Rapin, who inspired in me a passion for the mystery and complexity of pediatric neurology and who entertained my difficult questions (even when she didn't like them). Dr. Tieraona Low Dog, who encouraged me as an herbalist and healer at pivotal moments, and who has been a loving friend and brilliant colleague. Dr. Rocio Alarcon, who generously shares her heartwork in realms seen and unseen.

Thank you to my friends, colleagues, and other members of my amazing team: my fabulous agent Janis Donnaud, the ever-patient Rachel Holtzman, and my dedicated editor Leslie Meredith, and the entire team at Atria, who made it possible to bring this book into being. To Oly, for her intuition and huge heart. Elaina, Xania, Rosemarie, and Donna, whose unending support made it possible for me to be a mother and practicing doctor as well as an author. To the sisters of my heart: Brenda, Gail, Denice, Jaclyn, Inbal, Ariela, the Big Mouths, the Riverdale Chevra, and my dear fellow Ecuador Journeyers for ongoing love and encouragement. To Dr. Robert Naviaux, Geri Brewster, Dr. Stephan Cowan, Dr. Susan Blum, Dr. Michael Finkelstein, Dr. Martha Herbert, Kathie Swift, Dr. Nico Moshe, Dr. Jennifer Madan-Cohen, Anat Baniel, my University of Arizona

PIM classmates, and many others for being kindred spirits in my professional life.

Thank you to my family: my mother, who insisted that I eat a rainbow on my plate every night, planted an annual garden with me, took me to the National Arboretum often, and ensured with blood, sweat, and tears that I became an articulate writer; my father, whom I miss every day, and who deeply believed that I could do absolutely anything I set my mind to; my grandfather, who foretold that I'd become a doctor before anyone else suspected it, and my grandmother, who cooked all my favorite foods from scratch; my father's ten siblings, who understand the intersection of food, spices, and love like nobody else and who infused me with traditional cooking knowledge; Bill, who has pushed his usual food boundaries when in my home; as well as my husband's loving family.

Most of all, my husband, Avni, and my muses Margalit, Elan, and Erez: you've supported me unconditionally, nurtured my ideas, kept me grounded, and sacrificed so much of our family time so that I could write this book. I'm blessed to be able to learn from you and love you every day.

# NOTES

## PART I: Welcome to the Dirt Cure

1. http://www.cdc.gov/nchs/data/nhsr/nhsr065.pdf
2. http://www.consumerreports.org/cro/2013/12/are-too-many-kids-taking-antipsychotic-drugs/index.htm
3. http://www.cdc.gov/features/childrensmentalhealth/; http://www.ncbi.nlm.nih.gov/pubmed/24796725
4. http://www.ncbi.nlm.nih.gov/pubmed/19934770
5. http://jama.jamanetwork.com/article.aspx?articleid=1866098
6. http://www.aaaai.org/about-the-aaaai/newsroom/asthma-statistics.aspx
7. http://www.ncbi.nlm.nih.gov/pubmed/25038753
8. http://www.ncbi.nlm.nih.gov/m/pubmed/25838260
9. http://www.ncbi.nlm.nih.gov/pubmed/25584915
10. http://www.ncbi.nlm.nih.gov/pubmed/25404284
11. http://www.ncbi.nlm.nih.gov/pubmed/17683018
12. http://www.nature.com/ncomms/2015/150630/ncomms8486/abs/ncomms8486.html
13. http://www.ncbi.nlm.nih.gov/pubmed/18394317

## CHAPTER 1: Where True Health Begins

1. http://www.sciencedirect.com/science/article/pii/S0021755713000028; http://pediatrics.aappublications.org/content/127/3/580; http://www.clinicaltherapeutics.com/article/S0149-2918(06)00121-4/abstract
2. http://m.jleukbio.org/content/90/5/951.abstract
3. http://pediatrics.aappublications.org/content/127/3/580.full
4. http://www.nature.com/ncomms/2015/150512/ncomms8000/full/ncomms8000.html
5. http://www.ncbi.nlm.nih.gov/pmc/articles/PMC2822875
6. http://www.ncbi.nlm.nih.gov/pubmed/21727249
7. http://www.hngn.com/articles/30407/20140504/environmental-factors-increase-risk-of-autism-by-50-percent.htm
8. http://www.ncbi.nlm.nih.gov/pmc/articles/PMC4440679/
9. http://www.ncbi.nlm.nih.gov/pubmed/23608919
10. http://m.cpj.sagepub.com/content/early/2010/11/24/0009922810384728.abstract

11. http://www.thelancet.com/journals/laneur/article/PIIS1474-4422(13)70278-3 /abstract

12. http://www.ncbi.nlm.nih.gov/pmc/articles/PMC3166669/

13. http://www.ncbi.nlm.nih.gov/pubmed/12415039

14. http://www.ncbi.nlm.nih.gov/pubmed/10634297

15. http://www.ncbi.nlm.nih.gov/pmc/articles/PMC3166669/

16. http://www.ncbi.nlm.nih.gov/pubmed/24575806

17. http://jama.jamanetwork.com/article.aspx?articleid=1788456

## CHAPTER 2: Learning to Listen to the Body:
## What Symptoms Tell You

1. Boyle, C. A., S. Boulet, L. A. Schieve, R. A. Cohen, S. J. Blumberg, M. Yeargin-Allsopp, S. Visser, M. D. Kogan. Trends in the prevalence of developmental disabilities in U.S. children, 1997-2008. *Pediatrics*, 2011 Jun;127(6):1034–42.

2. Alessi-Severini, S., et al. Ten years of antipsychotic prescribing to children: a Canadian population-based study. *Canadian Journal of Psychiatry*, 2012 Jan;57(1):52–58.

3. Ibid.

4. http://www.latimes.com/science/sciencenow/la-sci-sn-antidepressants-selfharm-age-20140429-story.html

5. http://www.nytimes.com/2013/04/01/health/more-diagnoses-of-hyperactivity-causing-concern.html?pagewanted=all

6. Bach, J. F. The effect of infections on susceptibility to autoimmune and allergic diseases. *New England Journal of Medicine*, 2002 Sep 19;347(12):911–20.

7. http://www.nature.com/ni/journal/v15/n4/full/ni.2847.html

8. McBride, J. T. The association of acetaminophen and asthma prevalence and severity. *Pediatrics*, 2011 Dec;128(6):1181–85.

9. http://www.ncbi.nlm.nih.gov/pubmed/24322007

10. http://www.ncbi.nlm.nih.gov/pubmed/25251831

11. http://www.ncbi.nlm.nih.gov/pubmed/15878691

12. http://www.ncbi.nlm.nih.gov/pubmed/25956491

13. http://www.ncbi.nlm.nih.gov/pmc/articles/PMC2504411/

14. http://www.fda.gov/ForConsumers/ConsumerUpdates/ucm453610.htm

15. http://www.ncbi.nlm.nih.gov/pubmed/24646587

16. http://www.sciencedaily.com/releases/2011/02/110220193013.htm

## CHAPTER 3: Healthy Body, Healthy Brain

1. http://www.ncbi.nlm.nih.gov/pubmed/22940212

2. http://www.ncbi.nlm.nih.gov/pubmed/21392369

3. http://www.ncbi.nlm.nih.gov/pmc/articles/PMC2886850/

4. http://www.ncbi.nlm.nih.gov/m/pubmed/25731162/

5. http://www.nature.com/nature/journal/v519/n7541/full/nature14232.html; http://www.ncbi.nlm.nih.gov/pmc/articles/PMC3677668/

6. http://www.ncbi.nlm.nih.gov/pubmed/21370495

7. http://www.ncbi.nlm.nih.gov/pubmed/15228837
8. http://www.ncbi.nlm.nih.gov/pmc/articles/PMC2515351/
9. http://www.ncbi.nlm.nih.gov/pubmed/26092910
10. http://www.ncbi.nlm.nih.gov/pmc/articles/PMC1069066/
11. http://www.ncbi.nlm.nih.gov/pmc/articles/PMC1774411/
12. http://www.ncbi.nlm.nih.gov/pmc/articles/PMC3440091/
13. http://advances.sciencemag.org/content/1/3/e1500183
14. http://www.sciencedaily.com/releases/2014/08/140825152016.htm
15. http://www.ncbi.nlm.nih.gov/pubmed/21866137
16. Chen., Y., and M. J. Blaser. *Archives of Internal Medicine,* 2007;167:821–27.
17. http://www.ncbi.nlm.nih.gov/pubmed/25712154
18. http://www.ncbi.nlm.nih.gov/pubmed/25410903
19. http://www.ncbi.nlm.nih.gov/pubmed/?term=25656764
20. Weinstock, J. V., et al. *Gut,* 2004;52:7–8.
21. Wang, Y., and J. K. Pfeiffer. *Nature,* Dec 2014;516:42–43.
22. http://www.ncbi.nlm.nih.gov/pubmed/25409145
23. http://www.nature.com/nature/journal/v447/n7142/abs/nature05762.html
24. http://www.ncbi.nlm.nih.gov/pmc/articles/PMC2951028/
25. http://www.ncbi.nlm.nih.gov/pubmed/24574393
26. http://www.ncbi.nlm.nih.gov/pubmed/25996182
27. http://www.ncbi.nlm.nih.gov/pubmed/19203112
28. http://www.ncbi.nlm.nih.gov/pubmed/25575816
29. http://www.ncbi.nlm.nih.gov/pubmed/25394505
30. http://www.ncbi.nlm.nih.gov/pubmed/26122188
31. http://www.nature.com/mi/journal/v3/n5/full/mi201020a.html
32. http://www.ncbi.nlm.nih.gov/pubmed/25677705
33. http://www.ncbi.nlm.nih.gov/pubmed/14669332
34. http://www.ncbi.nlm.nih.gov/pubmed/21040780
35. http://www.ncbi.nlm.nih.gov/pubmed/21885731
36. http://www.sciencedirect.com/science/article/pii/S003193840800382X
37. http://www.ncbi.nlm.nih.gov/pmc/articles/PMC3788166/
38. Ibid.
39. http://www.ncbi.nlm.nih.gov/pubmed/21988661
40. http://www.ncbi.nlm.nih.gov/pmc/articles/PMC1856434/
41. Ibid.
42. http://www.ncbi.nlm.nih.gov/pubmed/1549382
43. https://www.sciencenews.org/article/inconstant-gardener?mode=magazine&context=188379
44. http://www.ncbi.nlm.nih.gov/pubmed/25311587
45. http://www.ncbi.nlm.nih.gov/pubmed/23877071
46. http://www.ncbi.nlm.nih.gov/pubmed/25404894
47. http://www.ncbi.nlm.nih.gov/pubmed/23404112
48. http://www.ncbi.nlm.nih.gov/pubmed/24299259
49. http://www.ncbi.nlm.nih.gov/pubmed/21881466

50. http://www.ncbi.nlm.nih.gov/pubmed/25602622
51. http://www.ncbi.nlm.nih.gov/pubmed/25142572
52. http://www.ncbi.nlm.nih.gov/pubmed/25239737
53. http://www.ncbi.nlm.nih.gov/pubmed/20170845
54. Ibid.
55. http://www.ncbi.nlm.nih.gov/pubmed/24505898
56. http://www.ncbi.nlm.nih.gov/pubmed/23825301
57. http://www.thelancet.com/journals/lanneurol/article/PIIS1474-4422(13)70278-3/abstract
58. http://www.pnas.org/content/107/26/11971
59. AAP. *Pediatrics*, 2012;129(8):e827–e841.cs 2012;129(8):e827–e841.
60. http://www.ncbi.nlm.nih.gov/pmc/articles/PMC4350908/
61. http://www.ncbi.nlm.nih.gov/pmc/articles/PMC4083661/
62. http://www.ncbi.nlm.nih.gov/pmc/articles/PMC4349412/
63. http://aem.asm.org/content/75/4/965.full
64. http://www.biomedcentral.com/content/pdf/1758-907X-1-7.pdf

## CHAPTER 4: Time to Clean Up

1. http://www.ncbi.nlm.nih.gov/m/pubmed/14754581/
2. http://www.ncbi.nlm.nih.gov/pmc/articles/PMC3237378/
3. http://toxsci.oxfordjournals.org/content/early/2013/05/22/toxsci.kft102.full
4. http://www.ncbi.nlm.nih.gov/pubmed/24606795
5. http://www.ncbi.nlm.nih.gov/pubmed/23981537
6. http://www.ncbi.nlm.nih.gov/m/pubmed/26343190/
7. http://www.ncbi.nlm.nih.gov/pubmed/26017680
8. http://www.ncbi.nlm.nih.gov/pubmed/26371195
9. http://www.ncbi.nlm.nih.gov/m/pubmed/21905454/
10. http://www.ncbi.nlm.nih.gov/pmc/articles/PMC3114825/
11. http://www.ncbi.nlm.nih.gov/pubmed/23516405

## PART II: Step One: Heal

## CHAPTER 5: Food Allergens and Sensitivities: How "Healthy" Foods Can Hurt

1. http://www.jacionline.org/article/S0091-6749(14)00899-9/abstract
2. http://www.cdc.gov/nchs/fastats/delivery.htm
3. http://www.ncbi.nlm.nih.gov/pubmed/25452656
4. http://www.ncbi.nlm.nih.gov/m/pubmed/26325665/
5. http://www.ncbi.nlm.nih.gov/m/pubmed/26113704/; http://www.ncbi.nlm.nih.gov/pubmed/26265016
6. http://pediatrics.aappublications.org/content/134/Supplement_1/S21.abstract
7. http://www.ncbi.nlm.nih.gov/pubmed/26126682
8. http://www.ncbi.nlm.nih.gov/pubmed/24973272
9. http://www.nature.com/nature/journal/v516/n7529/abs/nature13960.html

10. http://www.nytimes.com/2014/11/19/science/viruses-as-a-cure.html
11. http://www.ncbi.nlm.nih.gov/pubmed/16387585; http://www.ncbi.nlm.nih.gov/pubmed/19255001
12. http://www.ncbi.nlm.nih.gov/pubmed/10436392; http://www.ncbi.nlm.nih.gov/pubmed/11706842; http://www.ncbi.nlm.nih.gov/pubmed/7977735; http://online.liebertpub.com/doi/abs/10.1089/088318700750070411
13. http://www.ncbi.nlm.nih.gov/pubmed/10436392
14. http://www.ncbi.nlm.nih.gov/pubmed/19682267; http://www.ncbi.nlm.nih.gov/pubmed/19174791
15. http://www.sciencedirect.com/science/article/pii/S0194599804001305
16. http://www.ncbi.nlm.nih.gov/pubmed/20168232
17. http://www.ncbi.nlm.nih.gov/pubmed/24573125
18. http://www.sciencedirect.com/science/article/pii/S0196070903001182
19. http://www.ncbi.nlm.nih.gov/pubmed/16403684
20. http://ajcn.nutrition.org/content/79/5/727.full
21. http://www.ncbi.nlm.nih.gov/pubmed/10479881
22. http://www.ncbi.nlm.nih.gov/pubmed/22294663
23. http://www.ncbi.nlm.nih.gov/pubmed/24266677
24. http://www.ncbi.nlm.nih.gov/pubmed/25168224
25. http://www.ers.usda.gov/media/1282246/err162.pdf
26. http://www.nejm.org/doi/full/10.1056/NEJM199603143341103
27. http://digitalcommons.unl.edu/cgi/viewcontent.cgi?article=1028 &context=foodscidiss
28. http://www.nature.com/nbt/journal/v22/n2/abs/nbt934.html
29. http://www.nature.com/nbt/journal/v22/n2/full/nbt0204-170.html
30. http://www.ncbi.nlm.nih.gov/pmc/articles/PMC1364539/
31. http://onlinelibrary.wiley.com/doi/10.1002/jat.2712/abstract
32. http://www.ncbi.nlm.nih.gov/pubmed/21338670
33. http://www.ncbi.nlm.nih.gov/pubmed/23224412
34. http://www.thelancet.com/journals/lanonc/article/PIIS1470-2045(15)70134-8/abstract
35. http://www.ncbi.nlm.nih.gov/pubmed/23756170
36. http://apps.who.int/iris/bitstream/10665/43624/1/9241665203_eng.pdf; http://www.ncbi.nlm.nih.gov/pmc/articles/PMC3945755/
37. http://www.ncbi.nlm.nih.gov/pubmed/20180575; http://www.ncbi.nlm.nih.gov/pubmed/22591574; http://www.agweb.com/assets/import/files/58p20-22.pdf; http://www.greenpasture.org/documentFiles/3.pdf
38. http://www.ncbi.nlm.nih.gov/pubmed/20350266; http://www.ncbi.nlm.nih.gov/pubmed/24983973; http://www.ncbi.nlm.nih.gov/pubmed/23319082; http://www.ncbi.nlm.nih.gov/pubmed/21127082
39. http://www.ncbi.nlm.nih.gov/pubmed/23886227
40. http://www.medicalnewstoday.com/articles/264854.php
41. http://www.ncbi.nlm.nih.gov/pubmed/24251558
42. http://www.ncbi.nlm.nih.gov/pubmed/7868571
43. http://www.ncbi.nlm.nih.gov/pubmed/11903088

44. http://www.ncbi.nlm.nih.gov/pubmed/16366404

45. http://www.ncbi.nlm.nih.gov/pubmed/22294663

46. http://www.ncbi.nlm.nih.gov/pubmed/15870662; http://www.ncbi.nlm.nih.gov/pubmed/19348719; http://www.ncbi.nlm.nih.gov/pmc/articles/PMC3916846/

47. http://www.ncbi.nlm.nih.gov/pubmed/12161033

48. http://www.ncbi.nlm.nih.gov/pubmed/20406576; http://www.ncbi.nlm.nih.gov/pmc/articles/PMC3540005/

49. http://www.ncbi.nlm.nih.gov/pubmed/25311313

50. http://www.ncbi.nlm.nih.gov/pubmed/22237879; http://www.ncbi.nlm.nih.gov/pubmed/25583468; http://www.gastrojournal.org/article/S0016-5085(15)30192-X/abstract

51. http://www.enveurope.com/content/24/1/24

52. http://www.ncbi.nlm.nih.gov/pmc/articles/PMC3945755/

53. http://www.ncbi.nlm.nih.gov/pubmed/23396248; http://www.ncbi.nlm.nih.gov/pubmed/24985121

54. http://www.ncbi.nlm.nih.gov/pubmed/24505898

55. http://www.ncbi.nlm.nih.gov/pubmed/24533607

56. http://www.ncbi.nlm.nih.gov/pubmed/24505898

57. http://www.ncbi.nlm.nih.gov/pubmed/25457448

58. http://www.ncbi.nlm.nih.gov/pubmed/24566676

59. http://www.ncbi.nlm.nih.gov/pubmed/16194732; http://www.ncbi.nlm.nih.gov/pubmed/2390052; http://www.ncbi.nlm.nih.gov/pubmed/24813861; http://www.ncbi.nlm.nih.gov/pubmed/22845673

60. http://www.ncbi.nlm.nih.gov/pubmed/23666039

61. http://www.ncbi.nlm.nih.gov/pubmed/26150853; http://www.ncbi.nlm.nih.gov/pubmed/26486282

62. http://www.ncbi.nlm.nih.gov/pubmed/24048168; http://www.ncbi.nlm.nih.gov/pubmed/25925932; http://www.ncbi.nlm.nih.gov/pubmed/24369326

63. http://www.ncbi.nlm.nih.gov/pubmed/26198999

64. http://www.ncbi.nlm.nih.gov/pubmed/23030231

## CHAPTER 6: Artificial Food: Flavorings, Dyes, Preservatives, and Other Toxic Additives

1. http://www.ncbi.nlm.nih.gov/pubmed/21130826

2. http://www.ncbi.nlm.nih.gov/pubmed/25551610

3. http://www.ncbi.nlm.nih.gov/pubmed/25009784

4. http://www.ncbi.nlm.nih.gov/pubmed/24556450

5. McCann, D., A. Barrett, A. Cooper, D. Crumpler, L. Dalen, K. Grimshaw, E. Kitchin, K. Lok, L. Porteous, and E. Prince. Food additives and hyperactive behaviour in 3-year-old and 8/9-year-old children in the community: a randomised, double-blinded, placebo-controlled trial. *Lancet*, 2007 Nov 3; 370(9598):1560–67.

6. El-Wahab, H. M., and G. S. Moram. Toxic effects of some synthetic food colorants and/or flavor additives on male rats. *Toxicology and Industrial Health*, 2013 Mar;29(2):224–32.

7. Axon, A., F. E. May, L. E. Gaughan, F. M. Williams, P. G. Blain, and M. C. Wright. Tartrazine and sunset yellow are xenoestrogens in a new screening assay to identify modulators of human oestrogen receptor transcriptional activity. *Toxicology,* 2012 Aug 16;298(1–3):40–51

8. Tanaka, T., O. Takahashi, S. Oishi, and A. Ogata. Effects of tartrazine on exploratory behavior in a three-generation toxicity study in mice. *Reproducitve Toxicology,* 2008 Oct;26(2):156–63.

9. Noorafshan, A., M. Erfanizadeh, and S. Karbalay-Doust. Sodium benzoate, a food preservative, induces anxiety and motor impairment in rats. *Neurosciences* (Riyadh), 2014 Jan;19(1):24–28.

10. http://cspinet.org/new/pdf/food-dyes-rainbow-of-risks.pdf

11. http://cpj.sagepub.com/content/54/4/309

12. http://cpj.sagepub.com/content/53/2/133

13. http://www.ncbi.nlm.nih.gov/pubmed/25431840

14. http://www.ncbi.nlm.nih.gov/pubmed/20043888

15. http://www.ncbi.nlm.nih.gov/pubmed/15925301

16. http://www.ncbi.nlm.nih.gov/pubmed/25683673

17. http://www.truthinlabeling.org/hiddensources.html

18. Ibid.

19. http://www.scientificamerican.com/article/soda-chemical-cloudy-health-history/

20. http://www.fda.gov/forconsumers/consumerupdates/ucm048951.htm

21. http://www.fda.gov/downloads/AdvisoryCommittees/CommitteesMeeting Materials/FoodAdvisoryCommittee/UCM273033.pdf

22. http://www.ncbi.nlm.nih.gov/m/pubmed/20551163/

23. http://www.fda.gov/downloads/AdvisoryCommittees/CommitteesMeeting Materials/FoodAdvisoryCommittee/UCM273033.pdf

24. This sort of reaction may well extend to a similar population of the adult population, whose response to food additives simply hasn't been studied.

25. http://www.latimes.com/nation/la-na-sugar-limits-20150317-story.html

## CHAPTER 7: Sickly Sweets: Sugar and Sweeteners

1. http://www.cdc.gov/nchs/data/databriefs/db71.htm

2. http://www.medscape.com/viewarticle/732212

3. http://www.nytimes.com/2014/05/04/us/study-reveals-sizable-increase-in -diabetes-among-children.html?smid=tw-share

4. http://well.blogs.nytimes.com/2014/06/13/threat-grows-from-liver-illness-tied -to-obesity/

5. http://www.ncbi.nlm.nih.gov/pubmed/23482247

6. http://www.ncbi.nlm.nih.gov/pubmed/23390127

7. http://www.sciencedaily.com/releases/2014/11/141104141731.htm

8. Azadbakht, L., and A. Esmaillzadeh. Dietary patterns and attention deficit hyperactivity disorder among Iranian children. *Nutrition,* 2012 Mar;28(3):242–49.

9. Lenoir, M., F. Serre, L. Cantin, and S. H. Ahmed. Intense Sweetness Surpasses Cocaine Reward. *PLoS ONE,* 2007;2(8): e698.

10. http://drhyman.com/blog/2011/02/04/food-addiction-could-it-explain-why -70-percent-of-america-is-fat/#close

11. http://www.ncbi.nlm.nih.gov/pmc/articles/PMC2235907/

12. *Neuroreport,* 2001 Nov 16; 12(16):3549–52.

13. http://www.ncbi.nlm.nih.gov/pubmed/12055324/

14. Stevens, B., J. Yamada, G. Y. Lee, and A. Ohlsson. Sucrose for analgesia in new-born infants undergoing painful procedures. *Cochrane Database of Systematic Reviews,* 2013 Jan 31;1:CD001069.

15. Johnson, C. C. Sucrose Analgesia During the First Week of Life in Neonates Younger Than 31 Weeks' Postconceptional Age. *Pediatrics,* September 2002;110 (3):523–28.

16. http://www.ncbi.nlm.nih.gov/pubmed/25692302

17. http://www.ncbi.nlm.nih.gov/m/pubmed/1013192/

18. Moss, Michael. *Salt Sugar Fat: How the Food Giants Hooked Us.* Random House Trade Paperbacks (New York), 2014.

19. Ibid.

20. http://abcnews.go.com/Health/Business/story?id=962115

21. https://www.ftc.gov/news-events/press-releases/2009/04/kellogg-settles-ftc -charges-ads-frosted-mini-wheats-were-false

22. http://www.cerealsettlement.com/index

23. http://rodalewellness.com/health/sugar-marketing

24. http://www.ucsusa.org/center-for-science-and-democracy/sugar-industry-under mines-public-health-policy.html

25. Alexander, Anne, *The Sugar Smart Diet: Stop Cravings and Lose Weight While Still Enjoying the Sweets You Love!* (Emmaus, PA: Rodale, 2014).

26. http://ajcn.nutrition.org/content/79/4/537.abstract

27. Monzavi-Karbassi, B., R. J. Hine, J. S. Stanley, V. P. Ramani, J. Carcel-Trullols, T. L. Whitehead, T. Kelly, E. R. Siegel, C. Artaud, S. Shaaf, R. Saha, F. Jousheghany, R. Henry-Tillman, and T. Kieber-Emmons. Fructose as a carbon source induces an aggressive phenotype in MDA-MB-468 breast tumor cells. *International Journal of Oncology,* 2010 Sep;37(3):615–22.

28. http://www.ncbi.nlm.nih.gov/m/pubmed/10766253/

29. http://www.ncbi.nlm.nih.gov/m/pubmed/9568685/

30. http://www.ncbi.nlm.nih.gov/pmc/articles/PMC2235907/

31. http://www.ncbi.nlm.nih.gov/m/pubmed/15181085/

32. http://www.ncbi.nlm.nih.gov/pubmed/?term=25965509

33. http://www.ncbi.nlm.nih.gov/pubmed/19171026

34. http://www.motherjones.com/environment/2009/07/corn-syrups-mercury -surprise

35. Simintzi, I., K. H. Schulpis, P. Angelogianni, C. Liapi, and S. Tsakiris. l-Cysteine and glutathione restore the modulation of rat frontal cortex Na+, K+-ATPase activity induced by aspartame metabolites. *Food and Chemical Toxicology,* 2008 Jun;46(6):2074–79.

36. Humphries, P., E. Pretorius, and H. Naudé. Direct and indirect cellular

effects of aspartame on the brain. *European Journal of Clinical Nutrition,* 2008 Apr;62(4):451–62.

37. Sharma, R. P., and R. A. Coulombe. Effects of repeated doses of aspartame on serotonin and its metabolite in various regions of the mouse brain. *Food and Chemical Toxicology,* 1987;25(8):565–68.

38. Toru, K., T. Mlmura, Y. Takasakl, and M. Ichlmura. Dietary aspartame with protein on plasma and brain amino acids, brain monoamines, and behavior in rats. *Physiology Behavior,* 1986;(36):765.

39. Kussie, P. H., S. Gorina, and V. Marechal, et al., Structure of the MCM2 oncoprotein bound to the p53 tumor suppressor transactivation domain. *Science,* 1996;(274):948–53.

40. Soffritti, M., F. Belpoggi, D. D. Esposti, L. Falcioni, and L. Bua. Consequences of exposure to carcinogens beginning during developmental life. *Basic & Clinical Pharmacology & Toxicology,* 2008 Feb;102(2):118–24.

41. http://www.ncbi.nlm.nih.gov/pubmed/25609450

42. http://www.ncbi.nlm.nih.gov/pubmed/15798075/

43. http://www.ncbi.nlm.nih.gov/m/pubmed/15166298/

44. http://www.ncbi.nlm.nih.gov/pubmed/23701749

45. http://www.nature.com/nature/journal/v514/n7521/full/nature13793.html

46. http://www.cell.com/cell-host-microbe/abstract/S1931-3128(15)00021-9

47. Roberts, H. J. Does aspartame cause human brain cancer? *Journal of Advanced Medicine,* 1991; (4): 231–41.

48. Shephard, S. E., K. Wakabayaski, and M. Nagao. Mutagenic activity of peptides and the artificial sweetener aspartame after nitrosation. *Food Chemical Toxicology,* 1993(31): 323–29.

49. Olney, J. W., N. B. Farber, E. Spitznagel, and L. N. Robins. Increasing brain tumor rates: is there a link to aspartame? *Journal of Neuropathology & Experimantal Neurology,* 1996 Nov;55(11):1115–23.

50. Camfield, P., C. S. Camfield, J. M. Dooley, K. Gordon, S. Jollymore, and D. F. Weaver. Aspartame exacerbates EEG spike-wave discharge in children with generalized absence epilepsy: a double-blind controlled study. *Neurology,* 1992 May;42(5):1000–3

51. Rowan, A. J., B. A. Shaywitz, L. Tuchman, J. A. French, D. Luciano, and C. M. Sullivan. Aspartame and seizure susceptibility: results of a clinical study in reportedly sensitive individuals. *Epilepsia,* 1995 Mar;36(3):270–75.

52. Wurtman, R. J. Aspartame: possible effect on seizure susceptibility. *Lancet* 1985;2:1060 (letter).

53. Walton, R. G. Seizure and mania after high intake of aspartame. *Psychosomatics,* 1986 Mar;27(3):218, 220.

54. Van den Eeden, S. K., T. D. Koepsell, and W. T. Longstreth, Jr., et al. Aspartame ingestion and headaches: a randomized crossover trial. *Neurology,* 1994;44: 1787–93.

55. Loehler, S. M., and A. Glaros. The effect of aspartame on migraine headache. *Headache,* 1988;28:10–14.

56. Millichap, J. G., and M. M. Yee. The diet factor in pediatric and adolescent migraine. *Pediatric Neurology,* 2003 Jan;28(1):9–15.

57. Lipton, R. B., L. C. Newman, J. S. Cohen, and S. Solomon. Aspartame as a dietary trigger of headache. *Headache,* 1989 Feb;29(2):90–92.

58. http://pubs.acs.org/doi/abs/10.1021/es504769c

## PART III: Step Two: Nourish

1. This is why traditional growers always planted beans in combination or rotation with other types of plants, so that nitrogen would be plentiful in the soil for all plants.

2. http://www.hindawi.com/journals/jt/2012/862764/

3. http://www.ncbi.nlm.nih.gov/pubmed/15151947

4. http://www.ncbi.nlm.nih.gov/pmc/articles/PMC3981853/

5. http://www.sciencedaily.com/releases/2007/04/070402102001.htm

6. http://www.ncbi.nlm.nih.gov/pubmed/23454729

7. http://www.ncbi.nlm.nih.gov/pubmed/26339029/

## CHAPTER 8: Soil Power: Organic Fruits, Vegetables, and Plants

1. http://www.ncbi.nlm.nih.gov/pubmed/24947126

2. http://www.ncbi.nlm.nih.gov/pubmed/21123457

3. http://www.ncbi.nlm.nih.gov/pubmed/21098643

4. http://www.ncbi.nlm.nih.gov/pubmed/25876645

5. http://www.ncbi.nlm.nih.gov/pubmed/25635978

6. http://www.ncbi.nlm.nih.gov/pubmed/19042940

7. http://www.ncbi.nlm.nih.gov/pubmed/24481133

8. http://www.ncbi.nlm.nih.gov/pubmed/24459829

9. http://www.nottingham.ac.uk/news/pressreleases/2015/march/ancientbiotics—-a-medieval-remedy-for-modern-day-superbugs.aspx

10. http://www.ncbi.nlm.nih.gov/pubmed/22972323

11. http://www.ncbi.nlm.nih.gov/pubmed/25395702

12. http://www.ncbi.nlm.nih.gov/pubmed/25744406

13. http://www.ncbi.nlm.nih.gov/pubmed/25491608

14. http://www.ncbi.nlm.nih.gov/pubmed/25586902

15. http://www.ncbi.nlm.nih.gov/pubmed/25774338

16. http://www.ncbi.nlm.nih.gov/pubmed/24245576

17. http://www.ncbi.nlm.nih.gov/pubmed/24364759

18. http://www.ncbi.nlm.nih.gov/pubmed/25159039

19. http://www.ncbi.nlm.nih.gov/pubmed/25192721

20. http://www.ncbi.nlm.nih.gov/pubmed/25102117

21. http://www.ncbi.nlm.nih.gov/pubmed/25019218

22. http://www.ncbi.nlm.nih.gov/pubmed/23810671

23. http://www.ncbi.nlm.nih.gov/pubmed/24532027

24. http://www.ncbi.nlm.nih.gov/pubmed/21259333

25. http://www.ncbi.nlm.nih.gov/pubmed/25054107

26. http://www.ncbi.nlm.nih.gov/pubmed/18566435

27. http://www.ncbi.nlm.nih.gov/pubmed/25054107
28. http://www.ncbi.nlm.nih.gov/pubmed/18566435
29. http://www.ncbi.nlm.nih.gov/pubmed/22537070
30. http://www.ncbi.nlm.nih.gov/m/pubmed/26269198/
31. http://www.ncbi.nlm.nih.gov/m/pubmed/25313065/
32. http://www.ncbi.nlm.nih.gov/pubmed/21245306
33. http://www.ncbi.nlm.nih.gov/pubmed/24317433
34. http://www.ncbi.nlm.nih.gov/pubmed/25222709
35. http://www.ncbi.nlm.nih.gov/pubmed/24700279
36. http://www.ncbi.nlm.nih.gov/pubmed/24506007
37. http://www.ncbi.nlm.nih.gov/pubmed/24940315
38. http://www.ncbi.nlm.nih.gov/pubmed/19179623
39. http://www.nature.com/nm/journal/v16/n11/abs/nm.2237.html
40. http://www.ncbi.nlm.nih.gov/pubmed/25785234
41. http://www.ncbi.nlm.nih.gov/pubmed/24671262
42. http://www.ncbi.nlm.nih.gov/pmc/articles/PMC3041787/
43. http://www.ncbi.nlm.nih.gov/m/pubmed/20478945/
44. *Acta Paediatrica*, 2012 Aug;101(8):811–18.
45. http://www.ncbi.nlm.nih.gov/pubmed/23367522
46. Harari, R., et al. *Environmental Health Perspective*, 2010 Jun;118(6):890–96.
47. http://www.ncbi.nlm.nih.gov/pubmed/15997102
48. Sagiv, S. K., et al. *American Journal of Epidemiology*, 2010 Mar 1;171(5):593–601.
49. http://www.ncbi.nlm.nih.gov/pubmed/18226078
50. http://www.ncbi.nlm.nih.gov/pubmed/25063718
51. http://www.ncbi.nlm.nih.gov/pubmed/24726197
52. http://www.ncbi.nlm.nih.gov/pubmed/?term=dichlorophenol+food+allergies
53. http://www.mindfully.org/Pesticide/Preschool-Exposed-Mexico-Guillette.htm
54. http://www.ncbi.nlm.nih.gov/pmc/articles/PMC1241395/pdf/ehp0111-000377.pdf
55. http://pediatrics.aappublications.org/content/early/2010/05/17/peds.2009-3058.full.pdf
56. http://www.sciencedirect.com/science/article/pii/S001393511400067X
57. http://www.ncbi.nlm.nih.gov/pmc/articles/PMC1367841/
58. Allen, Will. *The War on Bugs*, (White River Junction, VT: Chelsea Green Publishing, 2007), page 78.
59. Ibid., 79; *Agricultural Chemical*, 1964;72:132.
60. http://www.the-open-mind.com/more-than-half-of-breakfast-cereals-exceed-limits-for-arsenic/
61. http://www.consumerreports.org/cro/magazine/2012/01/arsenic-in-your-juice/index.htm
62. http://www.consumerreports.org/cro/magazine/2015/01/how-much-arsenic-is-in-your-rice/index.htm
63. http://www.ncbi.nlm.nih.gov/pubmed/24134670
64. http://www.ncbi.nlm.nih.gov/pubmed/23817957
65. http://www.ewg.org/foodnews/dirty_dozen_list.php
66. http://www.ewg.org/foodnews/clean_fifteen_list.php

## CHAPTER 9: Unlocking Seeds: Nutritional Powerhouses

1. http://www.ncbi.nlm.nih.gov/pubmed/1627021; http://www.ncbi.nlm.nih.gov/pmc/articles/PMC3257681/
2. http://www.ncbi.nlm.nih.gov/pubmed/25599007; http://www.ncbi.nlm.nih.gov/pubmed/11122711; http://www.ncbi.nlm.nih.gov/pmc/articles/PMC28714/
3. http://www.ncbi.nlm.nih.gov/pubmed/25646339
4. http://www.ncbi.nlm.nih.gov/pubmed/25833976
5. http://www.ncbi.nlm.nih.gov/m/pubmed/24920033
6. http://www.ncbi.nlm.nih.gov/pubmed/14574348; http://www.ncbi.nlm.nih.gov/pubmed/25097630
7. http://www.ncbi.nlm.nih.gov/pubmed/23122211; http://www.ncbi.nlm.nih.gov/m/pubmed/18716179/
8. http://www.ncbi.nlm.nih.gov/pubmed/21489570; http://www.ncbi.nlm.nih.gov/pubmed/24084509
9. http://www.ncbi.nlm.nih.gov/pubmed/23321679
10. http://www.ncbi.nlm.nih.gov/pubmed/24871475
11. http://ucfoodsafety.ucdavis.edu/files/162415.pdf
12. Murano, Peter. *Food Irradiation: A Sourcebook.* ed. Dr. Elsa Murano (Iowa State University: Blackwell Pub Professional, 1995).
13. http://www.ncbi.nlm.nih.gov/pubmed/25694676; http://www.ncbi.nlm.nih.gov/m/pubmed/19774556/
14. http://www.ncbi.nlm.nih.gov/pubmed/20715598; http://www.ncbi.nlm.nih.gov/m/pubmed/16929240
15. http://www.ncbi.nlm.nih.gov/pubmed/25341870; http://www.ncbi.nlm.nih.gov/pubmed/14672293; http://www.ncbi.nlm.nih.gov/pubmed/21508424
16. http://ajcn.nutrition.org/content/47/2/270.full.pdf
17. http://www.ncbi.nlm.nih.gov/pubmed/2998440
18. http://www.ncbi.nlm.nih.gov/pubmed/11110854; http://www.ncbi.nlm.nih.gov/pubmed/12036813; http://www.ncbi.nlm.nih.gov/pubmed/19321589
19. http://www.ncbi.nlm.nih.gov/pubmed/10625946; http://www.ncbi.nlm.nih.gov/pmc/articles/PMC3876062; http://www.ncbi.nlm.nih.gov/pubmed/24260736
20. http://www.ncbi.nlm.nih.gov/pubmed/23551617; http://www.ncbi.nlm.nih.gov/pubmed/19674804; http://www.ncbi.nlm.nih.gov/pubmed/26384212
21. http://www.sciencedirect.com/science/article/pii/S0308814608002513; http://www.sciencedirect.com/science/article/pii/S0308814608014945; http://www.ncbi.nlm.nih.gov/pubmed/24050000
22. http://www.ncbi.nlm.nih.gov/pubmed/12499338; http://www.ncbi.nlm.nih.gov/pubmed/18460487; http://www.ncbi.nlm.nih.gov/pubmed/16366727
23. http://www.ncbi.nlm.nih.gov/m/pubmed/20597543/
24. http://www.ncbi.nlm.nih.gov/pubmed/16672077
25. http://www.ncbi.nlm.nih.gov/pubmed/24898231
26. http://www.ncbi.nlm.nih.gov/pubmed/23167584; http://www.ncbi.nlm.nih.gov/pubmed/22594854; http://www.ncbi.nlm.nih.gov/pubmed/20715598

27. Bernasek, 5th World Congress on Breads and Cereals, Dresden, 1970 (cited in Aubert, 1989), http://eap.mcgill.ca/publications/EAP35.htm

28. http://www.ncbi.nlm.nih.gov/pubmed/19723572

29. http://www.ncbi.nlm.nih.gov/pubmed/23194529

30. http://www.ncbi.nlm.nih.gov/pubmed/22017795

31. http://www.ncbi.nlm.nih.gov/pubmed/23057788

32. http://www.ncbi.nlm.nih.gov/pubmed/18680953

33. http://www.ncbi.nlm.nih.gov/pubmed/14766592

34. Aubert, Claude. "Pain au levain ou pain a la levure?" *Les quatre saisons du jardinage* 25(Mar/Apr 1984):57–60.

35. http://www.ncbi.nlm.nih.gov/pubmed/22307223

36. http://www.ncbi.nlm.nih.gov/pubmed/22474577

37. http://ajcn.nutrition.org/content/79/5/774.full

38. http://www.cdc.gov/nchs/pressroom/04news/calorie.htm

39. http://www.ncbi.nlm.nih.gov/pmc/articles/PMC3854723

40. http://www.ncbi.nlm.nih.gov/pubmed/23030231

41. http://www.ncbi.nlm.nih.gov/pubmed/24048168

42. http://www.ncbi.nlm.nih.gov/pubmed/24302835

43. http://www.ncbi.nlm.nih.gov/pubmed/22474577

44. http://pompeo.house.gov/uploadedfiles/safeandaccuratefoodlabellingactof2014.pdf

45. Including citric acid, aspartame, amino acids, sodium ascorbate, and flavorings.

46. Farmers Cope with Roundup-Resistant Weeds. *New York Times,* May 3, 2010.

47. Ge, X., D. D'avignon, J. Ackerman, and R. Sammons. Rapid vacuolar sequestration: the horseweed glyphosate resistance mechanism, *Pest Management Science,* 2010;66(4).

48. http://farmindustrynews.com/ag-technology-solution-center/glyphosate -resistant-weed-problem-extends-more-species-more-farms

49. Majewski, M. S., et al. "Pesticides in Mississippi air and rain: A comparison between 1995 and 2007," *Environmental Toxicology and Chemistry,* 2014;33(6): 1283–93.

50. Sundaram, A., and K.M.S. Sundaram. Solubility products of six metal-glyphosate complexes in water and forestry soils, and their influence on glyphosate toxicity to plants. *Journal of Environmental Science and Health,* Part B 1997, 32, 583–98.

51. http://www.omicsonline.org/open-access/detection-of-glyphosate-residues-in -animals-and-humans-2161-0525.1000210.pdf

52. Benachour, N., and G. E. Séralini. Glyphosate formulations induce apoptosis and necrosis in human umbilical, embryonic, and placental cells. *Chemical Research in Toxicology,* 2009 Jan;22(1):97–105.

53. Marc, J., et al. A glyphosate-based pesticide impinges on transcription. *Toxicology and Applied Pharmacology,* 2005;203(1):1–8.

54. http://onlinelibrary.wiley.com/doi/10.1002/(SICI)1098-2280(1998)31:1%3 C55::AID-EM8%3E3.0.CO;2-A/abstract

55. Romano, R. M., M. A. Romano, M. M. Bernardi, P. V. Furtado, and C. A. Oliveira. "Prepubertal exposure to commercial formulation of the herbicide glyphosate alters testosterone levels and testicular morphology." *Archives of Toxicology,* 2009.

56. http://www.ncbi.nlm.nih.gov/pubmed/11391760

57. Garry, V. F., M. E. Harkins, L. L. Erickson, L. K. Long-Simpson, S. E. Holland, and B. L. Burroughs. "Birth defects, season of conception, and sex of children born to pesticide applicators living in the Red River Valley of Minnesota, USA." *Environmental Health Perspective,* 2002 Jun;110 Suppl 3:441–49.

58. http://responsibletechnology.org/glutenintroduction

59. http://www.mdpi.com/1099-4300/15/4/1416

60. http://omicsonline.org/open-access/detection-of-glyphosate-residues-in-animals -and-humans-2161-0525.1000210.pdf

61. http://www.ncbi.nlm.nih.gov/m/pubmed/26537666; http://www.ncbi.nlm.nih .gov/m/pubmed/22337346

62. Ordlee, J., et al. Identification of a Brazil-Nut Allergen in Transgenic Soybeans. *New England Journal of Medicine,* March 14, 1996.

63. U.S. Food and Drug Administration. Statement of policy: Foods derived from new plant varieties. *FDA Federal Register,* 29 May 1992;57(104):229.

64. Kahl, L. Memorandum to Dr. James Maryanski, FDA biotechnology coordinator, about the Federal Register document: "Statement of policy: Foods from genetically modified plants." U.S. Food & Drug Administration, 8 January 1992.

65. Guest, G. B. Memorandum to Dr. James Maryanski, biotechnology coordinator: Regulation of transgenic plants, FDA Draft Federal Register Notice on Food Biotechnology. U.S. Department of Health & Human Services, 5 February 1992.

66. Matthews, E. J. Memorandum to Toxicology Section of the Biotechnology Working Group: "Safety of whole food plants transformed by technology methods." U.S. Food & Drug Administration. October 28 1991.

67. Shibko, S. L. Memorandum to James H. Maryanski, biotechnology coordinator, CFSAN: Revision of toxicology section of the "Statement of policy: Foods derived from genetically modified plants." U.S. Food & Drug Administration. 1992.

68. Pribyl, L. J. Comments on the March 18, 1992, version of the Biotechnology Document. U.S. Food & Drug Administration, March 18, 1992.

69. Sudduth, M. A. Genetically engineered foods, fears and facts: An interview with FDA's Jim Maryanski. *FDA Consumer,* January–February 1993; 11–14. http:// web.archive.org/web/20090202053904/http:/www.fda.gov/bbs/topics/consumer /Con00191.html

70. http://www.ncbi.nlm.nih.gov/pubmed/26133768

71. http://www.nytimes.com/2015/09/06/us/food-industry-enlisted-academics-in -gmo-lobbying-war-emails-show.html

72. Freese, W., and D. Schubert. Safety testing and regulation of genetically engineered foods. *Biotechnology & Genetic Engineering Reviews,* 2004:299–324.

73.

| Monsanto Position | Individual | Federal Position |
| --- | --- | --- |
| Senior vice president for clinical affairs at G.D. Searle and Co. (merged with Monsanto) | Michael A. Friedman | Acting commissioner of the FDA |

| | | |
|---|---|---|
| Consultant to Searle's public relations firm (merged with Monsanto) | Arthur Hull Hayes | Previously FDA commissioner |
| Top Monsanto scientist, oversaw approval of rBGH | Margaret Miller | Appointed deputy director of FDA, 1991 |
| Worked on Monsanto-funded rBGH in connection with Cornell University | Suzanne Sechen | FDA reviewer on scientific data |
| Attorney for Monsanto for 7 years, previous head of Monsanto Washington, D.C., office | Michael Taylor | Former FDA deputy commissioner for policy. In 2010 appointed senior advisor to FDA commissioner |
| Former Monsanto lawyer | Clarence Thomas | Appointed to U.S. Supreme Court in 1991 |
| Served on Board of Directors at Calgene, a Monsanto Biotech subsidiary | Anne Veneman | Appointed head of USDA in 2001 |
| Retired senior vice president for public policy at Monsanto | Dr. Virginia Weldon | Previously, member of FDA's Metabolism and Endocrine Advisory Committee |
| Vice president, Public and Government Affairs | Linda Fisher | Deputy Administrator, EPA |
| Manager, New Technologies | Linda Watrud | USDA, EPA |
| Director, Monsanto Danforth Center | Roger Beachy | Director USDA, NIFA |

74. http://www.mindfully.org/Farm/Green-Revolution-Revolving.htm
75. Harris, G. New official named with portfolio to unite agencies and improve food safety. *New York Times*, 13 January 2010. http://www.nytimes.com/2010/01/14/health/policy/14fda.html
76. Bittman, M. Why aren't GMO foods labeled? *New York Times*, 15 February 2011. http://opinionator.blogs.nytimes.com/2011/02/15/why-arent-g-m-o-foods-labeled/
77. U.S. Food and Drug Administration. Meet Michael R. Taylor, J. D., deputy commissioner for foods, 2011. http://www.fda.gov/AboutFDA/CentersOffices/OfficeofFoods/ucm196721.htm
78. http://www.nytimes.com/2001/01/25/business/redesigning-nature-hard-lessons-learned-biotechnology-food-lab-debacle.html?sec=health
79. http://www.sciencedirect.com/science/article/pii/S0929139312002466

80. http://www.nature.com/srep/2014/140709/srep05634/full/srep05634.html

81. Huber, D. What about glyphosate-induced manganese deficiency? *Journal of Fluid Mechanics,* 2007;20–22.

82. Zobiole, L.H.S., R. S. de Oliviera, D. M. Huber, J. Constantin, C. de Castro, et al. Glyphosate reduces shoot concentration of mineral nutrients in glyphosate resistant soybeans. *Plant and Soil,* 2009;328:57–69.

83. http://gmoanswers.com/ask/uk's-daily-mail-reports-an%C2%A0estimated-125000 -farmers-have-committed-suicide%C2%A0because-crop-failure

84. http://www.theguardian.com/global-development/gallery/2014/may/05/india -cotton-suicides-farmer-deaths-gm-seeds

85. http://www.huffingtonpost.com/2014/07/10/gmo-labels-congress_n_5576255 .html

## CHAPTER 10: Meet Your Meat

1. http://advances.nutrition.org/content/4/4/453.abstract

2. *Canadian Journal of Animal Science,* 1999 Sep;79(3):391–15.

3. http://www.ncbi.nlm.nih.gov/pubmed/12019607

4. http://www.ncbi.nlm.nih.gov/pubmed/20807460

5. http://www.ncbi.nlm.nih.gov/pubmed/19935865

6. Ip, C., J. A. Scimeca, et al. Conjugated linoleic acid. A powerful anti-carcinogen from animal fat sources. *Cancer* 1994;74(3 suppl):1050–54.

7. Aro, A., S. Mannisto, I. Salminen, M. L. Ovaskainen, V. Kataja, and M. Uusitupa. Inverse Association between Dietary and Serum Conjugated Linoleic Acid and Risk of Breast Cancer in Postmenopausal Women. *Nutrition and Cancer,* 2000;38,(2):151–57.

8. http://www.ncbi.nlm.nih.gov/m/pubmed/16183568/

9. Duckett, S. K., et al. Effects of winter stocker growth rate and finishing system on: III. Tissue proximate, fatty acid, vitamin and cholesterol content. *Journal of Animal Science,* June 2009.

10. Kruggel, W. G., "Influence of sex and diet on lutein in lamb fat." *Journal of Animal Science,* 1982;54:970–75.

11. Mutetikka, D. B., and D. C. Mahan. Effect of pasture, confinement, and diet fortification with vitamin E and selenium on reproducing gilts and their progeny. *Journal of Animal Science,* 1993;71:3211.

12. http://www.cafothebook.org/

13. "By-Product Feedstuffs in Dairy Cattle Diets in the Upper Midwest," College of Agricultural and Life Sciences at the University of Wisconsin at Madison, 2008.

14. http://www.omicsonline.org/open-access/detection-of-glyphosate-in-malformed -piglets-2161-0525.1000230.pdf; http://www.truth-out.org/opinion/item/25426 -one-little-piggy-had-birth

15. http://www.ncbi.nlm.nih.gov/pubmed/26133768

16. http://www.ncbi.nlm.nih.gov/pubmed/25448876

17. http://www.ncbi.nlm.nih.gov/pubmed/24930125

18. http://www.ncbi.nlm.nih.gov/pubmed/24719846

19. http://www.enveurope.com/content/26/1/14
20. https://www.tgen.org/news/archive/2011-media-releases/nationwide-study.aspx#.VO01lrPF-SY
21. http://www.cdc.gov/drugresistance/threat-report-2013/
22. http://www.ncbi.nlm.nih.gov/pmc/articles/PMC3553221/
23. http://www.foodproductiondaily.com/Safety-Regulation/US-contests-EU-chicken-restrictions
24. http://www.nytimes.com/2013/10/02/business/fda-bans-three-arsenic-drugs-used-in-poultry-and-pig-feeds.html?_r=0
25. http://www.fda.gov/AnimalVeterinary/SafetyHealth/ProductSafetyInformation/ucm055436.htm
26. https://www.aasv.org/shap/issues/v7n1/v7n1p29.pdf
27. http://www.ncbi.nlm.nih.gov/pubmed/22063148

## CHAPTER 11: Milk: Pasture-ization over Pasteurization

1. http://www.ncbi.nlm.nih.gov/pubmed/19747410
2. Vileisis, Ann, *Kitchen Literacy* (Island Press, 2010).
3. http://ucanr.edu/sites/UCCE_LR/files/152030.pdf
4. http://www.ncbi.nlm.nih.gov/pubmed/11049070
5. http://www.ncbi.nlm.nih.gov/pubmed/21875744
6. http://www.ncbi.nlm.nih.gov/pubmed/25441645
7. http://www.ncbi.nlm.nih.gov/pubmed/23041676
8. http://www.ncbi.nlm.nih.gov/pubmed/22846753
9. http://www.ncbi.nlm.nih.gov/pubmed/23993223
10. http://www.fda.gov/Food/ResourcesForYou/consumers/ucm079516.htm
11. http://www.cdc.gov/breastfeeding/recommendations/handling_breastmilk.htm; http://www.ncbi.nlm.nih.gov/m/pubmed/1557249; http://www.ncbi.nlm.nih.gov/pubmed/18784324; http://www.ncbi.nlm.nih.gov/pubmed/2723294
12. http://www.ncbi.nlm.nih.gov/pubmed/25731162
13. http://www.ncbi.nlm.nih.gov/pubmed/25512686
14. http://www.ncbi.nlm.nih.gov/pubmed/25310757
15. http://www.ncbi.nlm.nih.gov/pubmed/25213053
16. http://www.ncbi.nlm.nih.gov/pubmed/15015834
17. http://m.motherjones.com/tom-philpott/2014/05/nanotech-food-safety-fda-nano-material
18. http://onlinelibrary.wiley.com/doi/10.1002/bies.20708/abstract
19. http://www.ncbi.nlm.nih.gov/pubmed/24932525
20. http://www.ncbi.nlm.nih.gov/pubmed/25634802
21. http://www.ncbi.nlm.nih.gov/pubmed/25987426
22. http://www.ncbi.nlm.nih.gov/pubmed/15939853
23. http://www.sciencedirect.com/science/article/pii/030881469390171B
24. http://onlinelibrary.wiley.com/doi/10.1002/mnfr.200600303/abstract
25. http://pediatrics.aappublications.org/content/early/2010/08/09/peds.2009-3079.abstract

26. http://www.ncbi.nlm.nih.gov/pubmed/11758913
27. http://www.nytimes.com/1998/10/25/magazine/playing-god-in-the-garden.html?pagewanted=5
28. http://www.motherjones.com/environment/2014/03/a1-milk-a2-milk-america

## CHAPTER 12: Knowing the Chicken Before the Egg

1. Nicol, Christine (Bristol University professor of animal welfare). The Intelligent Hen. http://www.dailymail.co.uk/sciencetech/article-2344198/Chickens-smarter-human-toddlers-Studies-suggest-animals-master-numeracy-basic-engineering.html#ixzz3HLqzi7C8
2. Lopez-Bote, C. J., et al. Effect of free-range feeding on omega-3 fatty acids and alpha-tocopherol content and oxidative stability of eggs. *Animal Feed Science and Technology*, 1998;72:33–40.
3. http://www.ncbi.nlm.nih.gov/pubmed/23775487
4. http://www.ncbi.nlm.nih.gov/m/pubmed/25572556
5. http://www.ncbi.nlm.nih.gov/m/pubmed/26288263
6. http://advances.nutrition.org/content/4/4/453.full/
7. http://www.ncbi.nlm.nih.gov/pubmed/25713056
8. http://pediatrics.aappublications.org/content/135/1/e196
9. http://www.ncbi.nlm.nih.gov/pubmed/24558199
10. http://www.ncbi.nlm.nih.gov/m/pubmed/10648274/
11. http://www.ncbi.nlm.nih.gov/pmc/articles/PMC3066069/
12. http://www.hindawi.com/journals/cholesterol/2012/292598/
13. http://www.ncbi.nlm.nih.gov/pubmed/25223281
14. http://www.ncbi.nlm.nih.gov/pubmed/24723866
15. http://www.ncbi.nlm.nih.gov/pubmed/25482392
16. http://www.ncbi.nlm.nih.gov/pubmed/25457283
17. http://www.ncbi.nlm.nih.gov/pubmed/3553287
18. http://www.ncbi.nlm.nih.gov/pubmed/2170516
19. http://www.ncbi.nlm.nih.gov/pubmed/2564950
20. http://www.ncbi.nlm.nih.gov/pubmed/1607898
21. http://www.ncbi.nlm.nih.gov/pubmed/2170516
22. http://www.ncbi.nlm.nih.gov/pubmed/7246527

Krumholz, H. M., et al. Lack of association between cholesterol and coronary heart disease mortality and morbidity and all-cause mortality in persons older than 70 years. *JAMA*, 1994 Nov 2;272(17):1335–40.

Weverling-Rijnsburger, A.W., et al. High-density vs. low-density lipoprotein cholesterol as the risk factor for coronary artery disease and stroke in old age. *Arch Intern Med*. 2003;163(13):1549–54.

Jonsson, A., H. Sigvaldason, and N. Sigfusson. Total cholesterol and mortality after age 80 years. *Lancet*, 1997 Dec 13;350(9093):1778–79.

Räihä, I., J. Marniemi, P. Puukka, T. Toikka, C. Ehnholm, and L. Sourander. Effect of serum lipids, lipoproteins, and apolipoproteins on vascular and nonvascular mortality in the elderly. *Arteriosclerosis, Thrombosis, and Vascular Biology,* 1997 Jul;17(7):1224–32.

Behar, S., et al. Low total cholesterol is associated with high total mortality in patients with coronary heart disease. The Bezafibrate Infarction Prevention (BIP) Study Group. *European Heart Journal,* 1997 Jan;18(1):52–59.

Fried, L. P., et al. Risk factors for 5-year mortality in older adults: the Cardiovascular Health Study. *JAMA,* 1998 Feb 25;279(8):585–92.

Chyou, P. H. and E. D. Eaker. Serum cholesterol concentrations and all-cause mortality in older people. *Age Ageing,* 2000 Jan;29(1):69–74.

Schatz, I. J., et al. Cholesterol and all-cause mortality in elderly people from the Honolulu Heart Program: a cohort study. *Lancet,* 2001 Aug 4;358(9279):351–55.

Weverling-Rijnsburger, A. W., et al. High-density vs low-density lipoprotein cholesterol as the risk factor for coronary artery disease and stroke in old age. *Arch Intern Med.* 2003;163(13):1549–54.

Onder, G., et al., Serum cholesterol levels and in-hospital mortality in the elderly. *American Journal of Medicine,* 2003;115(4):265–71.

Casiglia, E., et al. Total cholesterol and mortality in the elderly. *Journal of Internal Medicine,* 2003 Oct;254(4):353–62.

Psaty, B. M., et al. The association between lipid levels and the risks of incident myocardial infarction, stroke, and total mortality: The Cardiovascular Health Study. *Journal of American Geriatric Society,* 2004 Oct;52(10):1639–47.

Ulmer, H., et al. Why Eve is not Adam: prospective follow-up in 149650 women and men of cholesterol and other risk factors related to cardiovascular and all-cause mortality. *Journal of Women's Health,* 2004 Jan-Feb;13(1):41–53.

Schupf, N., R. Costa, J. Luchsinger, M. X. Tang, J. H. Lee, and R. Mayeux. Relationship between plasma lipids and all-cause mortality in nondemented elderly. *Journal of the American Geriatric Society,* 2005 Feb;53(2):219–26.

Akerblom, J. L., et al. Relation of plasma lipids to all-cause mortality in Caucasian, African-American and Hispanic elders. *Age Ageing,* 2008; 37:207–13.

Newson, R. S., et al. Association between serum cholesterol and noncardiovascular mortality in older age. *Journal of the American Geriatric Society,* 2011; 59:1779–85.

Bathum, L., R. Depont Christensen, L. Engers Pedersen, P. Lyngsie Pedersen, J. Larsen, and J. Nexøe. Association of lipoprotein levels with mortality in subjects aged 50 + without previous diabetes or cardiovascular disease: A population-based register study. *Scandinavian Journal of Primary Health Care,* 2013;31:172–80.

23. http://www.ncbi.nlm.nih.gov/pubmed/25602855; http://www.ncbi.nlm.nih.gov/pubmed/20470020; http://www.ncbi.nlm.nih.gov/pubmed/21160131

24. http://www.ncbi.nlm.nih.gov/pubmed/9343498

25. http://qjmed.oxfordjournals.org/content/96/12/927.full?ijkey=172mwKXqzgmtE&keytype=ref

26. http://www.ncbi.nlm.nih.gov/m/pubmed/8225591

27. http://www.ncbi.nlm.nih.gov/m/pubmed/18028461/

28.  http://www.ncbi.nlm.nih.gov/m/pubmed/1355411; http://www.ncbi.nlm.nih.gov
     /pmc/articles/PMC3750440

29.  http://www.ncbi.nlm.nih.gov/pmc/articles/PMC2386667; http://www.ncbi
     .nlm.nih.gov/pubmed/10217054; http://www.ncbi.nlm.nih.gov/pmc/articles
     /PMC3683816/

30.  http://www.ncbi.nlm.nih.gov/pubmed/22985435

31.  http://www.ncbi.nlm.nih.gov/pubmed/20876207

32.  http://www.ncbi.nlm.nih.gov/pubmed/22890407

33.  http://www.ncbi.nlm.nih.gov/pubmed/26110252

34.  http://www.ncbi.nlm.nih.gov/pubmed/26166555

35.  http://www.nytimes.com/2011/11/03/health/policy/health-guideline-panels
     -struggle-with-conflicts-of-interest.html?pagewanted=all&_r=2&

36.  "The Institute of Medicine (IOM), an independent organization of scientists that
     analyzes available data and provides advice on medical issues, recommends that
     chairs of guideline committees should have no conflicts of interest if possible, and
     that the entire panel should also be free of ties to industry; if that's not possible,
     then at least half of the members should meet this criterion. . . .

     Those policies stem from studies suggesting that biases do creep in to people's
     behaviors, whether consciously or not. In one study published earlier this year, for
     example, scientists compared the guidelines proposed by two different groups of
     experts for treating a blood clotting disorder; the panel in which 73 percent of
     members reported connections to pharmaceutical companies suggested stronger
     recommendations for turning to drug-based treatments compared to a panel in
     which none of the members had ties to industry." http://healthland.time
     .com/2013/11/22/conflicts-of-interest-cholesterol-panel-head-defends-members
     -ties-to-industry/

37.  Love, D., R. Halden, M. Davis, and K. Nachman. Feather Meal: A Previously
     Unrecognized Route for Reentry into the Food Supply of Multiple Pharmaceu-
     ticals and Personal Care Products (PPCPs). *Environmental Science & Technology*,
     2012;46(7):3795–3802.

## CHAPTER 13: Fish: From the Water

1.  Omega-3 for bipolar disorder: meta-analyses of use in mania and bipolar, *Journal
    of Clinical Psychiatry,* 2011 Aug 9.

2.  Reduced mania and depression in juvenile bipolar disorder associated with long-
    chain omega-3 polyunsaturated fatty acid supplementation. *European Journal of
    Clinical Nutrition,* 2009 Aug;63(8):1037–40.

3.  http://www.ncbi.nlm.nih.gov/pubmed/25373095

4.  http://www.ncbi.nlm.nih.gov/pubmed/21961774

5.  Supplementation of polyunsaturated fatty acids, magnesium, and zinc in children
    seeking medical advice for attention-deficit/hyperactivity problems, an observational
    cohort study. *Lipids in Health and Disease,* 2010;9:105.

6.  http://www.ncbi.nlm.nih.gov/pubmed/18511348

7.  http://www.ncbi.nlm.nih.gov/m/pubmed/26318793/

8. Dietary supplementation with fish oil rich in omega-3 polyunsaturated fatty acids in children with bronchial asthma. *European Respiratory Journal,* 2000 Nov;16(5):861–65.

9. Effects of n-3 fatty acids on autoimmunity and osteoporosis. *Front Biosci,* 2008 May 1;13:4015–20.

10. Seigneur, C., K. Vijayaraghavan, K. Lohman, P. Karamchandani, and C. Scott. Global source attribution for mercury deposition in the United States: *Environmental Science & Technology,* 2004, v. 38, no. 2, p. 555–69.

11. http://www.ncbi.nlm.nih.gov/m/pubmed/26109549/; http://www.ncbi.nlm.nih .gov/m/pubmed/25757069/

12. http://www.ncbi.nlm.nih.gov/m/pubmed/10430235/

13. http://www.ncbi.nlm.nih.gov/m/pubmed/25461680; http://www.ncbi.nlm.nih .gov/m/pubmed/24598815; http://www.ncbi.nlm.nih.gov/m/pubmed/24561639; http://www.ncbi.nlm.nih.gov/m/pubmed/24555651

14. http://www.ncbi.nlm.nih.gov/m/pubmed/15298193/

15. http://www.ncbi.nlm.nih.gov/m/pubmed/22425897; http://www.ncbi.nlm.nih .gov/m/pubmed/14760257/

16. Greenberg, Paul. *Four Fish: The Future of the Last Wild Food* (New York: Penguin, 2010).

17. Ibid.

## CHAPTER 14: Water: What We Drink

1. http://www.nytimes.com/2007/04/03/health/03iht-snwater.1.5126782.html ?pagewanted=all

2. http://www.who.int/mediacentre/factsheets/fs379/en/

3. http://www.sciencedaily.com/releases/2013/07/130722071947.htm

4. http://www.ncbi.nlm.nih.gov/pmc/articles/PMC1566656/pdf/envhper00512 -0121.pdf

5. http://www.safewater.org/PDFS/scientificresearch/humanhealtheffectsfrom chronicarsenicpoisoning-areview.pdf

6. http://www.ncbi.nlm.nih.gov/pubmed/23176881

7. http://www.theguardian.com/environment/2015/jul/05/fracking-injection -chemicals-drinking-water-transparency

8. http://www.theatlantic.com/health/archive/2012/03/for-pennsylvanias-doctors -a-gag-order-on-fracking-chemicals/255030/

9. http://www.law360.com/articles/553427/doctor-s-challenge-to-pa-fracking -gag-rule-gets-nixed

10. http://www.nature.com/ncomms/2015/150421/ncomms7728/full/ncomms7728. html

11. http://thinkprogress.org/climate/2015/05/05/3654388/california-drought-oil -wastewater-agriculture/

12. Leiba, N., et al. Environmental Working Group, 2011. "2011 Bottled Water Scorecard," http://static.ewg.org/reports/2010/bottledwater2010/pdf/2011 -bottledwater-scorecard-report.pdf; Olson, E. D., Natural Resources Defense

Council, 1999. "Bottled Water: Pure Drink or Pure Hype?" http://www.nrdc.org /water/drinking/bw/bwinx.asp

13. http://www.motherjones.com/environment/2014/03/tritan-certichem-eastman -bpa-free-plastic-safe?page=2

14. http://www.mnn.com/earth-matters/translating-uncle-sam/stories/what-is-the -great-pacific-ocean-garbage-patch

15. Ganio, M. S., D. J. Casa, L. E. Armstrong, and C. M. Maresh. Evidence-based approach to lingering hydration questions. *Clinics in Sports Medicine,* 2007;26(1):1–16.

16. http://www.ncbi.nlm.nih.gov/m/pubmed/11229668/

17. http://www.ncbi.nlm.nih.gov/m/pubmed/23968739/

18. http://www.ncbi.nlm.nih.gov/m/pubmed/17008578/

19. Bryson, Christopher. *The Fluoride Deception* (New York: Seven Stories Press, 2006).

20. Ibid.

21. http://www.ncbi.nlm.nih.gov/pmc/articles/PMC2001050/

22. http://www.accessdata.fda.gov/scripts/cdrh/cfdocs/cfcfr/cfrsearch.cfm?fr=355.10

23. http://www.fluoridealert.org/wp-content/uploads/fda-2005a.pdf

24. The level of fluoride in mother's milk is remarkably low (0.004 ppm) compared to a bottle-fed baby consuming fluoridated water (0.6–1.2 ppm). http://www .ncbi.nlm.nih.gov/pubmed/26449642; http://www.ncbi.nlm.nih.gov/pubmed /15587090

25. http://www.cdc.gov/nchs/data/databriefs/db53.htm

26. http://www.ncbi.nlm.nih.gov/pubmed/26319807; http://www.ncbi.nlm.nih.gov /pubmed/25164033; http://www.ncbi.nlm.nih.gov/pubmed/22369953; http:// www.ncbi.nlm.nih.gov/pubmed/11275672

27. http://www.ncbi.nlm.nih.gov/pubmed/11434994

28. http://www.ncbi.nlm.nih.gov/pubmed/22820538

29. http://www.thelancet.com/journals/laneur/article/PIIS1474-4422(13)70278-3 /abstract?cc= y

30. http://www.ncbi.nlm.nih.gov/pubmed/19054310

31. Yiamouyiannis, J. A. "Water Fluoridation and Tooth Decay: Results from the 1986– 87 National Survey of U.S. Schoolchildren." *Fluoride,* 1990;23:55–67.

32. https://iadr.confex.com/iadr/2006Orld/techprogram/abstract_73811.htm

33. http://www.ncbi.nlm.nih.gov/pubmed/22320287

34. http://www.ncbi.nlm.nih.gov/pubmed/26092033

35. http://www.ncbi.nlm.nih.gov/pubmed/15153698

36. http://www.ncbi.nlm.nih.gov/pmc/articles/PMC1615305/pdf/amjph00440 =0107.pdf

## CHAPTER 15: Simple Pleasures: Healthy Sweets, Fats, and Umami

1. http://www.ncbi.nlm.nih.gov/pubmed/19103324; http://www.ncbi.nlm.nih.gov /pubmed/18598178

2. http://www.ncbi.nlm.nih.gov/pubmed/24983789

3. http://www.ncbi.nlm.nih.gov/pubmed/21033720; http://www.ncbi.nlm.nih.gov /pubmed/21675726

4. http://www.ncbi.nlm.nih.gov/pubmed/20132041; http://cfs.nrcan.gc.ca /publications?id=28297

5. http://www.ncbi.nlm.nih.gov/pubmed/22147441; http://www.ncbi.nlm.nih.gov /pubmed/23122108

6. http://www.ncbi.nlm.nih.gov/m/pubmed/25647359

7. http://www.ncbi.nlm.nih.gov/pubmed/25819960; http://www.ncbi.nlm.nih.gov /pubmed/18377679

8. http://www.ncbi.nlm.nih.gov/pubmed/24005018; http://www.ncbi.nlm.nih.gov /pubmed/25757438

9. http://www.ncbi.nlm.nih.gov/pmc/articles/PMC3715094; http://www.science direct.com/science/article/pii/S1756464611000296

10. http://www.ncbi.nlm.nih.gov/pubmed/19103324

11. Paolisso, G., and M. Barbagallo. Hypertension, diabetes mellitus, and insulin resistance: the role of intracellular magnesium. *American Journal of Hypertension*, 1997;10:346–55.

12. Pikilidou, M. I., et al. Insulin sensitivity increase after calcium supplementation and change in intraplatelet calcium and sodium-hydrogen exchange in hypertensive patients with type 2 diabetes. *Diabetic Medicine*, 2009;26:211–19.

13. Chatterjee, R., et al. Potassium intake and risk of incident type 2 diabetes mellitus: the coronary artery risk development in young adults (CARDIA) study. *Diabetologia*, 2012;55:1295–1303.

14. http://www.ncbi.nlm.nih.gov/pubmed/19103324

15. http://www.ncbi.nlm.nih.gov/pubmed/24228787

16. http://www.ncbi.nlm.nih.gov/pubmed/15630260

17. http://www.ncbi.nlm.nih.gov/pubmed/24876885

18. http://www.ncbi.nlm.nih.gov/pubmed/21196761

19. http://www.ncbi.nlm.nih.gov/pubmed/18056558

20. http://www.ncbi.nlm.nih.gov/pubmed/24886260

21. http://www.ncbi.nlm.nih.gov/pubmed/24690749

22. http://www.ncbi.nlm.nih.gov/pubmed/22811614

23. http://www.ncbi.nlm.nih.gov/pubmed/24476150

24. http://www.ncbi.nlm.nih.gov/pubmed/23584372

25. http://www.ncbi.nlm.nih.gov/pmc/articles/PMC4075678

26. http://www.ncbi.nlm.nih.gov/pubmed/23256446

27. http://www.ncbi.nlm.nih.gov/pubmed/23111883

28. http://www.ncbi.nlm.nih.gov/pubmed/23102243

29. http://www.ncbi.nlm.nih.gov/pubmed/23971045

30. http://www.ncbi.nlm.nih.gov/pubmed/25258397

31. http://www.foodsafetynews.com/2011/11/tests-show-most-store-honey-isnt -honey/#.VFp6Vf1lUZ0

32. http://abcnews.go.com/Health/hide-sweet-surprising-places-find-high-fructose -corn/story?id=23257519

33. http://www.ncbi.nlm.nih.gov/pubmed/26456559

34. http://www.ncbi.nlm.nih.gov/pubmed/26351933; http://www.ncbi.nlm.nih.gov

/pubmed/25498862; http://www.ncbi.nlm.nih.gov/pubmed/25790022; http://www.ncbi.nlm.nih.gov/pubmed/26258079; http://www.ncbi.nlm.nih.gov/pubmed/26480301

35. http://www.ncbi.nlm.nih.gov/pubmed/26318151
36. http://www.ncbi.nlm.nih.gov/pubmed/25722654
37. http://www.ncbi.nlm.nih.gov/pubmed/25709792
38. http://www.ncbi.nlm.nih.gov/pubmed/25840667
39. http://www.ncbi.nlm.nih.gov/pubmed/11160540; http://www.ncbi.nlm.nih.gov/pubmed/19437058
40. http://www.ncbi.nlm.nih.gov/pubmed/26200659
41. Vileisis, Ann, *Kitchen Literacy* (Island Press, 2010).
42. http://www.ncbi.nlm.nih.gov/pubmed/26410780; http://www.ncbi.nlm.nih.gov/pubmed/25303528
43. http://www.ncbi.nlm.nih.gov/pubmed/25222131
44. http://www.ncbi.nlm.nih.gov/pubmed/25031459
45. http://www.ncbi.nlm.nih.gov/pubmed/25997382; http://www.ncbi.nlm.nih.gov/pubmed/23515148
46. http://www.ncbi.nlm.nih.gov/m/pubmed/17570262; http://www.ncbi.nlm.nih.gov/pubmed/23471488
47. http://olivecenter.ucdavis.edu/oil-testing
48. http://olivecenter.ucdavis.edu/research/files/report041211finalreduced.pdf
49. http://www.jisppd.com/article.asp?issn=0970-4388;year=2008;volume=26;issue=1;spage=12;epage=17;aulast=Asokan
50. http://www.ncbi.nlm.nih.gov/pubmed/21163558
51. http://www.ncbi.nlm.nih.gov/pubmed/24556122
52. http://www.ncbi.nlm.nih.gov/m/pubmed/19022225/
53. http://www.ncbi.nlm.nih.gov/m/pubmed/18990554/
54. http://www.ncbi.nlm.nih.gov/pubmed/15736917
55. http://www.ncbi.nlm.nih.gov/pubmed/17764919
56. http://www.ncbi.nlm.nih.gov/pubmed/24435467
57. http://www.hindawi.com/journals/isrn/2012/251632/
58. http://www.ncbi.nlm.nih.gov/pubmed/24506418
59. http://www.ncbi.nlm.nih.gov/pubmed/22050471
60. http://www.ncbi.nlm.nih.gov/pubmed/25332990
61. http://www.ncbi.nlm.nih.gov/pubmed/24494050
62. http://www.ncbi.nlm.nih.gov/pubmed/22207209
63. http://www.ncbi.nlm.nih.gov/pubmed/21242065

## PART IV: Step Three: Put It All Together

1. http://www.ncbi.nlm.nih.gov/pubmed/19211608; http://www.ncbi.nlm.nih.gov/pubmed/17652719
2. http://scholar.lib.vt.edu/theses/available/etd-05062011-114155/unrestricted/Parsons_AE_T_2011.pdf; http://eab.sagepub.com/content/32/6/775.abstract

## CHAPTER 16: Healing from the Inside Out: Cooking Better Food

1. http://www.ncbi.nlm.nih.gov/pubmed/23143785
2. http://www.ncbi.nlm.nih.gov/m/pubmed/26366755/
3. http://www.ncbi.nlm.nih.gov/m/pubmed/26500095
4. http://www.ncbi.nlm.nih.gov/m/pubmed/21112742
5. http://www.ncbi.nlm.nih.gov/pubmed/25675368/
6. http://www.ncbi.nlm.nih.gov/pubmed/12690999/
7. http://www.ncbi.nlm.nih.gov/pubmed/22647733;
   http://www.ncbi.nlm.nih.gov/pubmed/22946853
8. http://www.ncbi.nlm.nih.gov/pmc/articles/PMC2896222/
9. http://www.ncbi.nlm.nih.gov/pubmed/25000133
10. http://www.nytimes.com/2014/09/02/health/childhood-diet-habits-set-in
    -infancy-studies-suggest.html

## CHAPTER 17: Healing from the Outside In

1. http://www.ncbi.nlm.nih.gov/pubmed/24887352
2. Strife, S., and L. Downey. Childhood development and access to nature. A new direction for environmental inequality research. *Organ Environ,* 2009;22: 99–122.
3. Wells, N. M. At home with nature: Effects of "greenness" on children's cognitive functioning. *Environmental Behavior,* 2000;32:775–95.
4. http://journals.plos.org/plosone/article?id=10.1371/journal.pone.0108548
5. Berman, M. G., J. Jonides, and S. Kaplan. The cognitive benefits of interacting with nature. *Psychological Science,* 2008;19:1207–12.
6. http://www.pnas.org/content/112/26/7937
7. http://journals.plos.org/plosone/article?id=10.1371/journal.pone.0108548
8. http://www.sciencedirect.com/science/article/pii/S0272494415000328
9. http://www.pnas.org/content/early/2015/06/23/1510459112
10. http://www.sciencedirect.com/science/article/pii/S0272494415000195
11. http://www.ncbi.nlm.nih.gov/pubmed/24858508
12. http://www.ncbi.nlm.nih.gov/pubmed/24858507
13. http://www.ncbi.nlm.nih.gov/pubmed/24858504
14. http://www.ncbi.nlm.nih.gov/pubmed/22840583
15. http://www.ncbi.nlm.nih.gov/pubmed/15151947
16. http://www.ncbi.nlm.nih.gov/pubmed/23863507
17. http://www.ncbi.nlm.nih.gov/pmc/articles/PMC1868963/
18. http://www.ncbi.nlm.nih.gov/pubmed/23454729
19. Oschman, J. L. Perspective: assume a spherical cow: the role of free or mobile electrons in bodywork, energetic and movement therapies. *Journal of Bodywork and Movement Therapies,* 2008 Jan; 12(1):40–57.
20. http://www.ncbi.nlm.nih.gov/pmc/articles/PMC3265077/
21. http://www.ncbi.nlm.nih.gov/pubmed/24697969
22. http://ajcn.nutrition.org/content/85/6/1586.full
23. http://www.ncbi.nlm.nih.gov/pmc/articles/PMC3256339/

24. http://www.thelancet.com/journals/lancet/article/PIIS0140-6736(04)15649-3/abstract

25. http://www.ncbi.nlm.nih.gov/pubmed/25207378; http://www.ncbi.nlm.nih.gov/pubmed/23638051

26. http://www.ncbi.nlm.nih.gov/pubmed/22279374

27. http://www.ncbi.nlm.nih.gov/pubmed/15068032

28. http://www.ncbi.nlm.nih.gov/pubmed/11594062

29. http://www.ajpcr.com/Vol5Suppl3/1238.pdf

30. http://www.cdc.gov/biomonitoring/Lead_FactSheet.html

31. http://www.washingtonpost.com/blogs/early-lead/wp/2014/10/09/is-there-a-link-between-artificial-turf-and-cancer-in-soccer-goalies/

32. http://www.ncbi.nlm.nih.gov/pubmed/12690999

33. http://www.nature.com/jid/journal/v134/n11/full/jid2014273a.html

34. http://www.ncbi.nlm.nih.gov/pubmed/17030480; http://www.ncbi.nlm.nih.gov/pubmed/17913417

35. http://www.ncbi.nlm.nih.gov/pubmed/17913417

36. http://www.ncbi.nlm.nih.gov/pubmed/25821503

# INDEX

# ABOUT THE AUTHOR

Maya Shetreat-Klein, MD, is an integrative pediatric neurologist with a medical degree from Albert Einstein College of Medicine, where she was awarded the Edward Padow Award for Excellence in Pediatrics and graduated with a Special Distinction in Research in Child Neurology for her original work in autism. Dr. Shetreat-Klein completed the University of Arizona's two-year Fellowship in Integrative Medicine, founded by Andrew Weil, MD, and is now a member of the faculty. She has lectured nationally and internationally for both physicians and laypeople on topics such as children's health, autism, integrative medicine and nutrition, toxins, and neurological health. She practices in New York City, where she lives with her family.